# Hospital Emergency Management

# Hospital Emergency Management

A BIBLE FOR HOSPITAL EMERGENCY MANAGERS

• • •

*Dr. Robert J. Muller, M.D.*

**Hospital Emergency Management**

A Bible for Hospital Emergency Managers

ISBN-13: 9781537683560
ISBN-10: 153768356X
LCCN: 2016916897
CreateSpace Independent Publishing Platform
North Charleston, South Carolina

Address for Communications: 105 Smart Place, Slidell, Louisiana, 70458; rmullermd@aol.com

## Dedication

This book is dedicated to my wife *Susan* and my children, *Ryan* and *Matt*, who have stood by my side though out my life and have always provided their encouragements. I appreciate their support throughout my career and the meaning they have brought to my life to give me the drive and dedication to achieve my goals. I AM FOREVER GRATEFUL.
Love, Rob

## Table of Contents

# Author

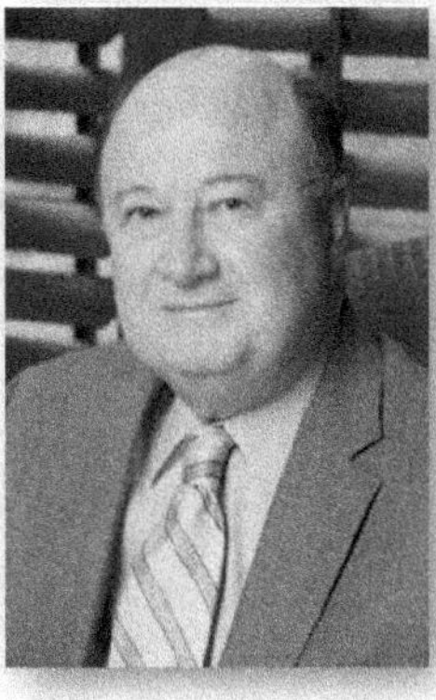

**Robert J. Muller, B.S., MSc., M.D., MBA/MHA, CEM, CFP, CHS, FACFE** is a physician with diverse interest, education and experience. He received his undergraduate education with a B. S. in Chemistry and Biology from St. Louis University; he has additional post graduate degrees from Emory University, and business degrees including a certificate and a MBA/MHA from Auburn University. He received his M.D. from Louisiana State University Medical Center in New Orleans.

He has received his Certified Emergency Management Credentials, being one of only twenty in Louisiana, and has completed over ninety certificate courses in emergency management from the Federal Emergency Management Agency. He is a certified Forensic Physician and certified and a Diplomat in Homeland Security and a Fellow of the American College of Forensic Examiners. He has received numerous search and rescue certifications, including being a certified instructor in the Incident Command System (ICS) used internationally by all fire and law enforcement agencies. He is a certified FEMA Level III Incident Commander.

Dr. Muller has extensive teaching experience having taught on all educational levels and is a frequent community lecturer on various topics and has taught in various fire and police academies on a local and federal level. He has given numerous seminars on Hurricane Planning and Business Continuity Planning and Preparation.

He has and/or currently serves as the medical director of numerous fire departments, the New Orleans Police Department, St. Tammany Parish Sheriff Department and Southeast Louisiana Search and Rescue as well as the New Orleans Lakefront Airport. He served as a Deputy Chief of the New Orleans Police Department in command of Search and Rescue, Hurricane Preparedness and Special Events. He has served as the deputy director of the St. Tammany Parish Office of Emergency Planning and as a deputy coroner in both Orleans and St. Tammany Parishes. He has served as the Designated Regional Coordinator of the Louisiana Department of Health and Hospitals, incorporating five parishes and 29 hospitals — a position he held during Hurricane Katrina.

Dr. Muller has served as a consultant to a national hospital chain and is president of his own consulting corporation.

Dr. Muller has 45 years of experience, education and training to formulate his expertise in Emergency Management.

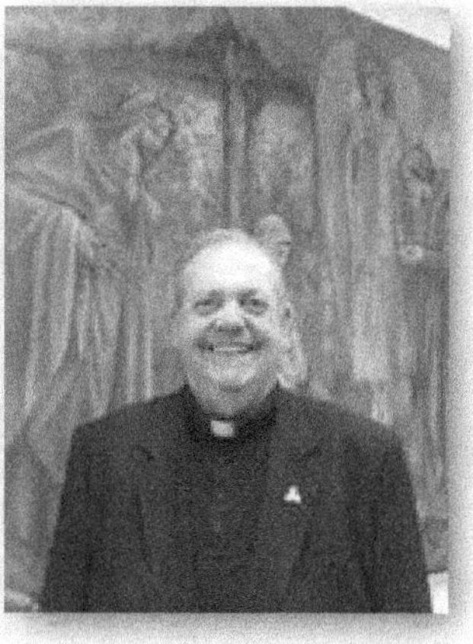

**Very Reverend Rodney P. Bourg, VF, BPS, MA, M.Div.** was born in New Orleans, Louisiana and grew up in St. Bernard Parish (County). Finished high school at Redemptorist High School and graduated from Loyola University in New Orleans with a bachelor's degree in Police Science and a Master's degree in Social Studies Education, while in college worked for the St. Bernard Parish Sheriff's Office as an EMT, Communications, Road Deputy, and in Administration.

After six years with the Sheriff's Office moved to Hyattsville, Maryland and went to work for the American Red Cross and Director of Safety Services and Disaster Operations. It was during this time that I felt called to be a priest.

In 1973 I entered Notre Dame Seminary in New Orleans and was ordained a Roman Catholic Priest in 1978. During my 37 years as a priest I have had a number of parochial assignments including parish work, teaching in the Seminary and presently the founding pastor of Most Holy Trinity Catholic Church.

Most Holy Trinity Parish was established immediately following Hurricane Katrina to accommodate the demographic shifts caused by the Hurricane. This required me to call upon all my previous training and skills to assist not only my new parishioners but many first responders and others to deal with the sense of lost, depression and anxiety that follows a major trauma.

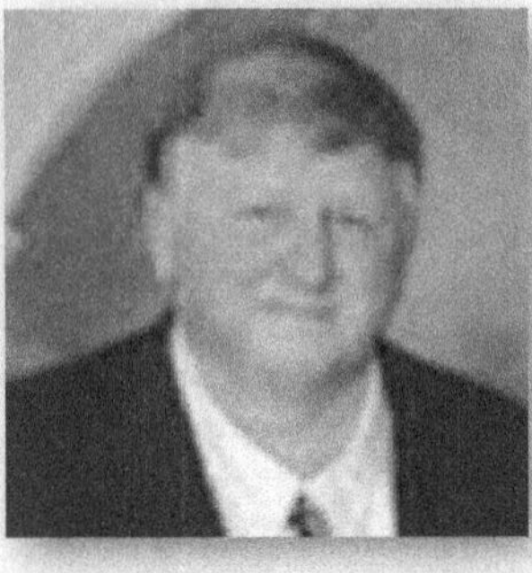

**John Curtis Brady** holds a Bachelor of Science degree from the University of Alabama, completed basic and advanced training in Infection Control from the Centers for Disease Control and Prevention. He is a Certified Infection Control Practitioner (CIC), a member of the Association for Professionals in Infection Control and Epidemiology as well as a past Vice-President and President of the New Orleans chapter of the organization.

Mr. Brady possesses a depth of experience in planning, organizing, and implementing infection control and prevention activities in healthcare facilities ranging from a 150 bed community hospital to an 800 bed Trauma Center. His efforts have achieved success in the development and application of specific interventions resulting in measurable reductions of specific hospital acquired infections. . He was an active participant in development of a comprehensive infection control software program for a large, national multihospital health system.

His experience includes active hospital infection control practice in South Louisiana during Hurricanes Katrina, Rita, Gustav and Isaac. This included pre-disaster planning, staff training, and an active member of Incident Command System as well as active involvement in post disaster recovery.

Mr. Brady is retired and currently a consultant in the area of hospital infection control and medical malpractice case review for hospital acquired infections.

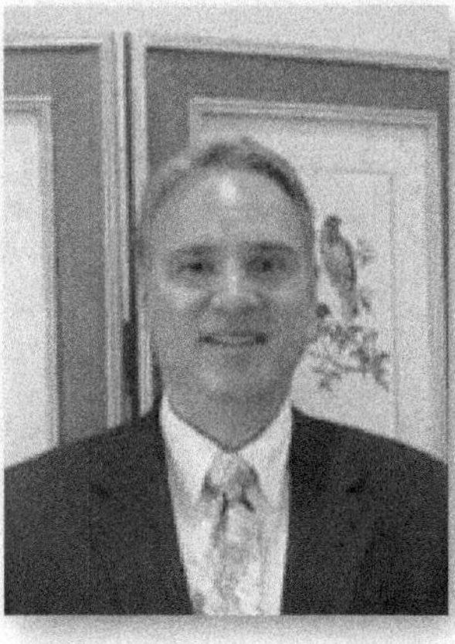

**Ernest P. Chiodo, M.D., J.D., M.P.H., M.S., M.B.A., C.I.H.** is a physician, attorney, biomedical engineer, epidemiologist, toxicologist, and Certified Industrial Hygienist. Dr. Chiodo received his medical, law, biomedical engineering, and toxicology degrees from Wayne State University. His Master of Public Health is from Harvard University. He received his Master of Science in Threat Response Management and his Master of Business Administration from the University of Chicago. He is board certified in internal medicine, occupational medicine, and public health and general preventive medicine. Dr. Chiodo serves as an adjunct professor of law at John Marshall Law School and Loyola University Law School in Chicago. He formerly served as the Medical Director and Manager of Medical and Public Health Services for the City of Detroit.

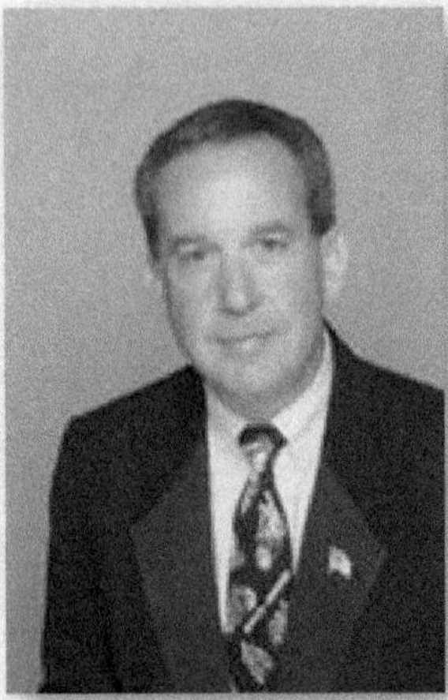

**Joseph E. DiCorpo, B.Sc., M.M.Sc., P.A.**, graduated from Fairfield University, Fairfield, Connecticut, with a Bachelor of Science, in June 1973, in Biology and Chemistry. He then attended Emory University School of Medicine, Atlanta, Georgia, where he obtained a Master of Medical Science, in June 1975, in Anesthesiology and Critical Care Medicine.

He is Board Certified in Anesthesiology and licensed to practice in Georgia by the Composite State Board of Medical Examiners, as a Physician Assistant Anesthetist.

He was Director of Critical Care Medicine for a Tertiary Referral Hospital in Georgia. Additionally, he was the Chief of EMS Programs in both Ohio (Statewide) and California (Local County Health Department) before returning to Atlanta in 1983. When he returned to Atlanta he was on the Faculty of Emory University School of Medicine in both Anesthesiology and Emergency Medicine for 6 years.

He has practiced Anesthesiology for 35 years and has personally performed over 250 Emergency Medical International Evacuations/Repatriations and has supervised hundreds of others over the years.

He now splits his time between being Chief Medical Officer for Medway Air Ambulance Service based in Atlanta, Georgia, and Chief Medical Consultant with Assist America, Inc., of Princeton, New Jersey.

**Michael J. Fagel, PhD., CEM**, has been involved in all phases of Emergency Management, Law Enforcement, EMS and Fire Rescue since the early 1970's. Fagel has held positions in numerous public safety agencies on the local and regional level.

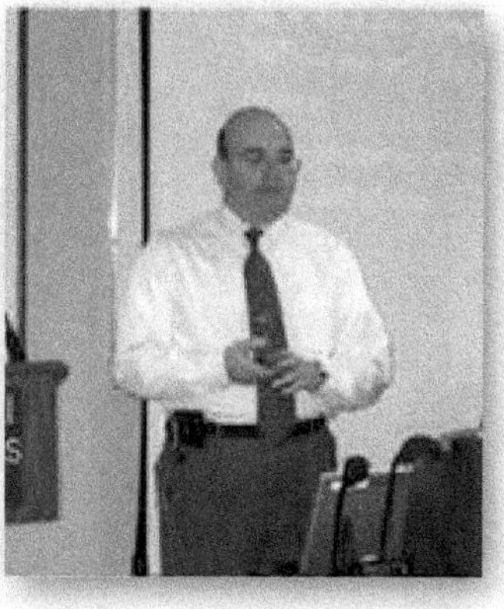

He has been a reservist for FEMA/DHS, and was deployed to the Oklahoma City Bombing in 1995, as well as the World Trade Center Attacks in 2001.

He has been deployed to the Middle East in 2005 -2007 to create a new FEMA like organization for a budding young American ally, as well as returning in 2011 and 12 to train military members from UAE, Kuwait and Jordan on Emergency Plans and procedures.

He currently teaches Homeland Security-Emergency Management at the Illinois Institute of Technology, Northern Illinois University, Eastern Kentucky University, Aurora University and Louisiana State University-National Center for Biomedical Research & Training. He also serves as an Instructor & Subject Matter Expert for the National Center for Security & Preparedness (NCSP) at the University of Albany.

Fagel serves in local governments as an elected and also an appointed official, and serves on Township, Fire District, 911 and Telecommunications advisory boards. He has published 5 textbooks on Emergency Management, Crisis Management, Emergency Operations Centers and Homeland Security. He may be reached at mjfagel@aol.com

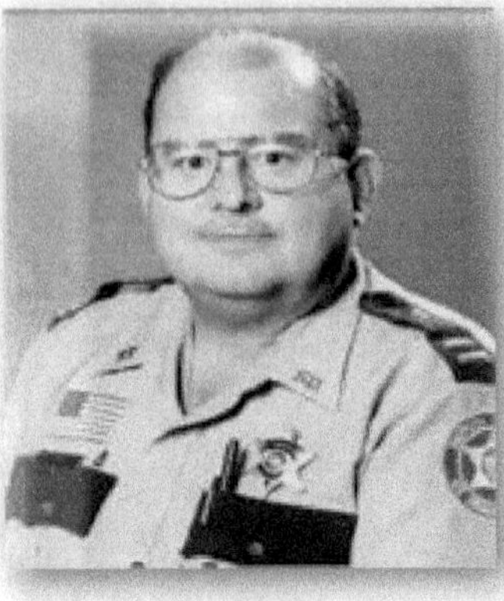

**Captain Ronald J. Frey**, Ret, served over forty years in law enforcement, working with multiple agencies within the New Orleans, Louisiana area. He retired from the ST. Tammany Parish Sheriff's Office as Director of their Forensic Crime Unit.

Captain Frey was the founding director of the Forensic Crime Unit for the ST. Tammany Parish Sheriff's Office and managed it for twenty one years until his retirement. Captain Frey came to the sheriff's office from the New Orleans Police Department's Crime Laboratory.

Prior to his career in forensics, Captain Frey was a member of the New Orleans Police Department Emergency Services Division. He is a graduate of the Tulane University School of Medicine Paramedic Training Program and a FEMA Instructor in Mass Fatality Incident Planning having trained at the Emergency Management Institute in Maryland.

He has served as a team member for the Louisiana Mass Fatality Task Force Training Team, and for the Louisiana State Office of Emergency Preparedness.

He has received forensic certification from the Miami-Dade Medical Examiner's Department Police-Medical Investigation of Death and the ST. Louis University Medical School Advanced Death Investigators programs; he has attended the National Fire Academy Fire Investigation program as well as the Southern Institute of Forensic Science in Scene Reconstruction, Arson, Fire related Death, Rape, Homicide, and Child Abuse training programs. Captain Frey has received several commendations for his work in forensic death investigation.

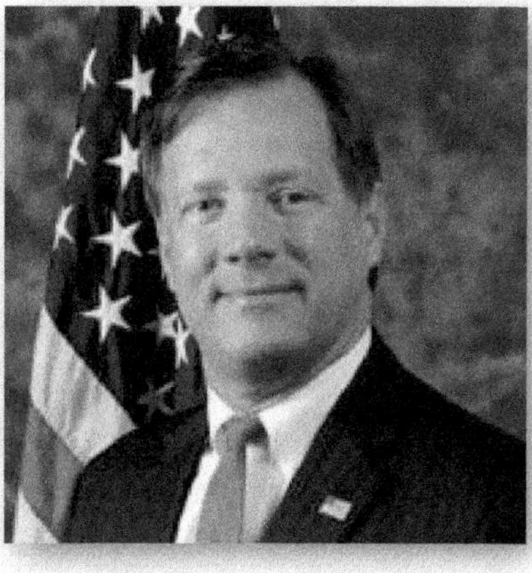

**Willard Hatcher** is a retired FBI Cyber agent with CISSP, GCIA, GCIH, GSEC certifications serving as Chief Information Security Officer practicing information security and HIPAA/PCI compliance at Ochsner Health Systems, a ten hospital and fifty clinic regional health care provider with over twenty thousand users and three hundred thousand patient visits annually.

He presently is the CISO for Ochsner Health Systems and Adjunct Professor at Tulane University. He had served as a FBI Special Agent for 22 years retiring as a supervisory special agent in 2012. During his career he has served in the FBI San Francisco and New Orleans offices as a SWAT team member, and in white collar crime, and as computer network investigator. He was one of the first FBI Cyber Agents starting in 1995 who focused on computer network intrusions into sensitive government or private financial networks.

A graduate of Florida State University as an accountant he has compiled numerous audits, computer security (CISSP, GCIA, GCIH, GSEC), physical security, and investigation courses. He has also developed and delivered international Cyber investigative professional courses for US government International Law Enforcement academies in Budapest and Bangkok.

Twitter: @Willhack
Linkedin: www.linkedin.com/in/willhatcher/

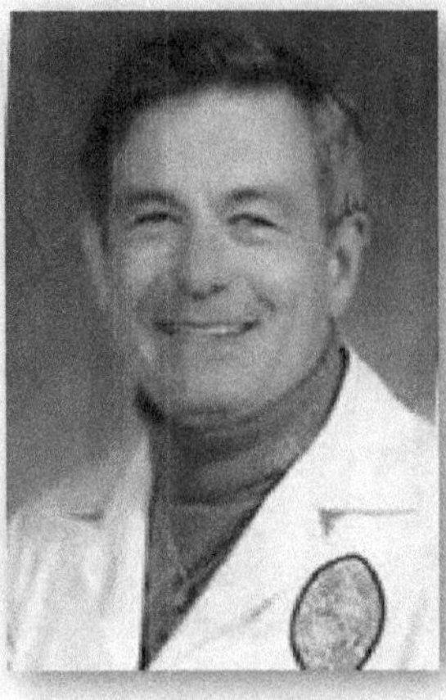

**Norman E. McSwain, Jr., MD, FACS,** was born in the hill country of Northern Alabama, half hillbilly and half redneck. He finished high school at Albertville High, went to college at The University of The South in Sewanee, Tennessee. Since a Cub Scout he knew he wanted to be a physician and a surgeon. He chose to return to Alabama at the University of Alabama, School of Medicine to learn medicine under Dr Tinsley Harrison (of *Harrison's Textbook of Medicine* fame) and Dr. Champ Lyons, in Surgery. Following graduation, he completed two years of surgical training at Bowman- Gray School of Medicine in Winston-Salem, North Carolina, then joined the Air Force (Berry Plan) and under the tutelage of Dr. Kermit Vandenbos preformed more than a thousand surgical procedures before he went to Grady Memorial Hospital in Atlanta to finish his initial education as a surgeon. He acquired more education about true patient care as a partner in private practice with Dr. Harrison Rogers (who later became President of the American Medical Association) for three years in Atlanta before he joined the clinical and academic faculty at the University of Kansas in Kansas City. While at the KUMC, he was given the responsibility of EMS education and system development for the State of Kansas. When he was recruited four years later to Tulane University School of Medicine, Department of Surgery, and Charity Hospital, he left behind 90% of the population of Kansas covered by paramedic quality care within ten minutes and one out of every five hundred Kansans (including the entire Kansas Highway Patrol) trained as an EMT- basic.

He joined the academic and clinical faculty at Tulane, but his main interest was in Charity Hospital and pre-hospital patient care. He came to New Orleans because he considered Charity Hospital to be one of the three most important trauma centers in the United States. After arriving in New Orleans and along with his work at Charity Hospital, he was recruited by the City of New Orleans to develop an EMS system for the city. He initiated both the EMT-Basic and EMT-Paramedic training within the New Orleans Police Department and a Citywide EMS System.

During this time he was recruited to the American College of Surgeons Committee on Trauma to assist in the development of the Advanced Trauma Life Support program. To fill the gap in the trauma team he worked with the ACS/COT and the National Association of EMTs to develop the Pre-Hospital Trauma Life Support program. Today, PHTLS has trained over half a million people in 45 countries. It is considered to be the world standard for pre-hospital trauma care. He has worked with the military and the Department of Defense to develop the Tactical Combat Casualty Care program for military medics.

Dr. McSwain is the only person in the history of the American College of Surgeons to receive all five of the major trauma awards:

- Committee on Trauma, Meritorious Achievement Award for State/Provincial Chairs, 2001
- Scudder Orator, 2001
- Committee on Trauma Millennium Commitment Award, 2000
- Surgeon's Award for Service to Safety, National Safety Council, 1998
- Advanced Trauma Life Support (ATLS) Meritorious Service
- Award, Committee on Trauma, 1989

For the past 30 years, he has provided care to severely injured police officers at Charity Hospital and while at Tulane, he has written or revised more than 25 textbooks; published more than 360 articles and traveled throughout the world giving more than 800 presentations. He has lectured in all of the 50 states, all provinces in Canada, most of the countries in Europe, most of the countries in Central America, and the upper part of South America. Japan, China, Australia, and New Zealand have also been places to which he has been invited to give lectures.

The major factors in these accomplishments have been the opportunity to see and care for patients and to learn and teach at Charity Hospital. Charity Hospital, until Hurricane Katrina, was considered by most to be one of the five top trauma centers in the United States. Charity Hospital continues to train medical students, residents and fellows in the skills and knowledge required to manage severely injured patients.

**Authors Note:**

Following completion of this chapter, Dr. McSwain suffered a massive cerebrovascular accident and expired several days later.

He will be sadly missed by all of his friends, the medical community, and the countless numbers of those lives he has saved through his surgery, treatment and innovative scientific discoveries and implementations. Dr. McSwain was a great friend, mentor and teacher who greatly enhanced my knowledge base and provided me with great insight. Rest in Peace Norman.

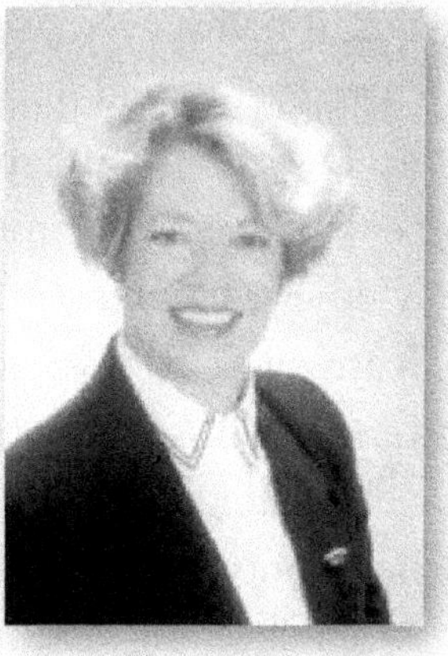

**Susan O'Brien, RN** is a 1967 graduate of Touro Infirmary School of Nursing and obtained a Bachelors of Health Administration from the University of St. Francis. She has over forty years of nursing experience. Her areas of expertise include Critical Care, Education, Quality Improvement, Accreditation and Administration. She served as the Director of Critical Care at Touro Infirmary and as the Assistant Director of Nursing at Sara Mayo Hospital. During her tenure at St. Charles General, she was appointed to the position of Director of Education and subsequently the Director of Quality and Risk Management. At St. Charles General Hospital, Susan also served as the Chief Nursing Officer for over twenty years. Susan was the Chief Nursing Officer at Northshore Regional Medical Center (NSRMC) and she served as an ethics instructor for the Tenet Corporate Ethics Program for over ten years. In addition, she also served as chairperson for the National Tenet Corporate Nurse Executive Committee.

Susan's honors include the rating of #1 in Employee Satisfaction in the Tenet Healthcare System, #2 in Physician Satisfaction in the Tenet Healthcare System, JCAHO Accreditation with Commendation, four Corporate Nurse Executive Leadership awards and was the first recipient of the Nightingale Award for Nursing Administrator of the Year awarded by the Louisiana State Nurses Association. She has served on multiple boards including Junior Achievement, NO/AIDS Task Force, Delgado Charity School of Nursing Advisory Board and the Louisiana Technical College Advisory Board.

Susan has served as a Chief Nursing Officer in hospitals for over thirty years and during her career she gained extensive experience in Disaster Management. Her most recent experience included serving as the Chief Nursing Officer at Northshore Regional Medical Center (NSRMC) before, during and after Hurricane Katrina. NSRMC served as a major evacuation center for New Orleans hospitals, receiving up to seventy-five helicopters a day delivering rescued patients and victims of the flooding and other horrendous conditions. Disaster management of this magnitude was a challenging and very rewarding experience.

Currently, Susan serves as an Accreditation Coordinator for a large managed care organization.

**E. Michael O'Bryan, MD MHA** attended LSU in Baton Rouge as an undergraduate and received the MD degree from LSU School of Medicine in New Orleans, Louisiana. Following medical school, he served a rotating internship at Earl K Long Hospital in Baton Rouge, a LSU affiliated facility, followed by a surgical residency at Charity Hospital, New Orleans. He, as well, served a fellowship in Surgery at the Lahey Clinic, Boston, MA.

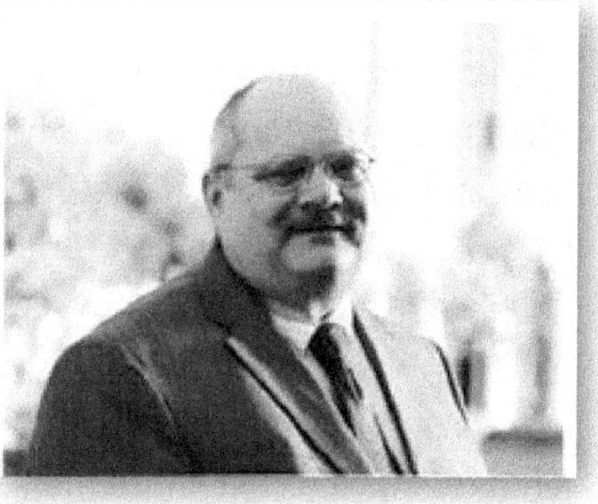

After 17 years of surgical practice as a member of Northshore Surgical Affiliates he returned to Tulane University and procured a degree of Masters of Health Administration through the School of Health Systems Management. In 1999 he accepted a position as Assistant Administrator of NorthShore Regional Medical Center in Slidell, LA and eventually became Chief Operating Officer and later moved into the position of Chief Executive Officer of that facility.

He became the Chief Executive Officer of Ochsner Medical Center, West Bank in 2006 and served in that capacity until retirement in 2010. During his career he has been a member of the American College of Surgeons, Surgical Society of Louisiana, American College of Healthcare Executives, and American College of Physician Executives, Louisiana Hospital Association, Louisiana State Medical Society and St. Tammany Parish Medical Society.

He has served on the boards of East St. Tammany Parish Chamber of Commerce and the Algiers Economic Development Foundation. He has also has been a member of the board of the Metropolitan Hospital Council of New Orleans and served as the Chairman of that organization in 2009.

**Author Note:**

Mike O'Bryan died suddenly early this year and will be missed by all those who knew him. He was a great surgeon as well as a hospital administrator, but most of all, a great friend.

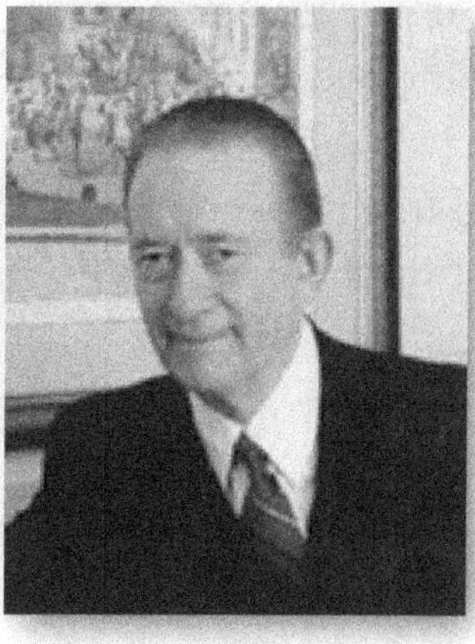

**Kenneth Rhea, MD**, is a native of Indiana having spent his professional life in southern states. His professional background includes engineering at GM Institute of Technology (GMIT) in Flint, Michigan, a Bachelor of Arts (BA) Degree from Westminster College, and his Doctorate in Medicine (MD) from Vanderbilt University School of Medicine. After Surgical Internship at Indiana University Medical Center, his medical background includes residencies in neurosurgery, ophthalmology, and associated neuropathology research.

He served in the USN as the Senior Medical Officer for USN Nuclear Submarine Forces based in Spain. After returning to private practice he was Director of Medicine and Surgery at Texas Medical Care, and Director of Clinical Ophthalmology for South Texas Eye Physicians. Dr. Rhea has served as Deputy Sheriff and Medical Advisor to the Harris County Sheriff's Department Houston, Texas and is one of two physicians in the US holding the medical risk management credential of Fellow of the American Society for Healthcare Risk Management (FASHRM).

As a private risk and liability consultant to commercial organizations and medical practices Dr. Rhea has over 17 years developed and presented CME accredited educational risk and regulatory liability prevention Internet education and lectures to thousands of physicians in national and state physician professional organizations as well as Tulane and LSU residency programs. He has lectured and written extensively in areas of physician communications, medical electronic communications, medical risk management, and federal privacy and security regulations, e.g. HIPAA Privacy and Security Rules and EMR Meaningful Use.

Dr. Rhea and his wife Kathleen have been married 38 years, have two children, and live in Baton Rouge, Louisiana. Dr. Rhea can be reached through MER Consulting, LLC at krheamd@mdriskconsulting.com.

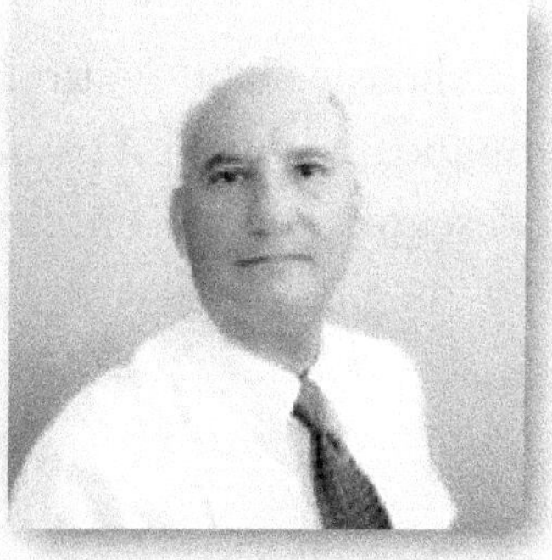

**Alfred F. Trappey, II, PhD** has an MBA, and received his PhD in Food Science from Louisiana State University. Since 2006, his working knowledge and applied use of the National Incident Management System (NIMS) was essential not only for documenting both federal and state procedural policies but also for re-establishing and protecting LSU Health Sciences Centers' critical research assets contained within its infrastructure.

Dr. Trappey's extensive background in emergency management training became evident in 2005 and 2008 by his direct involvement and decisive knowledge of LSU System entities affected by Hurricanes Katrina, Rita, Gustav and Ike. Dr. Trappey's knowledge of the National Incident Management System (NIMS) was essential for applying both federal and state procedural policies thus protecting and re-establishing LSU System's infrastructure. His expertise allowed for a coordinated and unified mobilization of local and state emergency administrators.

Dr. Trappey reports to the LSU Health Sciences Center Chancellor's Office and Office of Administrative, Community and Security Affairs and is responsible for developing and implementing programs and projects in emergency planning, training, response, recovery, and remediation for the LSU Health Sciences Center-System in Louisiana.

As the Emergency Management Specialist for the LSU Health Sciences Center Chancellor's Office and Office of Administrative, Community and Security Affairs since 2006, Dr. Trappey continues to be responsible for establishing and maintaining an "all comprehensive" mitigation and disaster recovery training protocols mandated by FEMA to protect LSU System entities; its medical research institutions, its people, resources and the environment.

## Acknowledgements

• • •

I GRATEFULLY ACKNOWLEDGE THE CONTRIBUTIONS of Ms. Misty Toruno for her time in working with me to complete and edit this manuscript on numerous occasions; Don Piatt and Curtis Brady for their help with proof reading and recommended changes, and Dr. Randolph Howes for his help and guidance during this process of publishing; to all the chapter authors for providing their expertise in this endeavor and their patience in awaiting the numerous changes in editing encountered during the publication process. Thank You ALL for making this publication a success.

**Robert J. Muller**

# Forward

• • •

By **Michael J. Fagel, PhD., CEM**

When Rob asked me to author a forward for his new book Hospital Emergency Management, I was elated to be able to help him with his new textbook.

We often look at "Emergencies or Disasters" through one filter, or one view point.... Ours!

There is an inherent risk in tunnel vison during any event planning, response, and of course Recovery.

Regardless of the event, we often hear and use the words "lessons learned", but, we usually make the same mistakes over and over again.

Take the time to thoroughly read EACH of these important chapters, and make notes while reading each one, and APPLY it to YOUR own situation, facility or organization. Be cautious to not fall into the trap of "That job belongs to another person, division or department, not me."

Rob has been through MANY historical events, and shares with you his keen insight as not only a practicing physician, but, using his management acumen to help make the right LOGICAL and non-emotional decision in regards to the aftermath of a disaster. The planning, practice and preparation that YOU DO NOW, can serve you, and the organization and community YOU serve tenfold by following the staid advice and counsel of what Rob has put together for you.

This book is not a "one and done" text book, IT IS A READY reference book that ALL hospital administrators should make part of the reference texts on their shelf for everyday use.

Rob takes some very practical approaches to common problems, and tries to put each element into a manageable perspective.

I have authored several textbooks, and Rob has taken some elements from our books, but, more importantly, REAL LIFE that makes his book invaluable.

As I tell my University Students, Emergency Management is an ART, a skill that takes years of honing and perfection. I have been deployed to many horrific events in my career, starting with the Oklahoma City Bombing in 1995, to the World Trade Center attacks in 2001, to Hurricane Sandy and active shooter events in between.

One thing is FOR CERTAIN, EVERY event is different, and, you will take ALL OF YOUR SKILLS, Knowledge and practice into EACH and every event to help bring it to a resolution.

I have been involved in Law Enforcement, Fire Rescue-EMS, Emergency Management at the Local and National Levels, as well as international deployments. I continually LEARN every single day, and never stop applying what I have learned.

Please take the time to study Dr. Rob Muller's book, understand it, and be prepared to implement these lessons learned and be better prepared.

Preparedness, Response, Recovery, it's UP to YOU!

Respectfully,
Michael J. Fagel, PhD., CEM
North Aurora, Illinois 2016

*Mike Fagel has served in various roles in law enforcement, fire, EMS and Emergency management for over 4 decades. Fagel served FEMA then DHS as a disaster safety officer for over ten years as a reservist. Fagel now teaches at Illinois Institute of Technology-Chicago, Northern Illinois University, Eastern Kentucky University and Louisiana State University. He is a subject matter expert for the National Center for Security & Preparedness in Albany, NY, as well as a Homeland security Analyst for Argonne National Laboratory in Chicago. Fagel serves on numerous public safety boards. He has authored 4 texts on Emergency Management, Crisis management, EOC Operations and planning. The views expressed herein are those of the author alone, and do not reflect the views of any federal state or local agency or organization. Fagel can be reached at mjfagel@aol.com*

## Preface

• • •

HAVING GONE THROUGH ONE OF the nation's greatest disaster, Hurricane Katrina, and serving as the Louisiana Department of Health and Hospitals Designated Regional Coordinator (responsible for coordinating 29 hospitals in several parishes in South East Louisiana), as well as the Incident Commander for a major hospital facility on the Northshore of Lake Pontchartrain, I realized just how totally unprepared most hospitals are to handle major disasters.

I served to coordinate hospital evacuation and redistribution of patients from the metropolitan New Orleans area during Katrina and for the placement and assignment of patients to numerous parishes/counties in Louisiana, Mississippi, Texas and Arkansas.

It was amazing yet sad to know that after so many years of planning meetings and discussions of disaster scenarios much went for naught; and when it was time to fish or cut bait, many of our facilities could not even get the bait to cut it!!!

Very little mitigation was done, after so much discussion and planning. The potential problems that could have easily been mitigated were actually ignored as if they would never happen ----- so why worry about them and even worse why spend any money in these mitigation efforts, as hospital budgets were best allocated to other areas of daily importance.

Problems such as generators and electrical connections being located in basements in already know low lying areas previously subject to flooding, or generators being placed at higher elevations but the fuel supply being located and drawn from flood prone sub elevations; no planning for flooding water evacuations, no planning for any type of evacuations (until post event); no planning for ongoing refueling, food, water and supplies. NO PLANNING --- WHY --- because of complacency --- an attitude that planning and money for mitigation was a waste --- because it will never happen.

It was truly amazing as well as very sad how all of this was ignored despite numerous fore warnings 20 years prior from numerous sources from the U.S. Corp of Engineers, the National Weather Service and the National Hurricane Center only to mention a few.

But because an event has NEVER happen before, is no criterion that an event will never happen in the future.

If you live in a disaster related area, i.e. hurricanes, tornados, earthquakes, or have a hospital down the road from a truck stop, main train line, or inter-state highway that carried hundreds of thousands of gallons of chemicals and explosives daily --- then you are prone that someday there will be a disaster of some magnitude --- someday --- do not ignore and hope the threat will somehow disappear. This is the ideal of vulnerability analysis and these should be taken seriously and not as an exercise in futility. The key word is **seriously**.

It is truly amazing how hospitals all have the flowery mission statements as to their existence to serve the community and for the well- being of patients and families, etc.; yet do not have WORKABLE disaster plans that have been exercised and tested with annual drills to illustrated their vulnerabilities and lack of preparedness. They have plans on paper — that's ALL.

Many hospitals are ready for day to day operations of patient care BUT have little if any preparedness for disaster and massive community emergency situations and mass fatality planning or surge situations.

It is only in the recent years that The Joint Commission has even had a requirement of emergency management planning within it member hospitals, and during their inspections review their planning requirements and annual drill completions --- but this again is far from the big picture of true preparedness and the inter and intra workability with the hospital as well as the community.

How does your hospital deal with it disaster communications issues? Are you relying on cell phones?

How does your hospital plan to interact with other healthcare facilities, nursing homes and clinics?

How does your hospital plan to deal with contamination from hazard materials?? Do you have a decontamination team? What is their make- up; what is their training, what equipment has been purchased for them; what interactions do they have in conjoined training with other agencies - local, state and federal?

How why? How to? How can? What makes it happen? All the answers are simple.

It takes PLANNING, MITIGATION and FUNDING.

If you do not have the desire, time, or someone with the knowledge or expertise, OR funding to complete to fruition, either all at once or in stages, then you are only making a cursory attempt at a serious problems and probably will not even begin to make a dent in the creation of serious disaster planning. You will become one of the many hospitals that have a plan that either is not feasible, workable or likely to succeed in an emergency situation.

It takes first and foremost commitment and the budget to make it workable in reality --- without that --- all you have is non-sensical paperwork.

If the hospital is serious about emergency management, then their first task should be to recruit someone with knowledge, training and experience in this field. This does not mean hiring someone that is retired from the military, as many hospitals do, assuming their past experiences includes emergency management, which is an incorrect assumption and most of these people have great difficulty within this role.

It is better to look for someone with strict emergency management experience and education. There are many new graduates coming out of degree programs, but the only problem is many of them have no experience, especially hospital management experience.

It may be better to consider someone within the hospital that knows the operations aspects, and train them in emergency management, which may be begun through on line courses at the Emergency Management Institute of FEMA in Emmitsberg, Maryland, then proceeding to an online degree or associate degree type program and the ultimate board certification in Emergency Management (CEM) though the International Association of Emergency Management.

If this is just totally not feasible for the budget, then it may be economically responsible to hire an emergency management consultant on contract for all aspects of EM for the hospital.

Whatever is decided as the best option for your particular hospital this phase is critically important to establish the right person for the job --- just as you would in involving a process for a CEO, COO, CFO and CNO or IT persons.

Again --- how serious are you and the hospital in correcting, preparing and mitigating for the future so your hospital is ready when the time comes.

The time is likely to come --- it is just when, how or where.

Remember the 5 P's utilized by the United States Secret Service: **P**roper **P**lanning **P**revents **P**oor **P**erformance.

## Book Praise

• • •

This is a book that should reside in every hospital administration office and have well-worn pages. It is written by an author who has academic credentials, as well as having the real life experience of "having been there done that". In 2005 I served as CEO of NorthShore Regional Medical Center in Slidell, Louisiana and had the opportunity to work with Rob during the weather event known as Hurricane Katrina. Rob served as our Director of Emergency Management for a number of years and his expertise and practical approach to disaster planning had us well prepared to address the challenges head on. This is a straightforward practical treatise on what works. I would encourage anyone to use it as a guide to format their own plan as it will be time well spent.

E. Michael O Bryan, M.D., MHA
CEO Tenet Healthcare Hospitals (Ret)
CEO Ochsner Medical Center, West Bank (Ret)

The marriage of the Author's history in Emergency Management coupled with his knowledge of how hospitals function clearly make this a must read for those responsible for the safety of patients under medical care. As someone who has dealt with the extremes of Mother Nature for 43 years, I know the only way to cope with surviving the storm is to have a detailed, well thought out, easily understood manual that outlines everybody's responsibility. This is not a book for the general population, rather, it is focused for those in hospital management and those associated with patient care. It is long overdue and should provide for an excellent easy read.

Bob Breck
Chief Meteorologist
WVUE-TV
New Orleans

As the founder and Commander of the Special Operations Division of the St. Tammany Parish, Louisiana, Sheriff's Department and Executive Director of SELSAR, (Southeast Louisiana Search and Rescue Organization), I have had the pleasure to have served with Dr. Rob Muller for over 20 years. His dynamic approach to Medical Incident Command is very unique and he is a trend setter, deploying modern and up to date strategies to the first responders as well as Hospitals throughout the Gulf South. Dr. Muller's book is an excellent asset to Emergency Management and Hospital Emergency Management and it is my pleasure to endorse it.

Lt. Colonel (Ret) William "Bill" Dobson, CMI, LPI
Commander Special Operations
St. Tammany Parish Sheriff's Department (Ret)

Dr. Muller has diligently presented a comprehensive assemblage of information for those involved in Hospital Emergency Management. His book will serve as an instructor's course in understanding and directing hospital emergencies. Personally, I have been privileged to know and work with Dr. Robert Muller for over the past thirty years and have gained great respect for his broad based knowledge of medicine, law enforcement, emergency medicine and hospital emergency management. For decades he has dedicated his talents towards working with a wide range of law enforcement agencies and with training of emergency management personal and first responders. His background is tailor made to author a book on Hospital Emergency Management. Although this is a complex subject, Dr. Muller presents a clear and methodical approach to dealing with all aspects of hospital emergency management structure and organization, HEICSs, EOCs and effective means of communications options. A book of this type can only be satisfactorily presented by Dr. Muller's decades of dedication to all aspects in the overall field of Hospital Emergency Management. He has accomplished that goal and this book should be a requirement for all hospital administrators and emergency facilities. Proudly, I highly recommend it.

Prof. Randolph M. Howes, MD, PhD
Adjunct Assistant Professor of Plastic Surgery, (RET.)
The Johns Hopkins Hospital, Baltimore, MD.
Professor of Surgery, Biophysics and Biochemistry,
Louisiana University of Medical Sciences (RET.)
Dean, Louisiana University of Medical Sciences (RET.)

# Introduction

• • •

EMERGENCY MANAGEMENT IS A VERY dynamic, ever changing field. Hospital Emergency Management poses multiple problems with varying daily scenarios but differs, in that continuity of care must be maintained without fail.

Hospitals may experience internal as well as external problems from electrical failure to weather related emergencies.

While it may seem logical that a hospital should be well prepared for these types of events, historically they have not, mainly due to lack of expertise in this field as well as budgetary constraints.

Only recently has The Joint Commission imposed standards for hospital emergency management; and now at the time of hospital inspections, mandates their presentation and review.

It is this new field of Hospital Emergency Management that we will address herein, and the approach will be in every aspect of hospital mitigation through recovery.

Hospitals and medical facilities of various types can be found universally and play a major role by their very nature and function, in the emergency response and recovery phases of all types of disasters.

While this book is based on United States hospitals, agencies and standards, many of the premises can be utilized worldwide in their adaptation. It is written to aid in preparation and as a guideline; it is not meant to be all inclusive, and mitigation and preparation is based on the particular locale, vulnerability, local hazards, structural engineering of facilities, local resources, and available response that comprise the entire global picture of the scenario. The book is not meant to be an all-inclusive source of information or training resource as it would be far too voluminous, but is meant to cover many of the basics and the details that are often overlooked.

The source of training should begin with the basics and then advance as required by the institutions' exposure, needs and budget. Obviously, the needs of a level one facility will far exceed those of a rural level three facility, although they both require the same basic planning and preparedness.

The contents of this book are based on many years of experience, many scenarios, and past events' history and are presented so that many past failures and lack of preparation need not be duplicated---for any reason. It is essential that we learn from history and the past mistakes of ourselves as well as others.

# Section One

• • •

# Administrative

CHAPTER 1

# Disaster Planning for Healthcare

• • •

**Robert J. Muller**

Disasters present their own set of paradigms that are unique in many ways but particularly so in hospital management and disaster planning. Each type of disaster presents its own individual challenges, but there are the same problems that likewise are affected by disasters in general.

Disasters all cause an increased response and flow of both victims and first response personnel depending on the nature of the disaster; likewise, hospitals are all faced with similar problems bases on the individual situations.

The most common are those related to the dichotomy of hospital personnel being torn between their own personal lives and family (including pets), and their responsibility and dedication to their medical job function.

In addition, other factors have to be taken into consideration, including loss of lifelines associated with the infrastructure and the actual physical destruction of the hospital structure.

The type of disaster ranging from those that are weather related to those that are community related from tornados to explosions and plane crashes all have several things in common in that they require planning, preparedness and readiness. Many disaster evolve and have some spatial time warnings associated with them, i.e. hurricanes, floods, wild fires; while other may have little to no warning time, i.e. earthquakes, tornados, explosions, accidents with multiple victims—buses, plane crashes, and the like.

The most common disaster in the United States is FLOODING which can include coastal, riverine, a dam failure and commonly urban drainage flooding.

Flooding in the United States causes the second most loss of life, and likewise the second most costly, first being hurricanes with earthquakes coming in third.

The significance of flooding for hospitals is the barrier that may be created by the area flooded and the locale of the hospital preventing or making more difficult access of victims and personnel to the facility. In addition, when waters recede, new health related problems may exist from such factors as residual mold, contaminated water and sewerage back-ups.

Tornados cause the most injuries, while severe heat waves cause the most fatalities.

What is the significance of these facts? Well, one has little or no warning and preparation phase while the other is usually well predicted allowing for adequate preparation.

What they all require in common is --- readiness.

Readiness is a factor that little thought is given many times as we discuss the big 5 of Planning, Preparation, Mitigation, Response and Recovery. We can execute all of the above and still not be ready when a disaster rapidly evolves if all facets are not coalesced into a concise package.

Many times these factors are simply carries out to meet The Joint Commission requirements and do not extend any further in the process of true readiness. If a tornado should strike in the next 15 minutes and the first action of a hospital is to pull and read the plan and what to do --- then readiness does not necessarily exists.

Readiness is knowing what to do, when and how; and having the necessary personnel available as well as supplies to deal with the situation in a timely manner.

Preparation for all types of disasters is imperative and usually is not found in areas where low probability exists even though there is a risk factor. A Tsunami on the West Coast or an earthquake in the southeast US? YES, risk exists but what is the probability!! It only takes once. Are southeast U.S. hospitals planned for an earthquake --- hurricanes yes --- but an earthquake!! What about coastal west coast hospitals are they in a possible path of destruction for a Tsunami or prepared to deal with a new set of circumstances associated with such an event.

Many years ago hurricane preparation in New York City was only a distant thought --- how that has changed now!

Whatever the hazard or vulnerability, medical facilities must plan for disruption of services via the numerous mechanisms such as communications, utilities, access channels, as well structural damage.

Facilities must be able to have continuity of function through self-sustaining mechanisms such as, adequate supplies, parts, fuel, food, water, cooking preparation and distributive services only to mention a few. All aspects must able to be sustained based on the various scenarios and evergreen contracts should be in place with specific understanding as to the need and response of those involved in order to be able to continuously function.

The new computer age presents additional problems in reestablishing functionality of facilities both from the point of patient electronic medical records as well as those to the administrative and business aspects of the facility; an alternate means must be planned in advance in order to continue function. Various systems that were in place prior to computerization may be needed for fall back.

Hospital should be part of some form of networking or conglomerate agreements with multiple other facilities to help sustain function. It is likewise imperative not only to network but to have various and multiple plans as to how networking can take place. Several hospitals within as defined area can be of no value to each other if they lack basic modalities of communication and access to each other. Alternate duplication of function to the nth degree is well within workable reason. There is no such thing as having too many alternate plans or "over planning".

If a facility is known to be in an area of increased vulnerability, a community education program should be initiated regarding patient involvement in their medical care and retention of some form of tangible medical care record either via hard copy or electronic discs or thumb drives.

Facilities should have plans to be able to sustain in part by having alternate locations both internal and external to the facility to be able to provide function; i.e. relocation of a cafeteria to a nearby school and use the current cafeteria location to gain valuable internal space to enhance the emergency room area or move the laboratory or add critical care areas, etc. Many options and scenarios should be looked at well in advance of the situation arising so that an easy and rapid transition may be made without further thought.

The significance of hospital disaster planning is reward in the future --- when it is most needed, thereby reducing stress levels and indicating the true mission statements of facilities in regard to the communities they serve.

CHAPTER 2

# Administrative and Command Structure

• • •

**Robert J. Muller**

Most hospitals are organized with a Chief Executive Officer (CEO) or Chief Administrative Office (CAO) as the lead executive in charge of the hospital. He/She may have various assistants depending on the size of the hospital and may include a Chief Operating Officer (COO), Chief Nursing Office (CNO), Human Resource Officer, and Chief Financial Officer (CFO). Many hospitals have a President and Vice Presidents in charge of various operational aspects. In smaller hospitals these functions may be combined.

Hospitals also have Department heads or chiefs, that are responsible for the operational aspects of sections of the hospital, and again depending upon size, may likewise be combined. Examples include, dietary, engineering, laboratory, X-Ray, cardiology, etc.

It is imperative that no matter what the particular hospital structure is called or what the composition, that it functions as an entire T**EAM**, and be structurally organized to be carried out in the most cost efficient manner.

It is imperative that the TEAM be trained in the Hospital Emergency Incident Command System **(HEICS**) and that each member of the team knows and understands their role and function within this structure.

Many hospitals choose to have the CEO or President assume the role of the Incident Commander (IC) within this structure and this may be a perfect fit for many hospitals.

I would suggest if the hospital has a designated emergency management person, that this person assume the role of the IC and the CEO be placed as general over seer of the entire hospital function; In this way he/she is able to roam the hospital for potential problems and not be held within the constraints of the Command Center.

Whoever is the IC; he/she must have the training and experience to carry out this very demanding and highly sensitive function and should possess at least ICS 200 level education.

The designated emergency manager is usually better trained in this function and thus better prepared to handle the scenarios, and has the knowhow for community liaison.

This is NOT a time for egos to dominate and this should all be predetermined by a command structure established in the planning phase long before any incident should arise. Remember the old saying, "the time to learn to dance is not fifteen minutes before the party".

See *Appendix for basic command structure templates that are available depending on the hospital needs and personnel training and experience.

CHAPTER 3

# Role of the CEO in Emergency Management

• • •

**Michael O'Bryan**

Health care facility CEOs come in all shapes, sizes, personalities, persuasions and philosophies and many different approaches to leadership work successfully. Within those philosophies there are varied opinions regarding the role of the CEO in Disaster Planning and its implementation during an event. There are those that feel delegation is appropriate and the real job is communication with the board, community, etc. There are those that would micromanage and see the role as being Incident Commander, CEO, Communicator, point person all rolled into one.

An entire book could be written on the CEO role in disasters, and it is certainly not the purpose of this chapter to exhaustively touch on all pertinent topics, but to provide an overview of the challenges most likely encountered.

If there was ever a time for leadership to be evident from the Chief Executive it is not only during an event but in the preparation and planning for such an occurrence. In everyday hospital life, be it JCAHO preparedness, operations, community and board relations the old Truman adage of "the buck stops here" applies and so it should in the realm of emergency preparedness and implementation.

Whether the CEO serves as Incident Commander or delegates that to a well prepared colleague, the CEO role is paramount to the many faceted duties during a manmade or natural disaster; and that all begins with the planning stage going back to the formulation of the Disaster Plan and the organization of the Incident Command System. Just as an executive has had insight and input into the periodic evaluations of his team, that insight is critical in assuring the right people are in the right positions in an emergency structure. A Chief Executive should have a good grasp of the hospital leadership and be able to ascertain whose talents and strengths would best fit into what positions on the ICS organizational chart. Along with the input of the Director of Emergency Preparedness, an organizational chart that reflects the strengths of each person named in the block will provide the basis for meeting any future disaster challenge.

An effective plan will take into account the requirements for a level of operability that is preplanned and tested. For an individual facility, that means evaluating the risk at hand from the external and internal environment at present. It also requires an ongoing adaptation of the plan to any changes in those environments that may occur. A hospital CEO should be clear on what the role of his/her facility is as it pertains to the community. As well there should be the assurance that the plan has been tested and revised as needed based on changing circumstances. It is too late to tweak the overall plan when the event is occurring. Not enough can be said about the benefit of preparation.

It is also incumbent upon the hospital leader to have a familiarity with the National Incident Management System (NIMS) and the Incident Command System (ICS). The level of the CEO involvement in each will depend upon the needs of the facility, and what role distribution is organized in the preparation process. At a minimum, though a working knowledge of both is necessary, even if the facility has an Emergency or Disaster Plan Director or Designated Regional Coordinator.

A comprehensive plan will take into account whether a facility will evacuate and under what circumstances or shelter in place under designated conditions. The CEO role will obviously have many commonalities but also differences in each. Having an opportunity to table top, drill or simulate these conditions will help focus the hospital leaders on what their challenges will be in each scenario.

The ability of a facility to fulfill its mission in a disastrous event will come down to how well it has planned and consequently how well it has prepared to enact that plan. It is paramount upon the CEO to be the leader that conveys the importance to this throughout the ranks of Directors and Staff.

In Louisiana there is an old saying that you may be at some time on a lonely Louisiana bayou known as Bayou Self. That is the event that needs to be planned for during preparation and disaster planning. Being by yourself can mean many things such as destruction of external communications, lack of supply routes for critical stores, security challenges, and a myriad of other scenarios in an actual disaster. Planning for the worst case should take into account that your facility may be very well be "on you own" for some number of hours, days or even weeks. And guess what, there will be situations that occur you did not think of; the goal is to have that list at an absolute minimum.

If there is one steadfast rule to serving as the CEO in a disaster it is that the person must commit to taking a very proactive role in communications. And although that applies externally and internally, the communication to and from the facility personnel must be a primary concern. Whatever the disaster type, the staff, including leadership structure, will be anxious and concerned not only for their patients and employees, but for their families who may be weathering the disaster near or far. Keeping this group of people as well informed as possible is critical and falls upon the CEO to provide the mechanism to disseminate current information as accurately and promptly as possible.

When people are in possession of information regarding current status, supply availability, what external support is or is not available, what the security status is, and what is known of the impact to the immediate environment, they will be much better equipped to carry out their individual functions. Fostering an open communication environment will serve to relieve as much of the "unknowns" as possible among the staff and allow them to concentrate on their immediate roles in the crisis.

A critical decision in planning is whether the CEO will serve as the Incident Commander or should that role fall to another staff member. This decision will take into account many factors. Obviously in smaller facilities with limited personnel, in all likelihood the CEO will fill this role. In larger facilities with greater resources, a distribution of talent that makes the most sense for that facility needs to be entertained. There are advantages and disadvantages of both structures and only the local factors within a facility can dictate which is the best for that organization. One of the advantages of delegating the Incident Commander role is that it allows the CEO more time to take in a broader view of the overall internal and external landscape of the event while the IC handles the ongoing operational matters in the command center. Based on circumstances wearing too many hats at some point can be a hindrance. And having the CEO free to coordinate with regional governmental authorities while confident that the operations are being adequately handled back in the Incident Command Center can be an advantage.

A major decision factor is having extreme confidence in one of the staff to act as the Incident Commander that has the proper training and knowledge. This can be of the utmost importance.

Regardless, both scenarios work and only local factors can dictate what is best for a given facility and organization.

With all of the responsibilities encountered on a day to day basis in facility management, it is sometimes difficult to set aside the proper time and energy for active involvement in the sometime lengthy ordeal of participating in meetings, planning sessions, etc., required to formulate an effective Disaster Plan and Incident Command System. With budgets, board preparations, negotiations, HR issues and a mix of other duties vying for an executive's attention it can be hard to put in the time to prepare for an event that may or may not occur. Just having a plan on paper and an organizational chart with all the blocks filled in is not enough. Will it work? That is the question and when it comes time to put that plan into operation, those periods involved in planning and testing will be paid back in multiples.

The existence of the plan is one thing, testing it is another, whether it be table top exercises or fully fledged community wide simulated disaster, it is incumbent upon the CEO to be as confident as possible that the plan will be realistic and effective when put into action. Participation in drills is paramount to tweaking the plan to meet the unique challenges and needs of the facility. Examining as many "what if" scenarios as possible in the process will serve well for future eventualities.

During an actual event, a CEO will be looked to for setting the groundwork for an environment in which teamwork is placed as a priority as never before. All pistons firing in the proper sequence makes an engine function effectively just as all parameters of a disaster plan would be coordinated to function in a rhythm that results in the entire team working as a unit. The CEO is the person that starts that engine and in activating the plan is put into a broader role of leadership that has not been needed on a day to day operational basis. This is true whether that person is the Incident Commander or not.

It is not the purpose of this chapter to go into the depths of the organizational chart for disaster management, that is done elsewhere, but to touch on the most likely challenges that an Executive Officer will encounter in the event of plan activation.

The first and one of the most important roles is that a CEO now becomes the source of information and communication of that information to the team members. Not enough can be said about how important this function is to the successful progression of the plan. Although it is impractical and probably not wise to share all information about what goes on in the command center, it is important that relevant information that affects those at the bedside as well as others on the front lines gets disseminated. Engineering, Security, Logistics, Purchasing, Finance, etc. need to be kept informed of the progression of events. Lack of knowledge at the staff level only creates an environment for speculation and anxiety. Sharing information such as environmental status, stores, security, plan for next 12 hours, etc. all serve to belay unknowns and empower the staff to worry less about that and concentrate on their current duties. The CEO needs to be acutely aware that everyone, no matter what staff level, is being affected by the event while serving on the front line.

This is not to say communication will be easy. In an event that wipes out cell, land line, radio, and satellite communications the facility will be on its own and rely on the disaster plan. This lack of communication with external sources can last for an indefinite period, so keeping the staff informed of the progress in reestablishing this is paramount. Remember, those folks have family members, friends, pets, etc. that are on the outside and will be concerned for their welfare. If a reasonable projection can be given as to when external communication will be in place it will most certainly ease some of the normal anxiety.

Internal communication to relay this type of information can best be accomplished by daily group meetings, the frequency of those meetings determined by the current status of the disaster. To meet as a group two or three times a day is not unusual in the early stages as assessments, planning implementation will be moving at a fairly rapid pace. Obviously there is no email, fax, pager or digital communication so whatever needs to be discussed will be done with management in attendance. If space allows, it is not a bad idea to invite any off duty personnel to attend as well. Keeping staff informed of important Incident Command discussions and planning for eventualities will go a long way in providing tools for the staff to perform at their best possible level.

In this forum the CEO will set the tone for what is to come. A realistic explanation of the situation, as best known, should be shared as well as what the plan for the next several hours will be. Many topics will be discussed in Incident Command; those that effect staff directly should be shared as honestly as possible. Such questions as: Are we safe? When will we have internal communication lines? What is the status of the area, city, state, etc.? Is the fuel status OK for the generators? Is adequate food available for patients and staff? Does Purchasing have adequate stores to see us through? When will we be able to communicate with family? Can we expect outside help? Will the relief staffing team be able to arrive at the planned time? What services are we prepared to offer the community? Is our census likely to change in either direction?

These are questions that will be going through the minds of all staff as they proceed to care for their patients and implement the planning in their respective departments. Answering the questions that can be and assuring answers to the unknowns will be made readily available as soon as possible will go a long way in helping staff focus on their assigned duties.

The frequency of these meetings can be adjusted as the initial challenges resolve, however, until some form of internal communication is reestablished that is available to everyone, at least daily debriefings should be in order. This can only be determined by the Incident Command team as the event progresses. Just as location, location, location is the byword in the real estate world; communication should be that of the Executive in a disaster setting.

Security is also extremely important. Everyone has heard of the lawlessness in New Orleans in the wake of Katrina. With the breakdown of social norms in a disaster environment security of staff and patients will be a major concern and one that the CEO should be intimately involved in. Immobilization of law enforcement by road blockages, destruction of their communication equipment, and other external duties of law enforcement may make their availability an issue for a health care facility. It is therefore incumbent upon the planning group that accommodations for the facility safety taken into account and is practical to implement should the plan be activated.

Perimeter security as well as building access needs to be well controlled for the safety of those in the facility as well as those seeking medical care during and after the event. The CEO should be well informed on all security issues in a real time basis, although the actual implementation will be delegated to the appropriate personnel. The status of security is one of those things that are of utmost importance to communicate to the staff as a whole. Fear for their own and patients' safety can definitely affect their ability to deliver care. Feeling "their backs are covered" will allow them to put aside one more concern that detracts from performance ability.

Most facilities have uniformed security that will initially serve this purpose. However, based upon the magnitude of the event, outside resources may need to be accessed to provide the level of security necessary over a protracted period of time. Prior arrangements with security services or law enforcement agencies should be considered in formulating the disaster plan. The staff during an event will be under a tremendous pressure and having to worry about their own safety or lawless events on the campus should not be a hindrance to them.

With the advent of a disaster, the CEO's responsibility for the financial health of the institution does not change. It is extremely important that Finance be an active department in the disaster plan and keep an accurate record of expenditures, losses, asset changes and any other fiscal events that affect the function of the facility during and after a disaster. Normally the Chief Financial Officer leads this effort and although not as high a priority as patient care, the CEO needs to assure that this important function is not allowed to go untended. Any potential for expense reimbursement post event will need complete and accurate documentation of the fiscal events that have occurred.

In the course of everyday hospital operations, one of the CEO's greatest responsibilities is Medical Staff relations. This is a unique relationship that is usually cultivated over a long period of time and must involve mutual trust to be effective. In the event of a disaster this becomes even more important and is critical for successful healthcare management of existing patients as well as those that may seek care as a consequence of the event. Those physicians who make up the initial response team will be those burdened with the most complex and challenging issues.

Their stay in that position could be very well for an extended period of time if the relief team cannot access the facility at the prescribed period. Their responsibility will be great in delivering medical care to existing patients but in triaging any patients arriving upon the campus seeking care. They may as well be called upon to act in a community wide triage fashion for mass causalities or evacuations from other facilities to theirs.

It is the CEO's responsibility to see that the clinical staff and Medical Staff have the tools they need to fulfill the mission. The Medical Staff will be practicing their profession under less than desirable conditions. Although a Vice President of Medical Affairs or Medical Director will be the most likely direct contact in an event, it is critical that they understand that the CEO is supporting that VPMA to make the challenging conditions as manageable as possible.

Medical staff representatives must be involved in the planning for disaster preparedness to answer such questions as: Will we have the capability to run operating rooms, and how many? What procedures will we be equipped to perform? Is the PACU functional and at what volume? What is the capacity and status of the MICU/SICU? What sort of volume is anticipated for the ED? These questions should be answered in the planning and drill sessions and fall seamlessly into the implementation of the plan with the leadership of the Medical Staff.

Medical protocols both to and from the facilities will have been worked out in planning stages as well. Obviously there is no plan that goes off without a hitch, however, having as many "what if" scenarios should have been worked through. The Medical Staff, with support of the CEO and Incident Commander, can be prepared and knowledgeable of what to expect and anticipate. The Medical Staff will look to the CEO to provide adequate staffing through direct reports of the various units that will be operational during and after an event.

The emergency department Medical Staff will need to be informed of as much information as possible on what to expect. They serve as the front line on intake and triage and it is critical that they have as much information as available in what to expect in terms of facility to facility transfers and any influx of patients seeking emergent care.

This once again illustrates the communications responsibility of the Chief Executive to assure that these folks have as much up to date knowledge as possible through whatever internal communications systems have been set up. That theme of communication never lessens as the course of events plays itself out.

The environmental assessment of the immediate local and regional area needs to occur as quickly as is feasible. The status of law enforcement, utility availability, other facility capabilities, transportation options, mobilization of regional emergency management resources, etc. needs to be garnered as quickly as possible and communicated to Incident Command. Ideally the CEO is the primary contact with the community emergency groups and participates in the local/regional meetings as soon as they are implemented. This can be delegated and most likely will be when conditions require the CEO's presence elsewhere, but with the Chief Executive being primarily involved, it is a message that the coordination efforts are at the highest levels of the stakeholders.

Taking ownership of this function also provides access to first-hand information regarding the status of conditions, support available, timetables etc. that needs to be communicated back to the facility in as real time a manner as possible.

This has been only a brief overview of what can be expected of a CEO's role in facility preparedness and execution, but there is one other thing that a hospital leader needs to be prepared for when a well thought out plan in implemented. And that is <u>prepare to be amazed</u>. Amazed at the resilience and dedication of the staff and the truly superhuman effort they put into caring for the facilities patients and meeting the many challenges thrown their way throughout the course of an event. Stories are merely anecdotal; however, I would like in closing to share a couple with you of what I witnessed as CEO of NorthShore Regional Medical Center in Slidell, LA during Hurricane Katrina.

We had a campus with a closed psychiatry hospital, an outpatient surgical center, an evacuated long term care facility and the acute care hospital. Being on the north shore of Lake Pontchartrain, we sustained mostly wind damage and with generator power were able to function under our plan. We also became the collection point for the evacuation of patients and staff of more severely damaged facilities on the south shore of the Metro New Orleans area. As a consequence our helipad was a flurry of activity with incoming patient transfers. By the time it was over the psych hospital, outpatient surgery suite, and long term care unit as well as the main hospital became acute patient care areas. Our census swelled from about 28 due to discharges and transfers in preparation for the event to over 400 at the peak of the incoming transfers.

To see a ninety pound nurse racing back and forth from the helipad pushing a gurney carrying a 300 pound patient at full speed to the triage area is truly amazing, not once or twice but many times. To have your Medical Staff who were stuck there, as the relief team could not access the area, work tirelessly day after day caring for current and incoming patients is amazing. To have your Performance Improvement physician and nurse director implement a system for assessing, tracking and recording the whereabouts and disposition of every patient that arrived during other facility evacuations is truly amazing.

With resolution of the event it may be tempting to say thank goodness it is over, but it is not over. At such time as is practical when the staff is rested and operations have returned to near normal it is critical to objectively debrief and form a constructive critique of what was done well and what could benefit from plan improvement. As soon as reasonable after the event this should take place in the time period where everyone's memory of the event is fresh. The CEO should convey to all concerned that this merely represents the ongoing planning process. Lessons learned will provide the alterations in the plan for next event, thus making the plan as it should be: a truly living document going through continuous improvement.

CHAPTER 4

# Emergency Operations Center (EOC)

● ● ●

**Robert J. Muller**

## Overview

The EOC must be organized to ensure the internal and external operations are able to function efficiently. It should be organized to serve as an effective Communication center, and information clearinghouse; a place to resolve confusion and conflict, and an authoritative source of information and decisions. It should also be designed so there is little disruption to current operational systems, converted rapidly, centrally located and exercised at least annually and be designed for totally **self-sustained operations** for at least 72-96 hours.

## Description

The hospital EOC can employ a variety of organization structures, depending on the breath and scope of the event.

1. Single Jurisdictional/ single agency involvement
2. Single Jurisdictional/ multiple agency involvement
3. Multi-Jurisdictional/ multi-agency involvement

The event will dictate what the magnitude of the response will be, and to what extent outside resources and personnel need to be utilized.

In a small community the hospital may become the focus of the EOC and be totally involved in the community response with other agencies. If this becomes the case always remember that the hospital needs to have its own operational center and NOT become a subdivision of a larger organizational response. If this should become the case, then form a hospital EOC and allow a section of the hospital (i.e. cafeteria) to be used for the community EOC if one has not been previously designated or an alternate location needs to be established from the previous established site. If this should become the case then a liaison officer or deputy liaison officer should be designated to the larger community EOC if necessary for continuity purposes.

## EOC Design

**Location**

1. Should be in same building as general operations unless precluded from doing so due to various reasons.
2. The location can be converted into an EOC rapidly by being converted for activation within 30 minutes. It should not be located within a potentially hazardous area or Bioterrorist target area.
3. An alternate (secondary) location should be planned and readily accessible. Secondary location should be away from the primary location in case of destruction, devastation, inability to access, etc., the primary location. The secondary

location should have a written SOP known to all applicable personnel as to when where, how to locate, report, and facilitate equipment transport and placement to said location.

4. The location should be internal or with special protected windows if an external perimeter placement location is necessitated.

**Size:**

1. A minimum of 50 square feet per EOC staff member assigned to the EOC is ideal, but with the known limited space within hospitals many variations of this suggestion can be made to work.
2. It must accommodate or be in the area of facilities for sleeping and eating in order to facilitate continuous operations. Suggested locations: Boardroom, Conference room, auditorium, etc.

**Equipment:**

1. Electrical power (alternative source- generator), fuel supply and life support (food, water, sewer, heating, air conditioning, etc.)
2. Emergency Communication equipment; easy runs for antenna access to rooftops, etc.
3. Protection against lightning, power surges, as well as all BT threats; Functional furniture, chairs, etc.
4. Set-up plan
5. Computer work-stations for laptop plug-in access; at least (1) Satellite computer connection
6. Redundancy of equipment in case of failure.
7. Telephone Connections- 8-10 lines.

**Necessary – Often Forgotten Equipment/ Supplies**

1. Paper products – plates, cups, plastic knives, forks, spoons.
2. Electrical Extension Cords – at least 10—15ft, 25ft and 50ft. lengths – depending on the need to connect to the emergency power supply.
3. Electrical strips and Table Fans.
4. Garbage cans/ garbage bags.
5. Emergency Lighting – temporary source i.e. battery style lights (Coleman Lamps); LED lighting most energy efficient for battery use.
6. Command Vests or Uniform Identifiable clothing for command center staff.
7. EOC Refrigerator – water, juices, drinks.
8. EOC Coffee Maker
9. Wall Maps & Flow Charts.
10. Bookshelves to house:
    EOC Plan
    Haz Mat Guide Book
    Master Telephone Directory
    BT Reference Material
    Supplier Reference Materials

## EOC Set-Up Criteria

**Keys:**

- Who has them?
- Where are they located?

**Furniture:**

- Where is it stored?

- Where does it go? Include an EOC floor plan that shows the furniture layout.
- Who is responsible for setting up the furniture?
- How are they altered?

**Communications:**

- If communication devices are not permanently installed in the EOC, where are they stored (phone sets, cellular phones, radio transceivers, intercom systems, scanners, etc.)?
- Where should they be located in the EOC?
- Where is the system connections located?
- Who is responsible for communications setup and how are they altered? (Have a backup plan)

**Display Services:**

- If display services are not permanently mounted, where are they stored?
- Where should they be located?
- Who is responsible for setting up the displays?

**Equipment and Supplies:**

- Where are the supplies and the equipment stored?
- Who is responsible for distribution of supplies?

***Same checklist would apply for deactivating the center.***

**Standard Operating Procedures (SOP)**

SOP should be formulated based on the specifics of the organization, but basics for all situations should be as follows:

Authority:

1. Define who has the authority to open the EOC and call out the staff.
2. Define who has the final authority in all disaster situations.

Conditions:

1. State under what conditions/ situations the EOC should be activated.
2. List and define the classes of Emergencies as pertained to the corporate or local structure and situations.

Alerting:

1. Define Call-out notification procedures.

Set Up:

1. Define and plan EOC set up; who is responsible for the set up tasks; as well who is responsible for the take down upon completion of the event.

Position Descriptions:

1. Written descriptions of each person's job duties should be included and part of the EOC plan book. See Annex under Incident Command Job Action sheets.

## Notification Procedures

Call out of command center personnel is usually done by the following:

1. Alert List
2. Notification Table
3. Cascade Notification System

Alert List
A roster of

- EOC positions
- Individuals occupying each positions
- Phone numbers

The alert list can contain cues for when the EOC members should report without a phone call, especially in situations where phone systems may be disabled.

Notification Table
This is a table formed based on EOC positions and types of emergencies as well as the severity of the emergency.

Cascade Notification System
This system is employed when there is limited notification/communication personnel available to activate an entire list. In this system, several key EOC members are notified who in turn notify other members. This system if instituted should be tied in two directions, both from the top down, and the bottom up, in case there is a one-way break in the system. This provides redundancy to the system.

## Staffing Requirements Matrix

Position: The title for a specific task or function.
Duties and Responsibilities: A description of the person's duties and responsibilities.

Sources and Qualification: The possible sources for procuring the services and desired qualifications.
Size/Composition/Number of Shifts: Provides details about when and how to staff up for a particular position.
Selective Priority: Indicates when personnel should be called in and who should be called first, etc.
Special Considerations: Describes any special considerations or situations of which you should be aware.

CHAPTER 5

# Welcome To the Emergency Operations Center

• • •

Robert J. Muller

So now the time is here. You have completed all the Incident Command System training on the basic and/or advanced level; you have been through training exercises from table tops to full scale; you have planned, rehearsed, memorized plans and scenarios BUT today is the REAL thing. How will you react; how will you respond; how will you perform? Will you be able respond; will you be able to put it all together to perform?

The Emergency Operations Center (EOC) must come together to deal with the emergency at hand and to deal with the current scenario. You are called to fulfill your role --- NOW and IMMEDIATE.

Where are you? What are you doing----can you immediately drop what you are doing and respond; or is there some delay before you complete your present task?

Where is your family and pets? Are they ok? Can you be away from them while you respond to the command center? Are they prepared to take care of themselves to deal with the possible crisis, especially if it involves the entire community? Have you prepared your family and employer for this day?

You arrive at the EOC and have reported in for your position --- you have your vest, you have logged in your tag. What do you do next?

Well here are a few hints, with a ten point plan, that may be of benefit, from someone who has been in your shoes many times before and in many different command positions.

If you are available for a command position, then you should always have a "Go Bag" (see Appendix) packed and ready to go --- in your office, home or the trunk of your car. It should contain all of your essential items both for personal use as well as that which may be needed to carry out you assigned function on the staff.

After initially reporting and receiving your current assignment, which may be changed later in the event, it is important to do several very basic things to acclimate yourself:

**First**; basic and simple --- introduce yourself to the members of the command center team and if you are in a joint command situation, establish the agencies represented and their role in the incident command structure.

**Second**; establish some of the basics until official briefings are given; set up your command position and make it homey. This will be your new temporary home for an unknown future period of time. Set up your laptop or position desktop computer; it you have your information on a thumb drive as many commanders do, insert it after making sure of the computer functionality and it is free of viruses; set up your telephones, cellphones, radio, pens, paper, ICS forms, etc. Welcome to your new home for the hours, days or weeks to come.

**Third**; evaluate the physical layout around you, especially if you are not familiar with your surroundings. If this is a large event, establish different possible locations the command center maybe relocated in case of an events that may force the present area to become inoperable. Also evaluate areas where other sections maybe located if the central command center is not large enough to accommodate all; i.e. finance and logistics. When possible the command staff and the operations section should all be within one area and not separated by walls. This all should be pre-planned well in advance. You should also familiarize yourself with the locations of restrooms, break areas, eating and sleeping locations.

**Fourth**; make sure you have at least a bottle of water and a few small snacks at your position; as the situation reaches a crescendo it may not allow for your absence for any extended period of time to seek nourishment.

**Fifth**; prepare your own notes and make your own sheet of those things that are important to your position, the event, and your role in carrying out your assignment. If you are the logistics chief, then you may want to begin to formulate your vendor contact list and make some phone calls to those you may want to put on alert. I recommend this be planned in advance and create a thumb drive with various folder categories with all possible pertinent information, contacts and telephone numbers that are ready for your viewing. (These should be updated on a regular basis to keep information current).

**Sixth**; prepare yourself in your position to report your status and anticipated plans at the IC briefing meetings. At the time of the initial staff meeting make sure that you are aware of all of the details of the event, and anticipate what is needed not only NOW, but in the near and distant future; initiate the process to prepare and deal with all of those events.

**Seventh**; make sure there is adequate security with the location, entrances and for the personnel of the command center. Establish protocols for entrance into the center to prevent the unauthorized flow of persons into the area that may cause distractions and prevent the necessary concentration of the staff.

**Eight**; as the events evolve, make sure you anticipate times for breaks, eating and sleeping; identify your replacement for any extended absences from your position and make sure he/she is thoroughly briefed as to your status of situations in progress.

**Ninth**; do not be afraid to ask for help from others, and they likewise the same from you. Remember no one is expected to know it all. A coalescence of information as well as the willingness of yourself and those around you helps to establish an "esprit de corps" within the group.

**Tenth**; remember the longer and event evolves, the more likely an internal conflict will develop with one or more coworkers. It never fails that someone(s) feels that you or another, including them, could be doing a better job at your position.

The prolonged stress of an event plays upon people's emotions, so don't be surprised if your best friend or coworker, all of a sudden becomes a raving maniac. It happens---it happens often. When it happens (not necessarily if it happens) be calm, cool, collected and well controlled and self-disciplined, rather than entering into a shouting match response. This is the best way to rapidly diffuse the situation and indicate your command of the situation rather than being an additional problem for other coworkers to have deal with and enter into arbitration.

This may also become a time for everyone on the staff to re-evaluate themselves and their stress levels and the need for additional time away from their position and the need for relief staff to be put into place to provide for much needed and appreciated breaks in the action.

The emergency operations command center is a dynamic place of constant change. The personnel must likewise be able to handle change --- sometime very rapid change. It is of the utmost importance that the command center be able to provide what it is designated to do--- provide the necessary guidance and support of an operation or event, as rapidly, efficiently and cost effective as possible with the preservation of life and property as its foremost goal. This goal is achieved through the knowledge, training and experience of its staff. The outcome of the operation is based on the preparedness of the staff --- the end point of its function is the individuals and their performance. Yes --- it is all about YOU!!

CHAPTER 6

# Managing Conflict

● ● ●

**Robert J. Muller**

In any event, when multiple talents and personalities are drawn together for a common goal fueled by a fervent intensity to achieve and succeed, **CONFLICT** is inevitable.

Conflict would not occur if two or more people did not care about something ------- something, usually, they feel they cannot get or something they feel that they cannot give.

The simplest way to reduce conflict is to stop caring --- this is also the **worse solution to the problem.** Learning how to disagree productively is a critical skill for people in an integrated emergency management system.

Positive results can be derived when conflict is handled effectively. Reaching a consensus is vital after all the views of the management team are heard and given fair consideration.

Conflict and disagreement is an innate and essential part of the process and occurs naturally when people are passionate about an issue; due to the fact the management team is comprised of many experts from different areas, many different viewpoints, as to the BEST modality to handle the crisis arise.

In any and all situations it is always best to have an amicable resolution to the conflict situation BUT also remember someone has to make the final decision which is in the best interest of all involved as well as the resolution of the situation in question. This will become the ultimate decision of the command staff and the incident commander.

It is important for the management team to build an atmosphere that is conducive to the expression as well as the resolution of different opinions after thorough investigation and application/consideration of all possible courses of action.

CHAPTER 7

# Communications

• • •

**Robert J. Muller**

THE KEY TO THE SUCCESSFUL operation of any Emergency Operation Center (EOC) is communications with contingency plans for multiple redundancies.

The following list should be a minimal of the type and kind of communication equipment necessary for successful continuous operations of the EOC:

1. Landline telephone system of 8-10 lines – supported by the local telephone company priority restoration* (TPS) agreement for the emergency restoration in case of loss contact.
2. Government Emergency Telephone System (GETS)*, (applied through a local United States Senator for government Satellite system access.) (Plastic Credit Cards are issued [following successful application and approval] with special telephone numbers that can be accessed thru landlines, cellular or satellite telephones; for nationwide connection.
3. Satellite Telephones- that are programmed into the building internal telephone system and have rooftop fixed antennae. The operation center should have are least 2, possibly as many as 4, OR the ability to add 2 more should the situation mandate additional needs. The cost factors

are minimal being about $1200-1500 for a fixed antennae internal system; Satellite access service is at $400-500 per year per phone for minimal usage (? 400 minutes/year).

4. Nextel /Verizon– Direct connect feature excellent in emergencies when cellular sites are jammed with excess traffic.
5. Amateur Radio (HAM)—excellent system for both long and short range contacts with hospitals as well as most government agencies. Antennas need to be roof mounted and able to be placed as part of the EOC set-up procedure. Only federally licensed HAM operators can use the equipment – the local HAM clubs usually will provide someone under a SOP agreement.
6. Cellular – Alternate means of communications in certain circumstances but have problems with weather related tower damage, as well as circuit (cells) overloading with excess traffic during emergencies.
7. Local Government Services Communications links for the area. This includes systems for communications with local police, fire, emergency operations, mayor's office, State EOC, etc. This would include systems of VHF, UHF, 700 & 800 MHz networks with good rooftop antenna systems. These systems would only be operable within a defined area dependent upon terrain, antenna height, radio frequency, power (watts), repeater systems, etc. These systems would require prior authorization from each of the agencies that frequency usage would be desired, i.e. P.D., F.D., State DPS, etc; Each of these system also require a federal license for use, unless the hospital system is part of a system that is already licensed, i.e. fire department, etc. This may be the better approach in many instances----make an agreement with these agencies that the hospital will purchase the specific communications equipment but it will be

maintained and licensed under the department from which it was issued. A local National Weather Service battery operated weather radio would be advisable for local weather conditions.

8. Internal Computer Access – modem, DSL and Broadband wireless access (3 different access redundancies).
9. One way Communication – Television and Radio, both standard AM/FM and Satellite should be available in the EOC to maintain utilization of the network capabilities to evaluate and report on the local emergency situations. The Weather Channel should also be available either by TV or computer.
10. Fax – one machine with a backup readily available from another source or other area.

For more and complete details on the subject of EOC, I refer you to my collogue Dr. Michael Fagel's book entitled "Principles of Emergency Management and EOC Operations," CRC Press, 2011

CHAPTER 8

# Hospital Blueprint for Disaster Management

• • •

**Susan O'Brien**

A HOSPITAL IS MANDATED BY The Joint Commission of Accreditation for Hospitals Organization (JCAHO) to establish an effective and efficient disaster plan that has been tested by the hospital on a routine basis. The hospital must participate in a community based disaster preparation program which in turn participates in a regional structured disaster preparedness program or committee, which may in turn request assistance through the Federal Emergency Management Agency (FEMA). Additionally, there are established laws and regulations which the hospital is required to meet on a 24 hour/7 day a week basis.

Every hospital faces some type of man–made and /or natural disaster. Man-made disasters include chemical spills, exposure to radiation, electrical system failure, etc. Natural disasters include but are not limited to weather conditions that create hurricanes, snow storms, earthquakes and flooding. Disaster preparedness is the key to success and requires the support of all of the hospital's staff and the community. The hospital leaders, medical staff, hospital managers and community leaders plan and coordinate disaster preparedness activities. The established JCAHO standards describe the specific steps the organization must complete to comply with the standards and meet the needs of patients, hospital and medical staff, board members and community needs. Standards are a level of achievement and quality which are considered minimally acceptable.

The hospital plan must evaluate and plan for the following:

- Maintaining or expanding services - At one point during Hurricane Katrina, we had over four hundred patients in our hospital which was licensed for less than 200 beds. Decisions were made about which patients could be safely transported to another hospital and which patients were too unstable for transport and required immediate admission into a hospital setting. This is called a medical surge and the hospital must establish plans to provide adequate medical evaluation and care during disasters that exceed the usual limits of normal hospital practices. This encompasses the ability of the hospital to survive and maintain or to recover operations which were compromised during a disaster.
- Conserving resources – Both staff and supplies must be addressed.
- Curtailing services – Once the humidity and temperature reaches a certain point, all OR and Delivery services are eliminated due to contamination of supplies unless the patient's condition is so dire and life threatening that intervention is indicated as an immediate need.
- Supplementing resources from outside the local community - During Hurricane Katrina, our national hospital system was able to recruit staff and obtain much needed supplies for continued operation. Huge generator trucks were sent to assist in supplying electricity and much welcomed air conditioning services. Normal routes were not available. Plans were made to fly supplemental staffing and

supplies to another state and transported via buses and trucks through open routes.

- Closing the hospital to new patients – This is not a reality when you are receiving patients from other hospitals which are without any services.
- Evaluate evacuation plans for completeness and potential outcomes of the plan as situations change. Planning and preparation for a worst case scenario must be considered.
- Total evacuation.

The hospital develops a Disaster Preparedness Plan or an Emergency Operations Plan based on a Hazard Vulnerability Analysis (HVA). The HVA is developed by hospital leaders, managers, medical staff and board members with the support of community leaders. The HVA provides information and builds the base for the development of the disaster plan. A hospital may develop several HVAs to comply with the standards. Some examples would include hurricane, flooding, external chemical spill, influx of patients, tornado, etc.

The HVA identifies the following:

- Potential emergencies that could affect the demand for hospital services or its ability to provide those services. These disasters could be in a geographically prone area. Earthquakes are a disaster threat in California but are not likely to pose a disaster threat in Florida.
- Defines mitigating activities designed to reduce the risk and potential damage from an emergency situation.
- Serves as a basic structure to develop activities that will organize and mobilize essential resources. The depth of this part of the HVA cannot be underestimated. Hospital staff, medical staff, hospital leaders and hospital departments

perform individualized HVA's which are reported to the appropriate committee to ensure collaboration across the organization and the community.

- Maintaining adequate resources and inventory must be addressed. Resources include personal protective equipment, water, fuel, all supplies needed on a daily basis, such as food and medications. The inventory list of what is available on site begins the process. The plan must also address the Incident Command Center including designation of needed members and physical placement of the command center with supplies, such as white boards, communication services, etc. Again, community leaders must participate in preparation of and recovery from a disaster.

The four phases of a disaster include mitigation, preparedness, response and recovery.

Communication and high visibility motivate the staff and provides a channel of communication of issues, barriers, etc., to ensure all standards, regulations and laws are met. The staff know what is working, what is not working, obstacles to achieve the goal of providing quality care despite the obstacles presented. Staff may avoid going through management layers to communicate, especially if they think the problem is "not important" but it may produce a "work around" which is less efficient or negatively impacts other areas of the hospital. Frequent "huddles" with the staff provide high visibility and excellent channels of communication.

Carefully consider your policy regarding the staff and their family members. Issues and or concerns can be identified during unit and departmental rounds. This policy must be in effect and communicated to all staff prior to a disaster to avoid any dissent during the early phases of the disaster. Carefully address and identify the staff and their family members that may stay at the hospital during the disaster as well as their limitations and needs, e.g. food, linen, medication, etc. Elder care may be a concern. Ensure that all elders who come to the hospital bring all appropriate medications and care items with them.

Develop a volunteer pool of visitors and family members to support hospital and professional staff. If the elevator system is damaged, not on emergency generator power or if emergency energy conservation is in place, this team of volunteers may provide to be a valuable asset in vertical transport. Food trays, linens, trash pickup and disposal and supplies must be provided. The most efficient process is to establish a line of volunteers to move the needed items as "everything that goes up, must come down". In this situation, patients are not being transferred for diagnostic testing, surgery, etc. Services become limited. For example, if the water pressure and or supply become an issue, this will result in no hemodialysis services for inpatients or community members who arrive at the hospital for care. The laboratory services became limited due to heat. Sensitive laboratory equipment is not reliable in excessive heat. Hospitals not affected will provide some support services if possible, but transportation of samples requires gasoline which at times may be limited.

In Louisiana we have an expression "when the water goes down, the snakes come up". Being surrounded by bayous, the lake, and other bodies of water was a cause for concern. A meeting with our Chief Pharmacist identified the types of snakes which frequent our area, if anti-venom is indicated, etc. Anti-venom is expensive, has a short shelf life and the dosage administered is calculated based on the patient's weight. Supplies were obtained; however, not a single dose of anti-venom was administered. A blue tent was set up outdoors and within close proximity to the E.R. for the administration of Tetanus Toxoid. After assessment and consent, over 4,000 doses of Tetanus Toxoid were administered free of charge. We also provided free bottled water and free formula. Many chain saw accidents were treated. Subsequently, our hospital presented education programs on chain saw safety based on this experience.

Staffing is always a major concern and takes patience, time and sometimes a bit of humor. Each hospital has a different approach on how to undertake staffing. The staff on duty is usually expected to respond to the disaster. It is essential for your team to address staffing, backup staffing, and contingency staffing plans in preparation for adequate provisions (water, food, linen, etc.) for everyone. This is a medical surge and the hospital should have plans to provide adequate medical evaluation and care during disasters that exceed the usual limits of normal hospital practices. This encompasses the ability of the hospital to survive and maintain or to recover operations which were compromised during a disaster.

Every hospital has a generator which provides limited essential electrical power. The generator is usually powered by diesel fuel from a tank that is maintained by support personnel and routine assessment. The amount of diesel fuel on hand and the ability to procure more fuel will affect what course of action the hospital takes over the next 24 hours. If the hospital generator is located in the basement and flooding occurs, all electrical services are lost. Fortunately, we had no flooding but the generator was located on the roof of our hospital. Total evacuation is always a reality; however, it certainly should be considered a last step. Plans for total evacuation should be frequently reviewed and revised as needed. A total evacuation can turn to shambles if not well planned and ready to implement on short notice.

Coordinated disaster protocols for transport must be identified in the Hospital Plan for Disaster. This includes EMS Services which are essential to transporting to another healthcare setting. During a disaster, local EMS services may not be operational or overwhelmed with requests. During Hurricane Katrina, dependence on local EMS was not sufficient to meet the need. Through coordination, EMS systems from other areas were designated to meet the hospital's needs. Several EMS units traveling to the disaster site were commandeered by other agencies and some were detained for gasoline which was siphoned off for other needs. That is how dire the situation can become.

If no definitive date is projected for the end of the disaster, the hospital must have vendor contractual arrangements in place to ensure delivery of adequate medications and supplies. Even with contractual agreements, the vendor may not be able to provide supplies. The response time of vendors after Hurricane Katrina was impressive. We never ran out of linens and even though food services were rather limited, we always had food.

Communication during and in the aftermath of a disaster is a challenge. The hospital may accomplish this via cell phones, land lines, bulletin boards, fax, satellite phones, text messaging, amateur radio, meetings and verbal exchanges. The disaster plan should outline the means of communication and various backup systems and plans on how hospitals communicate a disaster to external authorities, staff, medical staff, patients and families. The media should also be included in the hospital's plan. What information is appropriate for sharing with media and who should be identified as the hospital's spokesperson must be planned prior to the disaster. How and what information regarding patients must be addressed. It is usual and customary for transfer that identified parts of the medical record are appropriate for transfer. In "normal" times, these records would be copied. The recent introduction to the electronic medical record would eliminate copying but transfer of information electronically in a protected manner which ensures confidentiality may be compromised. All these usual policies may not be applicable in an overwhelming disaster situation. Patients arrived at our hospital with their entire medical record in plastic zip lock bags. As arrangements had been made to transfer stable patients to other facilities in our system, emergency power supported only one copy machine. The decision was made to transfer the paper record with the patient to another care setting. In regards to communication, the satellite phones were our savior.

In some situations the ability to track deaths and dignified care of remains may be a factor. Body bags and storage in the appropriate cooling setting may be a major issue. As such, appropriate processes need to be addressed. Coordination with local authorities and other facilities can assist in this process. Identification of organizational resources is of key importance in this process. Suggested resources include FEMA's National Incident Management System (NIMS) Implementation Activities for Hospitals and Healthcare Systems. http://www.fema.gov/pdf/emergency/nims/imp_hos.pdf

Security must be planned and carefully managed. Multiple entry points into the hospital create even more challenges. Employees may be needed to assist the security team to maintain a secure facility. Residents from nearby neighborhoods who have lost everything will seek refuge at the hospital for food, water, etc. The hospital must adopt a firm plan for intervention, e.g., water, formula, and tetanus toxoid was the adopted protocol during Hurricane Katrina. Certain supplies, especially food, must be conserved to feed staff and patients. Resources may be limited for an unknown period so thoughtful conservation must be addressed.

Hazardous waste must be contained and stored in a designated area. All hospitals must have a plan which addresses decontamination protocols and that these protocols have been practiced as part of an emergency drill.

Staffing from outside of the hospital's usual employee base may occur. If the disaster continues for a period of time, outside assistance becomes a necessity. The usual steps in credentialing healthcare providers may not be feasible; however, some systems must be utilized and an orientation to major hospital systems must be conducted and documented. It is expected that all documentation be completed within 72 hours or post disaster, whichever occurs first. All "volunteer" staff and professionals transported to the hospital are always under the supervision of regular hospital staff.

The physical transportation of this relief team must be planned. Despite all of the turmoil created by Hurricane Katrina, we were dependent on our hospital's corporate office for assistance and coordination with other hospitals to provide essential support systems to meet critical needs. Staff must oversee the practice of healthcare workers which are not members of your system. Healthcare and other support personnel must be readily identified. Disposable nametags will meet this need and must be a well-coordinated effort. Primary Source Verification may not be initially available; however, the disaster plan should describe what documents are needed from outside personnel.

This chapter does not review all standards, implementation, etc. The hospital's plan for disasters needs to be a living document, subject to revision at all times. Disaster plans do not always meet every situation in a severe and prolonged disaster. Certainly, it was recognized that some professional needs could only be met with supplemental staffing. For example, during Hurricane Katrina, the need for PBX operation was acute enough to necessitate supplemental assistance from individuals outside our hospital with this skill set.

The hospital represents a known relationship to the community. During Hurricane Katrina, people who had been on rooftops for days without food and water were rescued and transported via helicopter over a horrific scene of flooding, dead bodies and people crying out for help. These individuals needed to be treated with the utmost care and respect. Once they reached the safety of the hospital, most needed a gentle hand to guide them, listen to their stories and offer comfort. I encountered someone months later in a grocery, needless to say I did not recognize her but her feelings of our hospital and the comfort that she felt will never be forgotten in my lifetime.

Information sharing is an important process that a hospital must adopt. The process of information sharing should include:

- Facility operating status.
- Structural integrity of facility.
- Evacuation status and shelter abilities.
- Critical medical services.
- Critical healthcare services.
- Status of available staffing.
- ER status.

The hospital plan for disaster must include detailed plans for scheduling, triage, assessment, treatment, admission, transfer and discharge. All patients who have the potential for discharge should be scheduled for discharge prior to the disaster. This can be a cumbersome process if accountable parties, e.g. family, nursing home, etc. have already evacuated. It is essential for hospitals to initiate their disaster plan as early as possible. Some disasters are predictable such as hurricanes however, even that can change if the course of the hurricane changes or if an unexpected aftermath occurs. Chemical spills, train wrecks and tornados are examples of disasters which are unpredictable. The hospital plan for disaster must reflect the needs of such unexpected disasters.

A most challenging standard is providing the patients, staff and the community with mental health services during and after disasters. It is most improbable that psychiatric staff will be available in disaster situations. Social workers may be available to meet these needs initially, implement assessments and treatment plans. Many hospitals workers, patients and community members do not even know the status of their families, homes, etc. (Cell phones may not have reception as the towers which transmit signals may be lost due to wind, electrical issues, etc.) but continue to work diligently to meet patient needs and provide comfort to patients, families and co-workers. It is extraordinary to observe and participate in the ongoing processes during horrendous conditions.

Documentation cannot be overstated. The hospital's plan for disaster should assign a designee to document the successes, failures, identified issues and barriers and revise the plan as needed. Documentation of the arrival, assessment, treatment and disposition of patients must be performed.

Maintaining communication to all staff and others must be well planned. Leaders must adopt an attitude of calmness and reassurance as their attitudes during the disaster will cascade to staff, patients and families.

CHAPTER 9

# Decision Making

●●●

**Robert J. Muller**

THE DISASTER PLANNING PROCESS AND its importance has been stressed throughout this book.

Planning is the most vital aspect of emergency management and the warning period may range from just a few hours to days. All hazard planning will establish the template for disaster mitigation, response and recovery.

The only event that offers the emergency manager some degree of advanced notice is the weather related events of hurricanes and floods; and, sometime with much shorter notice --- tornados.

All other events with the probabilities of mass causalities and localized destruction, such as explosions, flash floods, earthquakes, Haz-Mat and terrorist events usually provide no lead time for warnings and preparation.

In the Gulf Coast and Atlantic coastal states, hurricane planning is a requirement due to its high vulnerability assessment value; and due to the prolonged time it takes for preparation and evacuation for the effects that can be caused due to local and regional devastation caused by this weather event. The planning has to be comprehensive and all-inclusive and will also provide an excellent All-Hazard template as well.

One of the very unique aspects about hurricane planning is that it is the only event that can be planned with decision- making time arcs, based on its many variables. This could also be said of wildland fires to some degree but without the numerous variables found in hurricane planning.

Due to these factors --- hurricane planning deserves special attention to understand the background and agencies that are vital, not only for it as an individual event, but also for the value as an All-Hazard template.

## Hurricane Forecasts

The Gulf Coast and Atlantic coast hurricane forecasting is a shared responsibility between the National Hurricane Center (NHC) and the local weather forecast offices (WFO) of the National Oceanographic and Atmospheric Association (NOAA).

The NHC covers the larger picture while the WFO analyses the NHC data and formulates local forecasts based on tidal data and potential impact to the area.

The NHC provides information on minimum central pressure (the lower, usually the stronger the hurricane), storm surge, rainfall, tornados and a predicted path.

## Location

The location of a hurricane is determined by the location of the storms eye. The eye is located by:

Satellite Imagery
Radar (when possible)
Reconnaissance aircraft (the famed Hurricane Hunters)

The accuracy with which each technology can pinpoint the storm depends on how well the storms eye is organized and defined. Each of these parameters have associated degrees of accuracy — generally being, the better organized and defined the greater the degree of accuracy.

The forecasting accuracy improves the closer the storm is to approaching landfall, with the 72 hour accuracy of a 300 mile margin error, compared to a 50 mile error at 12 hours.

## Storm Intensity

The well-known and well established Saffir-Simpson scale has been utilized for years and is generally based on the central barometric pressure of the storm, and predicted wind speed.

In 2012 the scale was revised and the parameter of barometric pressure was removed so that it is now called the Saffir-Simpson Wind Scale and also takes into consideration storm surge on the effects of the storm at landfall.

Storm intensity is most accurately measured by aircraft reconnaissance with accuracies of plus or minus 0-30 Knots and central pressures of plus or minus 3 millibars. (Due to this, a storm category can be inaccurately predicted).

These accuracies are predicated by the Hurricane Hunter aircraft dropping special devices called dropsones from a small shoot in the aircraft, and recording the data measurements in the aircraft as the dropsones fall to the ocean surface. Like the location predication, the accuracy of wind speeds varies with the storms area of central pressure.

## Hurricane "Products"

The NHC issues various types of advisories, forecasts and discussions and these are referred to as "products".

The main type of products are the public advisories, forecast, discussions and strike probabilities. All of these products are released on a scheduled basis in Zulu time. Zulu time compared to Eastern Daylight Time is 4 hours later. Z = 0600 (6 AM) is the same as 0200 EDT or 2 AM EDT.

Zulu time is also known as Greenwich Mean Time (GMT).

Tropical cyclone advisories are issued at 6 hour intervals (3 AM, 9 AM, 3 PM, 9 PM).

## Strike Probabilities

NHC tropical cyclone strike probabilities present the percentage chance that the center (eye) of the hurricane will pass within 65 miles of a specific location. The closer to land the more accurate the probability due to the fact the path deviation becomes smaller as it approaches a landfall.

## Weather Field Office (WFO)

The statements issued by the WFO are issued to augment the NHC advisories and are highly specific to the local area. They are designed to keep the local emergency manager, media and the general public up to date on the anticipated storm impacts.

## Watch and Warning Areas

Before selecting a warning area, hurricane forecasters consult and analyze several computer models to determine the storms' probable course.

Due to the fact the majority of storm damage occurs within a 125 mile swath, the forecasters select a warning area of approximately 300-miles in width (jump points) due to all of the error variables and to ensure that the potential population that is threatened is properly warned.

Remember in plotting and positioning, one degree equals 60 minutes and thus 6 minutes is 1/10 of a degree. One degree latitude equals 60 nautical miles (One nautical mile equals 1.15 land miles). Degrees of latitude are constant, whereas, degrees of longitude become closer toward the north as they converge.

## Storm Surge

Storm surge is an abnormal rise of water generated by a storm, over and above the predicted astronomical tides. Storm surge should not be confused with storm tide, which is defined as the water level rise due to the combination of storm surge and the astronomical tide. This rise in water level can cause extreme flooding in coastal areas particularly when storm surge coincides with normal high tide, resulting in storm tides reaching up to 25 feet or more in some cases.

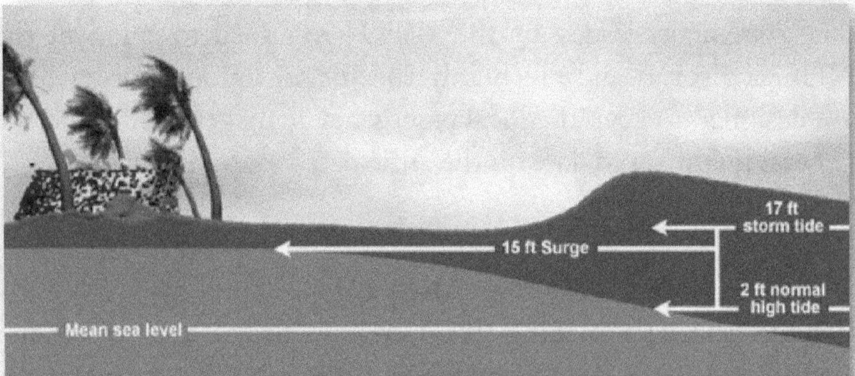


Storm Surge vs. Storm Tide
Source: www.nhc.gov

## Summary

Thus based on distance and forward motion speed, arcs can be created based on time factors, such as 72, 60, 48, 36, 24, 12 and 6 hour arcs. (These will only vary if there is significant change in forward speed or deviation of direction). These are usually termed as T-72, T-24, etc. and post storm events are termed as T+12, T+72, etc.

Planning then can be done based on the anticipated timing and the degree of time it takes to complete a task, such as a hospital evacuation. If a hospital evacuation takes 36 hours to complete, then a decision has to be made at a decision arc of 48 hours to begin that task and allow sufficient time before the storm begins to have an effect on your locale. (A storm plotter can be found on the National Hurricane Center web site www.nhc.gov/gccalc.shtm? to assist in decision arc planning).

Decisions made may eventually prove to be wrong and unnecessary --- but never the less the decision has to be made to properly achieve the task in the allowed time period.

For every decision made there is usually less than a 33% probability that it was necessary, or a 1 in 3 to 1 in 4; but still with these high probabilities one cannot afford to not make the "right" decision at the time.

Remember --- the only wrong decision is the one that turns out to endanger lives because of indifference and delay.

**Decisions are COSTLY but the loss of LIFE is priceless.**

CHAPTER 10

# The Joint Commission (TJC)

• • •

**Robert J. Muller**

"ENVIRONMENT OF CARE (EC) STANDARD EC.1.4 requires hospital, ambulatory care, behavioral health, home care, and long term care organizations to *develop* a management plan that ensures effective response to emergencies affecting the environment of care. Standard EC.2.4 requires these organizations to *implement* the emergency management plan. Standard EC.2.9.1 requires them to *execute* the plan by conducting emergency management drills. Although not required by JCAHO standards, it would be prudent for other types of health care organizations to plan for disasters given today's environment".

The requirements of standards EC.1.4 and EC.2.4 vary among the accreditation programs. Refer to your accreditation manual to identify what specifically is required of your organization. As part of the four phases of emergency management activities, organizations may be required to identify and implement processes to conduct a hazard vulnerability analysis; establish, in coordination with the community emergency planning, priorities among the potential emergencies identified in the analysis; identify procedures to mitigate, prepare for, respond to, and recover from the priority emergencies; define and integrate the organization's role with that of community emergency response agencies, including identifying a community command structure; define a common command structure (for all hazards)within the organization which links to the community structure; cooperate with health care organizations within a contiguous geographic area to establish a process to share information about the essential elements of a command structure and emergency control centers; names, roles, and phone numbers of individuals in the command structure; resources and assets to share or pool in a community emergency response; and timely identification and location of names of patients and deceased individuals following an emergency; describe how, when, and by whom the plan is activated; identify which personnel are responsible for which activities during emergencies; initiate response and recovery phases; notify external authorities of emergencies, including possible community emergencies such as evidence of a bioterrorist attack; notify care providers and other personnel when emergency procedures are initiated; identify personnel during emergencies; assign available personnel to cover all necessary positions under emergency conditions; manage patient/resident care activities, staff and family support activities, logistics of critical supplies, security, and communication with news media during emergencies; evacuate the facility if necessary; establish an alternate care site(s) that can meet patients' clinical needs; transfer patients/residents or transport and track patients/residents, staff, and equipment to an alternate care site as needed; communicate with the alternate care site; reestablish and/or continue operations following the disaster; provide alternate means of meeting essential building utility needs to provide continuous service; establish backup internal and external communication systems ; identify radioactive, biological, or chemical isolation and decontamination sites (ambulatory care and hospitals only); clarify alternate responsibilities of personnel, including to whom they report during a disaster, in a command structure consistent with that used by agencies in the local community; establish an orientation and education program for staff, including licensed independent practitioners, who participate in implementing the plan; monitor ongoing performance in drills and real emergencies; and determine how an annual evaluation of the plan's objective, scope, performance, and effectiveness will occur.

Methadone/LAAM clinics must also provide links with community agencies to ensure emergency dosing capabilities; 24-hour telephone answering capability to respond to facility and patient emergencies; and updated patient rosters and medication dosage logs that are accessible to the staff on call.

The emergency management standards also address the needs of your staff. In an actual emergency, staff will naturally be concerned for the safety and wellbeing of their colleagues and loved ones. Accordingly, standard EC.1.4 calls for the management of staff activities—including housing, transportation, and incident stress debriefing—and staff and family support activities.

(Ref: Joint Commission Perspectives)

CHAPTER 11

# Liability Issue

• • •

**Robert J. Muller**

By definition, a tort is defined as an intentional action that harms another person, business, or group for which there is a legal remedy. This can occur by actions or failure to act, thus causing harm directly or indirectly.

Two types of torts would directly apply to the hospital liability setting. Negligent liability occurs when an entity fails to do what other prudent entities have already done or established as a precedent under the same or similar circumstances. Warrant liability occurs when a promised or perceived promise service level is not delivered and harm results.

Four elements must be necessary in order to prove negligence.

- First, the existence of a duty that establishes a standard of conduct. By the very present of establishment of an Emergency Department, it would be our duty to be prepared for emergencies, including bioterrorism events; unless, a prior warning was issued to the public that we are NOT prepared to treat victims of bioterrorist emergencies.
- Second, a breach of duty or failure to carry out that standard of duty (an action or omission).

- Third, there is a direct or indirect connection between the act and the injury to the party as the legal cause of harm.
- Fourth, the actual loss or harm to the injured party.

In our hospital settings, the very nature of establishment of an entity as a general/medical hospital imparts on expectation of services to the public, whether they be real or perceived.

In the event these services are unable or incapable of being provided and a prior statement of warning has not been issued to those parties that would prudently expect to utilize these medical services, then the elements for liability would befall the hospital entity for breach of duty, etc.

Areas of Potential Liability

1. The lack of plans for a known hazard
2. Emergency plans that are out of date
3. Plans that are not based on realistic assumptions or inflate capabilities
4. Improper distribution of the planning document
5. Plan should be followed – situations that occur that are opposite or contrary to the plans without just cause can increase liability (**Plans are NOT static they are always dynamic.)** Documents are subject to constant change. A common plan axiom is to "plan for tomorrow with what you have and can do today".
6. Poor or absent training
   a. Public may seek judgments based on lack of training by hospital employees.
   b. Hospital employees may file suits against their employer if they are expected to perform functions for which they are not adequately trained or prepared. (example – use of hazardous material protective suits)

7. Failure to warn the public that a perceived or anticipated service is unavailable or is unable to be adequately provided.
8. Negligent operation of equipment and or services – Plans must be workable and training must fulfill the planned roles. Plans must be implemented in an effective way. Equipment must always be kept in good working order and maintenance and repairs should be well documented. Written procedure should be established to deal with defective equipment and its removal from service.

## Standards of Care

The Standard of Care is a common law notion that involves the basic issue of what is considered to be reasonable actions.

Planning, systems and response to disaster must change as the Standards of Care change and/or improve.

Standards of Care are based on what is reasonable care under the circumstances. These include: cost/benefit analysis, capabilities of in place systems, and capabilities of similar systems.

JACHO requirements generally establish guidelines for national recommended standards of care, but do not necessarily deal with local Standards of Care that may apply to local "ALL Hazard" assessments and disaster readiness.

## Summary

The issue of liability and the concerns surrounding it are extremely complex and highly variable. State statues, local ordinances, and issues regarding Standards of Care will vary by state and by community.

Due diligence through planning, mitigation, and training are of paramount importance to avoid liability and litigation.

## Recommendations

1. The hospitals that do not provide full service Emergency Departments post a disclaimer that the facility is not equipped to treat victims of disaster, including bioterrorism.
2. Full service hospitals with Emergency Departments should be properly planned, trained and equipped to adequately triage, treat and admit patients that are disaster victims including those of bioterrorism.

CHAPTER 12

# Legal Considerations for the Emergency Manager and Physician

• • •

**Ernest P. Chiodo**

There are a number of legal issues that must be considered by emergency department physicians and managers in preparing and dealing with responses to threats such as disasters, epidemics, and terrorist attacks. Emergency physicians and managers must be aware of legal issues that are likely to arise in a crisis. These issues include hoarding of vital supplies including medical supplies as well as prescriptions; provision of medical services by physicians distant to the local patient; the unique qualifications required for a physician to make public health decisions as opposed to medical decision; and the police powers possessed by public health organizations as opposed to medical organizations. While there are a wide range of legal issues that may be of interest to the threat response manager, the issues discussed in this chapter are not likely to be readily accessible in the general legal literature and the insights are crucial in a crisis. The legal issues will be consider from a United States federal, state, local and when appropriate international prospective.

## Supplies of Prescription Drugs

Obtaining adequate supplies of prescription drugs is likely to become difficult during a crisis. Even obtaining the prescriptions may become very difficult since licensed physicians are likely to be scarce during a crisis.

## Federal Legal Issues:

Medical licensure within the United States is conducted by the various states of the Union. Consequently, a prescription written by a physician in one state may not be deemed valid in another state. The various states in the United States have the right to protect the health of their citizens by means of controlling licensure of physicians to practice medicine within the borders of the State.

> *"The right of a physician to toil in his profession ... with all its sanctity and safeguards is not absolute. It must yield to the paramount right of government to protect the public health by any rational means."*
> Lawrence v. Board of Registration in medicine, 239 Mass. 424, 428, 132 N.E. 174 (1921).

This may result in difficulties in filling of prescriptions in states other than the state where the prescription was written. The licensure statutes of the states had the original propose of ensuring that physicians had the minimum scientific knowledge in order to safely practice (Legal Medicine. Fifth Edition. © 2001 by Mosby, Inc. St. Louis, Missouri. Page 70). However, in the case of *Hawke v. New York, 170 U.S. 189, 194 (1898)* the United States Supreme Court ruled that states have the right to use standards of behavior and ethics as factors in granting or removing physician licensure. Consequently, the various states have the power to control the practice of medicine within their borders through medical licensure. The writing of prescriptions in one state to be filled by the patient in another state may be deemed a clear violation of the right of the State where the prescription is filled to control the practice of medicine in that state.

In addition, during the time of an epidemic there may be migration of persons from colder areas of the United States to warmer areas in the mistaken brief that there is less risk of becoming infected with influenza. As a result, there may be abnormal stresses placed upon the supplies of non-influenza related medications that may be problematic for health delivery. For example, a state such as Florida may experience an abnormally large demand for medication needed to treat diabetes such as insulin. This may result in a lack of necessary medications for diabetics who usually live in Florida. Conversely, there may be an oversupply of insulin in a cold northern state such as Michigan where there may be a lower prevalence of diabetes due to a younger age demographic. The federal government may wish to control the supply of vital medical supplies across state borders. This control of the flow of medical supplies across state borders may be controlled by the federal government through the operation of the Interstate Commerce Act. Interstate and foreign commerce are defined as follows:

> *Commerce between a point in one State and a point in another State, between points in the same State, through another State or through a foreign country, between points in a foreign country or countries through the United States and a point in a foreign country or in a Territory or possession of the United states, but only insofar as such commerce takes place in the United States. The term "United States" means all the States and the District of Columbia.*
>
> 18 U.S.C.A. § 831.

Black's Law Dictionary. Fifth Edition. © 1979 West Publishing Co. St. Paul Minn. ISBN 0-8299-2041-2. Page 735.

Interstate commerce was defined in *Gibbons v. Ogden, 22 U.S. (9 Wheat.) 1, 6 L.Ed. 23* as follows:

> *Traffic, intercourse, commercial trading, or the transportation of persons or property between or among the several states of the Union, or from or between points in one state and points in another state; commerce between two states, or between places lying in different states.*
> Black's Law Dictionary. Fifth Edition. © 1979 West Publishing Co. St. Paul Minn. ISBN 0-8299-2041-2. Page 735.

*Furst v. Brewster, 282 U.S. 493, 51 S.Ct. 295, 296, 75 L.Ed. 478* further defines interstate commerce as "It comprehends all the component parts of commercial intercourse between different states." (Black's Law Dictionary. Fifth Edition. © 1979 West Publishing Co. St. Paul Minn. ISBN 0-8299-2041-2. Page 735.)

The Interstate Commerce Act provides for the following:

> *The act of congress of February 4, 1887 (49 U.S.C.A. § 1 et seq.), designed to regulate commerce between the states, and particularly the transportation of persons and property, by carriers, between interstate points, prescribing that charges for such transportation shall be reasonable and just, prohibiting unjust discrimination, rebates, draw-backs, preferences, poling of freights, etc., requiring schedules of rates to be published, establishing a commission to carry out the measures enacted, and prescribing the powers and duties of such commission and the procedure before it.*
> Black's Law Dictionary. Fifth Edition. © 1979 West publishing Co. St. Paul Minn. ISBN 0-8299-2041-2. Page 735.

Clearly the federal government has the power to have some degree of control over the flow of medical supplies and pharmaceuticals across state borders.

However, the federal government may not be able to control the flow of persons across state borders due to the privileges and immunity clause of the United States Constitution. Perhaps more importantly, the various states may not normally control the flow of United States citizens into their state from other states. The Privileges and Immunities Clause of the United States Constitution provides the following protections:

> *There are two Privileges and Immunities Clauses in the federal Constitution and Amendments, the first being found in Art. IV, and the second in the 14th Amendment, § 1, second clause, clause 1. The provision in Art. IV states that "The Citizens of each State shall be entitled to all Privileges and immunities of Citizens in the several States," while the 14th Amendment provides that "No state shall make or enforce any law which shall abridge the privileges or immunities of citizens of the United States.*
>
> *The purpose of these Clauses is to place the citizens of each State upon the same footing with citizens of other states, so far as the advantages resulting from citizenship in those states is concerned.*
>
> Black's Law Dictionary. Fifth Edition. © 1979 West publishing Co. St. Paul Minn. ISBN 0-8299-2041-2. Page 1079.

Consequently, there is likely to be a bar against actions by the governments of the various states in attempting to prevent entry of United States citizens into their state from another state. This bar may be effective even during the time of a crisis such as an avian influenza epidemic.

## State Legal Issues:

The various states within the United States regulate the prescriptive authority of the physicians, dentists, and nurse practitioners within each state. Consequently, one state may have a different law concerning prescriptive authority than another state. For example, one state may allow a nurse practitioner to write prescriptions while another state may not allow nurse practitioners to write prescriptions. As a result, a prescription written by a nurse practitioner in a state granting prescriptive authority to nurse practitioners will almost certainly not be honored in a state that does not grant nurse practitioners prescriptive authority. In addition, even if a practitioner such as a physician is of a profession that is granted prescriptive authority in two different states, the writing of a prescription by a physician licensed in one state with knowledge that the patient intends to fill the prescription in another state in which the physician is not licensed may be considered the unauthorized practice of medicine. It should be noted that the unauthorized practice of medicine is usually considered a felony. Consequently, prescriptions written by a physician in one state where the physician knows that during a crisis the prescription will be filled and dispensed in a foreign state may present issues concerning the unauthorized practice of medicine.

The unset of an epidemic may lead people to attempt to obtain medical advice and treatment in means other than through direct contact. There are likely to be attempts to obtain medical advice and treatment via electronic devices such as the telephone or the internet. The reasons for the desire to obtain medical treatment over a distance through electronic means are likely to be three fold. First, there will be reluctance by persons to attend physician offices where there will be an increased likelihood of coming into contact with sick persons who may be infected with an infection disease that is causing the crisis such as avian influenza. There may also be a reduction in the availability of physician services within the patient's immediate geographic area. This will cause patients to seek medical advice and treatment at a distance. The providers of this medical advice and treatment may be located across state borders. In addition, patients may seek the advice of specialists with particular expertise in the diagnosis and treatment of disease caused by the infectious agent of concern such as avian influenza. These considerations will encourage patients to seek medical care from physicians that may not be licensed to practice medicine within the state of residence of the patient. Physicians may also be drawn to provide care to patients at a distance who may not be located within the same state as the physician and who may have never been seen by the physician. The factors that will draw physicians into this telemedicine activity are also three fold. First, there may be commercial factors that may draw physicians into areas of practice in great demand. Due to the demand, these areas of specialized practice may be very lucrative. Physicians may also wish to provide medical care without the risk to their personal health due to infection that would arise with direct patient contract. In addition, there will be the admirable desire on the part of physicians to provide needed services to persons that may not have access to medical services in their own communities due to remote geography or other factors limiting access to care. The issue of telemedicine raises a number of legal concerns.

The first legal consideration concerning telemedicine services involves legal liability for medical malpractice. The case of *International Shoe v. State of Washington, 325 U.S. 310, 66 S.Ct. 154 (1945)* established the principle that in order for a state to have legal jurisdiction over a person, that person must have some minimal contacts with the state seeking the jurisdiction. Within the realm of medical malpractice, it generally considered that the physician can only be sued within the state where he provided the medical service even if the patient has a place of residence in another state (Legal Medicine. Fifth Edition. © 2001 by Mosby, Inc. St. Louis, Missouri. Page 238). However, in *Bullion v. Gillespie, 895 F. 2d 213 (5th Cir. 1990)* a physician was held to be subject to the jurisdiction of another state where the patient lived when it was shown that the physician attracted patients to his practice through nationally distributed marketing literature. In *Kenndy v. Freeman, 919 F. 2d 126 (10th Cir. 1990)* a physician was found to be subject to the jurisdiction of another state when he was involved in the reading of biopsy specimen sent by physicians located outside of his own state. It should also be noted that several states have forbidden the prescription of medications for patients where the only contact with the patient was through telemedicine (Legal Medicine. Fifth Edition. © 2001 by Mosby, Inc. St. Louis, Missouri. Page 238). *In re B.T. Taylor, M.D., Action report, Medical board of California (Oct 1999)*, the Board of Medicine of the State of California reprimanded a California physician when it received notification of a disciplinary action by the State of Colorado due to the physician having prescribed medications to patients in Colorado with whom the physician only had contact via the internet.

## Local Legal Issues:

Local governments may have concerns about stresses placed upon the healthcare delivery network in their areas. Public healthcare delivery services such as municipal and county health departments may be overwhelmed by the demands placed upon them by persons seeking prescriptions.

## International Legal Issues:

Each national government has the power and right to regulate the practice of medicine within its national borders. Prescriptions written in foreign countries are not likely to be honored in a nation other than the country of origin of the prescription. The public policy issues in this matter are similar to the concerns of the various states of the United States in preventing the unauthorized practice of medicine. It should be noted that the United States Supreme Court only ruled in 1973 that a requirement that a person be a citizen of the United States in order to obtain medical licensure is an unconstitutional discrimination (Legal Medicine. Fifth Edition. © 2001 by Mosby, Inc. St. Louis, Missouri. Page 71). It should not be surprising if foreign nations may consider the medical advice to its citizens or residents by a physician that is not a citizen of that nation is an unauthorized practice of medicine.

## Hoarding

During a crisis there may be concerns about hoarding of vital supplies and food stuffs by individuals and corporations. During past times of crisis there have been efforts by individuals and corporations to store large quantities of supplies.

## Federal Legal Issues:

The federal government implemented a program of rationing of foods and consumer goods during the Second World War. Rationing has not occurred to any extent during any military conflict involving the United States since the Second World War. The lack of need for rationing is a manifestation of the large surplus production capacity of the United States compared to the needs of the military during the time of active conflict. However, the collapse of the Soviet Union in the early 1990s occurred at a time of a major economic expansion in the United States. At that time there were thoughts that one of the reasons for the major economic expansion was the "war dividend" due the lack of further expenditures to fight the "Cold War".

Consequently, there is some evidence that the ability of the United States to maintain production at a level to counter a military treat has some limits even during times of normal economic functioning. The disruptions that would be anticipated to occur during a major crisis would be likely to place tremendous stresses upon the supply of foods and consumer goods. The plans of individuals and corporations to stock-up on food and other supplies may run afoul of the plans of the United States federal government. However, it should be noted that the Center for Disease control website does provide the same recommendations for the general public.

It should be noted that the U.S. Food and Drug Administration (FDA) has authority over foods as well as drugs sold within the United States. The earliest federal legislation that dealt with food and drugs was the Drug Importation Act of 1848 which was passed by the United States Congress in order to require the U.S. Customs Service to conduct inspections so as to stop the importation of adulterated drugs from overseas (Legal Medicine. Fifth Edition. © 2001 by Mosby, Inc. St. Louis, Missouri. Page 560). The first comprehensive Food and Drugs Act was enacted by the United States Congress under the Theodore Roosevelt administration on June 30, 1906 (Legal Medicine. Fifth Edition. © 2001 by Mosby, Inc. St. Louis, Missouri. Page 561). In 1938, the United States Congress passed the Federal Food, Drug, and Cosmetic Act (FDCA) (21 United States Code [U.S.C.] 321 to 394) (Legal Medicine. Fifth Edition. © 2001 by Mosby, Inc. St. Louis, Missouri. Page 561).

## State Legal Issues:

Each individual state within the United States may have concerns about stresses placed upon local sale and supply of food and consumer goods that may mirror the concerns of the federal government.

## Local Legal Issues:

The local governments such as counties and municipalities may have concerns about disruption of supplies that mirror the federal and state concerns.

## International Legal Issues:

Large corporations have employees in many countries throughout the world. The governments of each nation with employees of a corporation may have concerns about hoarding of food and consumer supplies. The hoarding of food and consumer goods in second and third world countries may place great stress upon the resources of these nations. Consequently, corporations that recommend that their employees store supplies of food and materials may be giving recommendations contrary to the mandates of the various nations in which the corporation has employees. In fact, during times of great national crisis, many nations have made hoarding of food and consumer goods a criminal act. During the Second World War persons that were involved in hoarding were often considered to be "Black Marketers".

> *"Black market" was the term given to the illegal trade in consumer goods, manufactured products and raw materials without regard to rationing or price fixing statutes, practiced because of the scarcity of goods. The constantly escalating game of bidding and the risks that the traders ran pushed prices up to unbelievable levels.*

The Historical Encyclopedia of World War II. © 1980 by Facts on File Inc. Greenwich House. New York. ISBN 0-517-431491. Page 57.

In Britain and the United States black marketers were subject to imprisonment. These hoarding activities were a capital offense in totalitarian regimes such as Nazi German and the Soviet Union.

## Hoarding of Nonprescription Drugs and Other Health Supplies

During a crisis, individuals and corporations may wish to stockpile nonprescription drugs and other health supplies that may be needed during the crisis. These supplies include toiletries, and products for personal and dental hygiene such as soap, deodorants, and tooth paste. Fluids with electrolytes may also be important in cases of dehydration due to diarrhea.

## Federal Legal Issues:

The public policy issues in this matter are essentially the same as in the recommendations for food and consumer goods since the issues for prescriptive authority do not apply.

## State Legal Issues:

The public policy issues in this matter at the state level are essentially the same in the case of the recommendations concerning food and consumer goods since the recommendation concerns non-prescription medications.

## Local Legal Issues:

Local authorities may have concerns about local distribution of the personal hygiene products because of the risk of disease spread with declines in hygiene. There may be a need for an increase in disease surveillance on the part of local health departments.

## Autonomy and Direction of Care

During a crisis questions will likely arise as to who will direct the care of person who become ill during the crisis.

## Federal Legal Issues:

In Western democracies including the United States there is the understanding that persons have the right to make their own decisions about matters influencing their health. This concept is termed *autonomy* from the Greek *auto nomos* which means self-rule. This means that in a medical setting that a patient has freedom of choice. (Legal Medicine. Fifth Edition. © 2001 by Mosby, Inc. St. Louis, Missouri. Page 291). In *Schoendorf v. Society of New York Hospital, 1914, 105 N.E. 92 (N.Y.C.A.)* Justice Cordozo stated that "Every human being of adult years and sound mind has a right to determine what shall be done with his own body."

## International Legal Issues:

In 1948 there was a Universal Declaration of Human Rights that were ultimately adopted by the World Medical Association and the World Health Organization. These measures were designed to prevent some of the great evils that occurred during World War II. The focus was to prevent human experimentation of the type that occurred during the Nazi regimen (Legal

Medicine. Fifth Edition. © 2001 by Mosby, Inc. St. Louis, Missouri. Page 291).

## Qualifications of Physicians Making Public Health Decisions

During a crisis, there will be a need for crucial public health policy decisions to be made by qualified physicians. However, the issue of what are the necessary qualifications for a physician to make public health policy decisions is often not known by most physicians. While the qualifications needed by a physician to properly determine public health policy and procedures is not strictly a legal matter, the failure of threat response managers to recognize what type of physician is qualified to provide public health guidance raises obvious liability concerns.

## Federal, state, local and international legal issues:

There is specialized training required for effective function of a physician as a public health official.

For example, the fundamental tools of public health officials are not part of the routine medical or nursing training. Epidemiology and biostatistics are crucial tools in the arsenal of any public health official. However, these disciplines are either not taught or provided only superficial coverage in most medical and nursing schools. In addition, course work in public health management is virtually non-existent in medical and nursing school curriculum. Public health related disciplines such as epidemiology and biostatistics are taught primarily in schools of public health. In addition, subject matter focused upon public health issues and identification and control of disease in populations of persons is not part of the specialty training of most physicians. Issues concerning public health are covered in training in the specialties under the American Board of Preventive Medicine. The American Board of Preventive Medicine requires that a physician have documented formal education in the following areas in order to qualify for the board certification examinations in the preventive medicine specialties.

> *In addition to the knowledge of basic and clinical sciences and the skills common to all physicians, the distinctive aspects of preventive medicine include knowledge and competence in:*
>
> 1. *Biostatistics,*
> 2. *Epidemiology,*
> 3. *Administration, including planning, organization, management, financing, and evaluation of health programs,*
> 4. *Environmental and occupational health,*
> 5. *Application of social and behavioral factors in health and disease,*
> 6. *Application of primary, secondary, and tertiary prevention measures within clinical medicine.*
>
> (The American College of Preventive Medicine Directory of Preventive Medicine Residency Programs in the United States and Canada. Fifth Edition. © 1988 American College of Preventive Medicine. Washington D.C. Page 1.)

The American College of Preventive Medicine defines the roles of preventive medicine specialists as follows:

> *The roles of preventive medicine specialists include serving as:*
>
> 1. *Health planners and administrators,*

2. *Teachers of preventive medicine,*
3. *Researchers in preventive medicine,*
4. *Clinicians applying preventive medicine in health care.*

(The American College of Preventive Medicine Directory of Preventive Medicine Residency Programs in the United States and Canada. Fifth Edition. © 1988 American College of Preventive Medicine. Washington D.C. Page 1.)

The American College of Preventive Medicine describes that setting in which preventive medicine is practiced as follows:

*The setting in which preventive medicine specialists may be found include:*

1. *Government organizations such as local, state, national, and international public health departments and other military and civilian agencies concerned with the health of populations,*
2. *Educational institutions such as schools of medicine, public health, and allied health,*
3. *Organized medical care programs in industry, other employment settings, and in the community, where clinical practice involves prevention and health maintenance,*
4. *Voluntary health agencies, professional health organizations, and related organizations.*

(The American College of Preventive Medicine Directory of Preventive Medicine Residency Programs in the United States and Canada. Fifth Edition. © 1988 American College of Preventive Medicine. Washington D.C. Page 1.)

The American Board of Preventive Medicine provides board certification to physicians in three areas of specialization. The American Board of Preventive Medicine specialties are *occupational medicine*, *aerospace medicine*, and *public health and general preventive medicine*.

*Occupational medicine* is the medical specialty that is primarily focused upon the diagnosis, prevention, and treatment of disease in persons in a work setting. The practice of *occupational medicine* requires skills that allow detection of disease in populations such as the work force of a company. An outbreak of an occupational disease that can arise due to poor industrial hygiene practices such as occupational asthma may not be apparent to a physician not trained in *occupational medicine*. Consequently, the medical directors of most major industrial corporations are board certified in *occupational medicine*.

*Aerospace medicine* is the area of board certification held by physicians involved in the medical aspects of air and space flight. The physicians working for NASA are usually board certified in *aerospace medicine*. The public health skills required to detect disease in populations rather than solely in individuals are crucial for the functioning of physicians working in *aerospace medicine*.

*Public health and general preventive medicine* is the medical specialty that is focused upon detection, prevention, and control of disease in large populations such as a large city, county, state, or nation. The CDC 'hot zone" doctors and the medical directors of major city and state health department are usually required to be board certified in *public health and general preventive medicine*.

Added to additional training required for physicians to function as public health officials, the healthcare system and public health systems differ in that public health systems have "police powers" while healthcare systems do not have "police powers".

Police powers are those powers that are necessary to function in a police capacity. The police powers of local public health officials in the State of Michigan in the event of an epidemic, emergency or case where quarantine is required are described in the Public Health Code of the State of Michigan (Act 368 of 1978, as amended) as follows:

> *333.2453 Epidemic; emergency order and procedures; involuntary detention and treatment.*
>
> *Sec. 2453. (1) If a local health officer determines that control of an epidemic is necessary to protect the public health, the local health officer may issue an emergency order to prohibit the gathering of people for any purpose and may establish procedures to be followed by persons, including a local governmental entity, during the epidemic to insure continuation of essential public health services and enforcement of health laws. Emergency procedures shall not be limited to this code.*
>
> *(2) A local health department or the department may provide for the involuntary detention and treatment of individuals with hazardous communicable disease in the manner prescribed in sections 5201 to 5238.*

The difference between a public health department and a hospital as part of a healthcare system is illustrated by what happens in the case of a person with a serious infectious disease such as tuberculosis. A hospital that has a patient with infectious tuberculosis who refuses to take anti-tubercular medication cannot force the person to take the medication. If the person with infectious tuberculosis wishes to leave the hospital and enter into the general community with the risk of spread of tuberculosis, the hospital must allow the infectious person to leave since the hospital is a non-public organization without police powers. In this situation the hospital must contact the local public health department which then exercises its police powers to detain the infectious individual and compels the person to take anti-tubercular medications.

The essence of the above dissertation is that the healthcare and public health systems are fundamentally different. The focus of the healthcare systems is on provision of healthcare services to individuals. The focus of the public health systems is detection and control of disease in populations. Public health systems have police powers. Healthcare systems do not have police powers. There is a fundamental difference in the training and therefore the mind set of physicians working in public health compared to physicians working in healthcare.

In summary, the threat response manager must be aware of legal issues that are likely to arise in a crisis. These issues include hoarding of vital supplies including medical supplies as well as prescriptions; provision of medical services by physicians distant to the local patient; the unique qualifications required for a physician to make public health decisions as opposed to medical decision; and the police powers possessed by public health organizations as opposed to medical organizations.

CHAPTER 13

# Federal Response Resources

• • •

Robert J. Muller

There are many federal resources available before, during and after a disaster. The important aspect is to know and understand what resources are available and at what point of the disaster they are available and what the resources functions are related to the hospital.

## Strategic National Stockpile

The Strategic National Stockpile (SNS) (http://www.bt.cdc.gov/stockpile/index.asp) is a national repository of critical medical supplies and equipment designed to supplement and resupply state and local public health agencies in the event of a national emergency within the United States or its territories and available 24/7/365. The SNS is managed by the CDC's Division of Strategic national Stockpile working in conjunction with state and local communities who have responsibilities for developing their own local plans for the receipt and distribution of the SNS supplies and equipment. The CDC deploys medical supplies and equipment, some of which is configured and packed as a 250-bed Federal medical Station but does not operate or staff mass casualty centers, clinics or hospitals.

The SNS contains multiple caches of medical supplies and equipment in warehouses across the countries that are mostly kept secret to the general public for obvious security reasons. The caches include antibiotics, chemical antidotes, antitoxins, life support medications, intravenous fluids for administration, ventilators, airway management supplies, and surgical items along with the deployable Federal Medical Station assets.

Items included in the SNS are based upon threat assessment, the vulnerability of the U.S. civilian population, and availability and ease of distribution of the supplies.

The SNS is activated by results from local or state public health agencies to the Governor's Office, who thereby request the SNS from the Center for Disease Control (CDC).

The supplies may be sent in a 12 hour push package which contains a broad range of products potentially needed in the early state of an emergency. These supplies are loaded immediately from the predetermined locations via trucks or aircraft and sent to pre-designated receiving, staging and storage sites, depending upon the situation and needs of the affected areas and communities.

The Federal Medical Station (FMS) may be deployed when treatment or quarantine capability is required. The FMS units are designed to provide low to mid-level acuity of care or quarantine for 250 patients and can be employed as a platform for use also as a special needs shelter or alternate care facility to augment the needs of local hospitals and medical facilities when they exceed their capacity. The FMS is intended to be installed within existing facilities such as warehouse, shopping center, etc. or tents, located near an existing hospital. Local, state officials are responsible for the receipt, storage and security and operation as well as the distribution of the SNS supplies and equipment once they arrive at the agreed upon site.

Along with the FMS the CDC will deploy its Technical Advisory Response Unit to provide technical assistance and advice in receiving and distributing supplies upon arrive at the receiving location.

The Cities Readiness Initiative program, begun in 2004, provides funding to 72 metropolitan areas throughout all 50 states to improve their operational capability to receive, distribute and dispense the SNS assets. This initiative aims to provide aid with medicines and supplies to designated cities entire populations within 48 hours of a disaster or critical situation. A list of the cities may be found at http://www.bt.cdc.gov/cri/.

## Federal Medical Response Teams

The Federal Government has several teams that are available for response under the Health and Hospital Services that can be quickly deployed to an area in disaster or critical situations: the U.S. Public Health Service Commissioned Officer Corp, and the National Disaster Medical System teams. They may also reach out to the Department of Veterans Affairs and the Department of Defense should more medical personnel be needed.

## United States Health Service Commissioned Office Corp

The U.S. Public Health Service (USPHS) Commissioned Officer Corp is one of the seven U.S. uniformed services, and is a source of, 6,000 public health professionals who are available to respond rapidly to an urgent public health challenge and health care emergencies. This group is led by the Surgeon General, and has 14 teams ready to be deployed including:

Five deployable Rapid Deployment Force Teams—each trained to manage and staff Federal Medical Shelters.

Four Applied Public Health Teams --- each with USPHS officers with experience in water safety, sewerage, solid waste and other environmental challenges; disease surveillance and public health communications.

Five Mental Health Teams --- each with USPHS officers who are subject matter experts to help assess and provide early intervention for mental health requirements in disaster settings.

## National Disaster Medical System

States that require additional manpower can obtain additional medical staff through pre-arranged mutual aid agreements with other states or jurisdictions and in addition through the National Disaster medical System (NDMS) (http://ndms.dhhs.gov), a federally coordinated system that provides medical services to aid local and state agencies respond to major emergencies and disasters, including acts of terrorism.

This system is made up of medical professionals who are specially trained and volunteer their services in emergency situations, to supplement local hospital systems.

NDMS becomes operational in two different situations: 1) the declaration of a National Emergency; 2) by request of a state or local government. These services are paid by the federal government's Public Assistance Program of the Stafford Act if a National Emergency is declared. If a National Emergency is not declared, then the state will have to reimburse NDMS for any service that may be requested. To request NDMS assistance, the state will work with the liaison staff at the Emergency Operations Center and the Joint Field Office to develop a medical assessment document that list the needs and why federal assistance is being requested. This request document is then sent on to the Federal Emergency

Management Agency for approval and action. As expected, this process may take days to weeks until fruition.

The five types of NDMS teams that maybe requested are:

1. Disaster Medical Assistance Teams (DEMAT)
2. Disaster Mortuary Operational Response Teams (DEMORT)
3. Veterinary Medical Assistance Teams (VMAT)
4. National Nurse Response Teams
5. National Pharmacy Response Teams

## Disaster Medical Assistance Teams

There are 26 teams across the country, each composed of 35 professional and paraprofessional personnel and logistical staff with another 20 additional teams being available on special request if necessary for the situation.

These teams include four National Medical Response Teams which are specially equipped and trained to deal with Weapons of Mass Destruction (WMD), and other specialized teams to handle specific needs such as burns crash injuries, pediatric emergencies and mental health.

These are all rapid response teams designed to supplement the local and/or state response personnel, until additional resources, federal, state or private can be activated and mobilized.

## Disaster Mortuary Operational Response Teams

There are ten regional teams that can be mobilized to provide assistance in recovery, identification and burial of victims. One national team is specially trained to handle events related to Weapons of Mass Destruction.

The team is composed of private citizens with areas of special expertise such as funeral directors, medical examiners, coroners and pathologists and there are two portable morgue units that can be deployed to the situational site.

## Veterinary Medical Assistance Team

There are five nationally deployable teams of private citizens who can provide care following major emergencies with such tasks as; medical treatment for rescued animals, farm animals and pets; the tracking and disease assessment in animals and animal decontamination.

This team is composed of clinical veterinarians, veterinary pathologist, veterinary technicians, microbiologists, virologists, epidemiologists and toxicologists.

## National Registered Nurse Team

The teams are formed with the intention of assisting with vaccination and providing specialized services in cases where the nursing force may be overwhelmed during a major emergency there are ten such teams with each consisting of approximately 200 civilian nurses, including specialized nurses in burn care.

## National Pharmacy Response Team

There are ten regional teams assembled to assist in emergency situations that may require a large number of pharmacy professionals, such as in medication preparations, inventory, etc. of mass vaccinations. This team is sponsored by the Joint Commission of Pharmacist Practitioners and work in partnership with Health and Human Resources.

## Federal Coordinating Centers

In addition to the five types of teams, NDMS also coordinates a network of about 200 hospitals to assist in disasters in conjunction with the National Disaster Medical System. These hospitals participation is voluntary, usually consist of facilities of 100 beds or more, and commit a number of acute care beds for NDMS patients in a disaster situation. Upon admission, the patient stay is guaranteed by the federal government. Many times patients are transported to unaffected areas NDMS hospitals by the Department of Defense.

## Medical Reserve Corps

These are teams of volunteers on a local or state level who have offered to contribute their skills and expertise following a disaster to enhance community needs. Most of these programs are coordinated through the state and/or local Department of Health and Hospitals. Many of these groups meet and train on a regular basis and likewise offer continuing medical education credits for training participation as well as call out in service time.

## American Red Cross and Faith Based Organizations

The ARC is a key player in responding to emergencies, disasters and public health situations. This is a nonprofit humanitarian organization staffed primarily by volunteers although they do have a staff of paid members likewise.

These organizations offer services such as emergency first aid, supportive counseling for victims and personnel to assist at temporary shelters, clinics, morgues, hospital and nursing homes; the assistance with food and sheltering and the provision of blood products.

CHAPTER 14

# Public Health Response Plan

• • •

**Michael Fagel**

The Emergency Management cycle is just as important to the Public Health Officer (PHO) as it is to any other person or agency that has a role dealing with incident response. It is only through planning and training, under the preparedness portion of the cycle that Public Health Officers will know how to adequately respond to a major incident that is clearly beyond the scope of a routine emergency. A PHO is not going to be involved in a routine emergency. These are almost always best handled by local fire, police, and EMS resources on a daily basis.

But for incidents beyond that, which are larger in scope, and then the Public Health Officer is going to be involved in a variety of different fashions. Moreover, the PHO must also be able to answer a variety of questions very quickly after an incident occurs to determine what kind of response is needed.

These questions listed below are among those that the Public Health Officer needs to think about, and will be expounded upon later in the chapter:

## What is the incident?

- The answer to this question will of course determine all courses of action related to the questions below. What might be a significant and sufficient response for one type of incident (such as coordinating to assist first responders in getting to an explosion scene as quickly as possible to perform rescue/recovery operations) may be completely inappropriate in a suspected hazardous materials incident, for example, where the first goal would be to identify the problem and clear as many people from the area as possible.

## When can the PHO help?

- An Incident Commander under ICS procedure is probably going to be in place already by the time the PHO gets word of a significant incident that will require his/her involvement and response. But when can the PHO help? Have training exercises and materials been developed that clearly indicate when the PHO will be a part of the emergency management effort? Are there resources that the PHO needs to call upon that won't be immediately available, such as supplies from the Strategic National Stockpile (SNS), that even with everything functioning properly, could see 12 hours pass before necessary medicines and supplies arrive to an affected area? How quickly can the PHO provide necessary resources to an incident commander if those resources need to come from outside his/her agency? For example, a medical or research doctor from outside the area that may have particular expertise in bird flu, other pandemic crises, or other biological/chemical agents that could be used in a terrorist incident or could be unleashed accidentally in a spill or accident.

## Who is Involved?

- When State and Federal resources are called in; who is the point of contact to make sure everything is delivered efficiently and effectively? Who does the PHO absolutely have to keep open lines of communication with in the wake of a major disaster or terrorist attack? Who coordinates the information gathering and dissemination in such a situation, making sure that the public is not overly panicked, not underestimating the gravity of the incident, and accurately informed of what their immediate, short-term, and long-term next steps should be?

## Your training plan in action

- This section will discuss a sample incident that could occur in your jurisdiction and provide a walkthrough of what actions must be taken, who must be contacted, and other important things to remember related to the Public Health Officer's role in an emergency response scenario. This will also help to summarize the information presented throughout the rest of this chapter.

## What is the Incident?

The type of incident at hand will always determine what sort of response is needed. The time to decide how to respond to incidents that vary in type and severity is NOT after the incident occurs. This is where the preparedness portion of the Emergency Management Cycle is critical.

As part of the training and preparedness process, the PHO must, through his/her agency and with the cooperation of other agencies and neighboring jurisdictions, lay out specific plans for how to respond to various types of incidents. Your department must understand the fundamental differences in responding during the aftermath of a tornado strike in your jurisdiction and a terrorist attack or other large scale explosion that causes not only casualties, but disruption of services and supplies that the public would view as basic needs.

While it may sound like painstaking work, the PHO must partner with those in his/her agency, surrounding jurisdictions, and other organizations to develop plans on how to handle each type of incident. For example, your agency may have the following types of plans (general examples):

- **Storm aftermath response**
  - This will cover how the PHO will be involved in Emergency Management responses to tornadoes, hurricanes, and even severe thunderstorms that may cause damage in critical areas such that a Public Health response is needed.

- **Natural disaster response**
  - If you work in an area that lies on or near fault lines, you must have a plan in place to deal with emergency response in the wake of an earthquake. Or, if you work in a coastal

area, plan for the possible response need in the wake of a tidal wave that could affect your jurisdiction – even if the earthquake or other event that causes the tidal wave occurs well away from your location, where you wouldn't normally be providing assistance in an emergency response.

## Non-natural disaster response (non-terrorist)

- How will the Public Health response be coordinated for disasters not caused by nature, but that can and do happen on a regular basis. Examples of this would include chemical plant explosions, train derailments (is a hazardous materials incident involved?), plane crashes or other similar incidents that could involve mass casualties, etc. These will be incidents that will involve large-scale work from first responders, but significant follow-up work by Public Health officials to deal with what could be a large number of dead or injured, and the aftereffects of a hazardous materials release in the event of the chemical plant explosion or transportation incidents.

## Terrorist Attack

- The difficulty for the PHO, and for everyone in Emergency Management, is that the exact form of the terrorist attack won't be known, of course, until after it's already occurred. Hurricanes can be forecast with a great degree of accuracy. Earthquakes, while predicting them is still proving to be difficult, have been well studied in terms of what kind of

> destruction they cause and what response is needed in order to help the most number of people in a timely, effective fashion. Even the minutes given by releasing a tornado warning just before one strikes can be beneficial in coordinating the necessary Emergency Response effort.
>
> There is no such advantage with terrorist attacks … however, by planning for all the other major types of events listed here, and by working with local, state, and Federal authorities to coordinate the Incident Command planning and the Public Health agency's role in such a response, the emergency response to a terrorist attack will be more efficient, effective, and will, in the end, save more lives.

This type of effort requires more than simple planning. It is always wise for the PHO to work in his/her agency to coordinate drills and exercises that will allow everyone who could be involved in a response the opportunity to practice for the real thing – keeping in mind that inevitably, the real thing will occur in some form. Training your agency for any kind of incident should definitely include training on how to utilize Personal Protective Equipment (PPE). In an emergency response, staff in your agency are either going to have to know how to function using this equipment, or they are going to have to quickly be able to teach someone else how to do so. It may also fall on the Public Health agency to train staff from other agencies and even volunteer organizations in how to use PPE, and such training should be offered as broadly as possible.

Another thing to think about is that first responders and everyone else who will be offering some sort of assistance after an incident have probably developed their own plans for how to do so, based on what the incident is. The Public Health facet of the response cannot ignore the plans of everyone else. The PHO should train those staff in his/her agency (and volunteers, if necessary) in the entire emergency operations plan for your jurisdiction. It is important that everyone is on the same page at all points during an emergency response to an incident. Success in this area prevents "turf wars" between agencies and jurisdictions over who is the right person or agency to carry out a particular part of a response. Another matter to think about is that the Public Health agency should be involved in, or create, a Continuity of Operations (COOP) plan, in the event of a disaster so significant that preplanned communication lines, incident command response and coordination are interrupted.

For the most part, the Public Health Officer/Agency is not going to be the lead in Incident Command. Instead, the PHO and his/her staff will be coordinating various aspects of the response that first responders, law enforcement and EMS crews are not going to have the time nor ability to deal with – resources, supplies, coordinating a volunteer effort, infrastructure, public information, and possibly mass evacuation. While Public Health is not going to be the lead, it should be involved at nearly all levels, and should coordinate with surrounding jurisdictions and necessary contacts at the local, state, and Federal levels to be able to respond efficiently no matter what type of incident is at hand.

Beyond the pre-incident training, there are questions that need to be answered immediately after an incident occurs related to a possible Public Health response. For example, if an incident occurs for which it is known going in that a Public Health response is required, is the incident significant enough that some abilities of the Public Health agency have been cut off? For example, you may need to have a plan for alternate communications with key staff that will participate in the Public Health response should electricity and communications (particularly cell phone communications) be cut off in the wake of an incident. Has the incident caused outages or damages to Public Health facilities? Will area hospitals become areas where rescue is needed instead of where victims are taken, such as what occurred in New Orleans in the aftermath of Hurricane Katrina? If Public Health operations have been affected, what is the backup plan that can be put into action and does such a plan require extra staff or volunteers of time and/or resources?

For Public Health staff training, a job aid is provided on the next page that can be used by incident in the planning process. Note that this job aid includes just general questions to go through by incident – conditions will of course vary by the severity, location, and scope of an incident. But this job aid can help Public Health officers determine who should be involved in an incident response, what coordination needs to take place with outside agencies and jurisdictions, what safety measures need to be taken and what other questions need to be asked immediately after an incident occurs so that the Public Health response can be efficient and effective. It is a starting point to effective planning that should also include instruction, exercises and coordination with other likely responders.

## Public Health Response Plan: Incident X

Purpose: To describe the means, organization, and process by which the Public Health agency in a jurisdiction will coordinate its role in an emergency response for this particular type of incident.

Type of Incident: (Brief description of the type of incident. This job aid can be used to draw out the necessary Public Health response for all types of incidents, based on the categories already mentioned.)

Staff Needed (with contact information and particular areas of expertise): (For each type of incident, list the Public Health staff in your agency that will be critical to the emergency response. Some staff will be needed no matter what the type of incident is, but they should still be listed here. Also list key people outside your agency that will be important contacts, such as the Emergency Operations coordinator; Police and Fire Chiefs; local, state, and Federal Government contacts; and key contacts from nearby jurisdictions)

Responsibilities for the staff listed above, based on the type of incident.

Supplies Needed: (For each type of incident, list key supplies that either the Public Health response will need to provide, or that will need to be procured from either volunteer organizations (blood from the Red Cross), outside jurisdictions (vehicles, blankets, food, etc.), or the Federal Government (Strategic National Stockpile (SNS)).

Emergency Operations Center Liaison: (Name and contact information for someone in your agency will be within the EOC to help coordinate Public Health efforts related to the overall effort. Liaison may change based on the type of incident that occurred and the type of expertise necessary – for example, upon the discovery of a Bird flu case(s) in the United States, it would be wise to have an EOC liaison with research knowledge in that area, and/or knowledge of pandemics, etc.

Lessons Learned: (Has your jurisdiction faced this kind of incident before? If so, what worked well, what didn't? What supplies and resources were found to be useful and whose expertise is required – even if that person is no longer in the area, the PHO may still need to call on him/her. Part of being prepared is learning from the past and this is a section that can provide a brief synopsis of the response to previous incidents – can be particularly useful in the case of train derailments, hurricanes, tornadoes, etc.

## When Can the PHO Help?

The type of response needed from a Public Health perspective varies by the amount of time that has elapsed after an incident occurs. What is needed from the Public Health function is different in the first 3 hours after an incident than it is after the first 12 hours, for example. In the first hours after an incident occurs, the most important function for the PHO and agency is, based on the training that has been performed and the exercises that the Public Health staff has went through, is to assess what the incident is (discussed above), then coordinate what the public health response is going to be.

The opening hours after an incident occurs are the time for the Public Health agency to coordinate with all necessary agencies and jurisdictions to determine the response. In the first hours, the Public Health agency should determine if their locality is affected (if the incident is beyond your jurisdiction's borders, for example), and how many people in your area could be affected. If the incident is in another jurisdiction, is it a significant enough of a disaster that it will still affect an increased portion of the population that you serve? A PHO will also need to know who the other responders are to the incident, as well as once in the area, who the Incident Commander is – if the Incident Command System has been set up at that point. You will also need to know if an EOC has been activated and if so or if it will be, provide information to the person in your agency who will work within the EOC to help coordinate the Public Health response to the disaster. Remember, Public Health will not lead the incident response except in rare cases, so this early coordination in the first 3 hours after an incident is critical to assuring a cooperative, efficient, and effective response plan.

As time passes from when the incident occurs, moving toward the period 3-6 hours afterward, there are additional responsibilities that the Public Health response must take on. This is done while continuing to carry out all the responsibilities with coordination and assessment that take place in the first few hours discussed above. This next period of time serves as the first window to begin seriously updating the public about what has taken place, what rescue and stability plans are in place and being activated, if an evacuation is necessary or any other instructions the public needs to heed, and set up means for Public Health functions to receive donations and other volunteer work that may be needed in a disaster. For example, if a disaster renders a significant need for donated blood – this will need to be communicated to the public by a Public Information Officer, with directions on where to go to do so (presuming the disaster hasn't made it unsafe to do so). This is almost an automatic in any kind of significant disaster, given the regularly reported shortages of many blood types on hand for organizations such as the American Red Cross.

Another critical function of this post-incident communication is providing direction for members of the public with special needs, or who are disabled, or otherwise unable to respond as needed after an incident occurs. There may be a specific Public Health need to order an evacuation of nursing homes and other large health-care facilities and this will need to be made public, as well. The PHO must also know the makeup of his/her community. Do you work in a largely diverse population area, where for many, English is not the first language? If so, you will need to have pre-planned for communicating in English, Spanish, and possibly other languages (depending on the area) to your community regarding the incident, what has occurred and what next steps the public should take. This is especially critical in the event that a mass evacuation has to be ordered, or, in the case of a biological or chemical incident, that you must order people to stay in the homes and take certain precautions so as to not be adversely affected.

During this time period, especially in the course of responding to a significant incident, there will be large, continuing coordination effort between agencies and jurisdictions. What may start as a local incident, depending on whether it's a terrorist attack or simply how many people are affected, may become an incident with state and Federal response interest. There will need to be people available from the Public Health agency to work with these officials for coordination purposes. During this time period, the local Public Health agency may also discover that due to the gravity of the incident, local supply resources and staffing needs are going to be insufficient for this level and response, and state and Federal assistance is going to be needed.

This is the type of effort that will continue as the response reaches the 12- to 16-hour marks after occurrence. By this point, the local Public Health agency will be working in tandem with various Federal agencies. Take the example of an epidemiological emergency, such as Bird Flu. According to the Centers for Disease Control web site, there have been only 2 U.S. cases of this disease since 1997, but there are cases currently being reported in Asia on a more increased basis. It is not going to be likely that the local Public Health agency, no matter how well-equipped and organized, is going to be able to handle such cases, or an outbreak, on its own. In such a case, the local Public Health agency is going to need to work with, at the very least, the Centers for Disease Control (CDC) and the Department of Health and Human Services (DHHS).

In addition, someone from the Public Health agency, probably the PHO, should be in contact with officials regarding the Strategic National Stockpile (SNS). Very rarely will a locality have sufficient supplies of medicines and such needed in the case of Bird Flu, or any significant epidemiological event, to handle the response, treatment, and possible vaccines on its own. The SNS was designed to be able to send needed supplies of medicines to localities within 12 hours of request. Beyond simply providing medicines, the SNS also houses supplies of antidotes, antitoxins, and medical/surgical items. It is specifically designed to bring necessary resources to localities that in most cases will not be expected to stock all such things – even though the public will need them in the case of specific types and degrees of disasters. Initial contact with SNS officials should be made within the first 6-12 hours after an incident has occurred or discovered, to assure the most rapid delivery of supplies and medicines to those in your community that will need them.

As part of the Public Health response, there are also other concerns to look at as the time beyond an event changes from hours to days. Is there an environmental impact that the disaster has caused, and if so, what Federal and state officials and agencies will need to be called in to assist in assessment, cleanup, and recovery? It is at this point in the recovery stage after an incident that the Public Health agency can also work in tandem with transportation, utility and government agencies to assess other needs. Is a mass evacuation center needed and if so, how will affected people be transported to that facility? Have transportation routes been affected such that calling for a mass evacuation may cause more chaos and distress than that of the incident? Are there other Federal agencies that have specialized teams which the Public Health agency needs to be in contact?

On the next page is a job aid that features things for the PHO to think about in the aftermath of an incident, at varying time intervals. While certain responsibilities are listed for certain time periods, keep in mind that as part of the response, those tasks that need to be taken care of early in a response will need to be continued as the response moves along, even as new responsibilities are added. This job aid should be used as part of training the entire Public Health agency staff, and shared with any volunteer organizations or other agencies that will be assisting as part of the Public Health response effort.

## Public Health Response: A Timeline

Purpose: To describe what, in general, actions should be taken in the aftermath of an incident to provide the most coordination with other local, state, and Federal responders and to best serve the public's needs.

0-3 Hours after Incident:

- Determine what localities are affected by the incident
- Determine what parts of the possible Public Health response have also been affected and/or cut off by the incident itself
- Coordinate with other local agencies and if necessary, Public Health agencies from other jurisdictions
- Determine who has been assigned as the Incident Commander Determine if an Emergency Operations Center is being opened
- If so, who from the Public Health office will be the liaison to the EOC?

3-6 Hours after Incident:

- Assign a Public Information Officer (PIO) to update the population on what has happened, the state of recovery, and any next steps they need to take (evacuation, vaccination, protecting their homes, etc.)
- Begin coordination of volunteer effort for donated blood, food, water, and other supplies Contact the Strategic National Stockpile if it's deemed necessary, based on the type of incident and medicinal supplies available in the locality

- Begin serious coordination with other jurisdictions and state and Federal agencies, as by this time there will be involvement from all levels of government depending on the severity and type of the incident

6-12 Hours after Incident and Beyond:

- Have shelters up and running for the public
- Have facilities available to handle mass casualties, if necessary
- Begin consulting with environmental, transportation, utility and facilities experts to determine what long-term plans are going to be needed for recovery, in addition to the short-term plans for continuing to deal with the aftermath of the incident for those with immediate needs
- Determine if any other specialized assistance from state or Federal agencies are necessary based on the severity/type of the incident
- Is a quarantine facility necessary in the case of Bird Flu or other biological, chemical attack/incident?

## Who is Involved?

As mentioned previously, the success of the Public Health agency's response to a disaster/incident will depend greatly on the cooperation of many people. And that involves more than just the other staff that makes up the agency and work for the lead Public Health Officer. This part of the chapter will look at particular people the PHO should look to for assistance and help in coordination, and note how these lines of communication should be opened well before any incident takes place, but rather during the Preparedness phase of the Emergency Management cycle. Trying to establish these contacts during the immediate aftermath of an incident will only make the overall response less efficient, along with making the Public Health response less effective.

The types of people that the Public Health Officer needs to contact after an incident will always depend on the incident itself. A chemical plant or refinery explosion that spreads flames, smoke, and potentially hazardous fumes over a densely populated region in your jurisdiction is not going to require the expertise of an epidemiologist. But you can't discount the contribution that person could make in the event of the discovery of a Bird Flu case in your jurisdiction, or something more standard, such as a disease outbreak of a malady that is well-known, but that arrives on a large scale. As another example, the PHO will probably have no need to call on supplies from the Strategic National Stockpile in the wake of a tornado, but there may be other disasters – ones that aren't necessarily biological or chemical related, but simply happen on a grand scale – that could require that sort of contact.

On the next page is a list of possible contacts that the PHO should have constantly open lines of communication with so that when an incident occurs, the PHO, his/her staff, the Incident Commander, or other entities can more effectively and efficiently coordinate the response by calling in all the necessary expertise.

Note, if you are in the Public Health agency in an urban area, or cover a large jurisdiction with a significant population, there may be even more agencies and contacts that you need to have to cover the communications lines for all possible incidents. The contacts listed below are suitable for any jurisdiction, but it is never unwise to add to it. The more prepared; the better.

## Public Health Response Plan: Contacts

Purpose: To generate as complete a list as possible of those who need to be called upon in the event of a disaster, either man-made or natural, that will lead to better coordination and a more efficient, effective emergency response. This list is designed to be useful for a Public Health Officer who is new to the job, or who may be on his first PHO assignment in a smaller locality. Some of the entries may seem elementary, but all are necessary and the time to open the line of communications is before an incident occurs, not after it.

- Local Police Chief/Sheriff/State Police Barracks
- Depending on the locality, these designations may differ, but open lines of communication with whoever is present.

- Local Ambulance services and EMS personnel.
- Are these personnel in your area volunteers? If they are, they will be responding to an incident from many different directions, and the PHO will not have a central place to call to reach all of them. Get necessary mobile/text/Blackberry contact information as soon as possible.

- All local and regional medical centers and emergency rooms
- While all incidents are local, the incident that happens in your jurisdiction may require resources from outside your area. In addition, incidents that occur far from your area, that you may think won't affect you, may require evacuation of the wounded to facilities in your area and you must be ready for this eventuality.

- Non-emergency health care personnel

- Any major incident is going to find the Public Health Officer in need of nurses and other care givers, as well as doctors who may have specific areas of biological, chemical, physical or environmental health expertise. Track down these contacts in your area and make sure they are aware that you will look to them as resources in the incident response process. As a new PHO, you may question whether you would ever need the assistance of the pandemic flu expert in your area. The answer to this question is yes, you do. The time to find that out is not AFTER the discovery of multiple Bird Flu cases in your jurisdiction, at which point every action and minute spent will be critical.

- State and Federal agencies that will be critical in an emergency response
- Examples include the Centers for Disease Control; officials who coordinate distribution of materials from the Strategic National Stockpile; the National Transportation Safety Board (for major train derailments and plane crashes); the Federal Emergency Management Administration (local and regional contacts); the Department of Health and Human Services and their Emergency Response Teams; specialized emergency response teams at both the state and Federal level; the Environmental Protection Agency, etc.

- Coroner's Office, both in your jurisdictions and others nearby.

- Local and state transportation departments
- Consider the scenario if the PHO has to order an evacuation from an area after an incident occurs. This contact is necessary in order to notify the public of safe escape routes and ones that should be absolutely avoided.

- Local and Regional Animal Control and Veterinarians
- The purpose of this is two-fold. The potential loss or displacement of pets is an issue in any incident. Note the victims of Hurricane Katrina who flat refused to evacuate their homes amid rising flood waters, all because they did not want to leave without their pet. The PHO can't be involved with this directly, but must know who to call in when the situation arises. On the other hand, some incidents will require the direct involvement of veterinarians, such as disease carried by birds or other animals that could cause a local epidemic.

- Local and regional Utilities
- The PHO will need to coordinate with these organizations to discuss possible power outages resulting from an incident, or if there are special instructions the public must follow in terms of drinking water, bathing water, etc., natural gas lines being turned off, etc.

- Volunteer organizations
- The PHO should establish strong lines of communication with local, state, and Federal volunteer organizations, such as the American Red Cross and the Salvation Army, as well as other community service organizations such as blood banks and shelters. This is often the public face of a response, in that requests for donated blood will be issued, and while the people affected by an incident will require assistance with supplies that these organizations can supply as part of the coordinated effort, others not directly affected by the incident will want to know where they can send donations and other assistance – or go volunteer themselves. This extra resource of human help in an emergency response can

never be discounted and it is important to know before an incident occurs how this is going to be coordinated from the Public Health perspective.

- Local, State and Federal Government Officials
- Beyond dealing with any particular agency at these levels, the PHO must have emergency contacts that can provide a direct link to those that will need to make key management decisions in an incident. Is the incident significant enough that the Federal Government is going to officially designate your jurisdiction as a Disaster Area? If so, what does this mean for you and the Public Health response to the incident? These are issues that have to be discussed and coordinated during the preparedness stage.

## Your Training Plan in Action

The final section of this chapter will carry you through the PHO's role in incident response based on a possible scenario. This scenario will deal with Bird Flu, and the confirmation of cases in your jurisdiction. Your first thought may be to read on only casually – after all, as of December 2005, this malady hadn't been reported as striking a human in the United States, and the likelihood that it would seems very small.

But in emergency management, this is exactly where the training process begins instead of ends. The key to successful emergency management coordination is planning for everything, to the point of having a Plan X when all the other plans have failed due to catastrophic conditions. Two cases of Bird Flu, as you will see in this scenario, do not instantly set off the kind of response effort you would have were a jetliner to crash in a densely populated residential neighborhood, such as what occurred outside New York City several years ago. However, the sequence of events and contacts that the PHO must work on and with is similar and every bit as important.

One factor to consider in a Bird Flu incident, or similar type of disease outbreak, is that the typical first responders won't necessarily be in play. Police, fire, and EMS, who will be first to the scene in a transit accident, derailment, plane crash or explosion, will not be the first ones called in upon the discovery of a Bird Flu case in your jurisdiction. Instead, the scenario would look something like this.

- The PHO is likely to be first made aware of this situation once the first patient who has been infected is in the hospital. There are several concerns that the PHO must consider at this point:
  - What medicines are available to treat the person infected in this particular case? You will discover this easily enough

through dealing with the primary caregivers at the medical center where the patient is checked into. Medication to assist the patient (though not cure the disease) is available currently.

- Who else in that medical center may be infected?
- Surely, the personnel at the medical center did everything possible to keep this patient away from possibly infecting others. But did they all take the kind of precautions necessary in this situation? Could the disease have spread to either a caregiver or another patient? How many patients have checked OUT of that facility in the time that this patient has been there, thus raising the possibility (no matter how small it may be) that the disease could be carried into the general population in your area?
- Contacts: You are lucky here in the sense that if there has been no spread, you have your incident zone, and many of the people you need to have on site to handle this situation are already in place. However, it is at this point that the PHO would have to contact:
- Local or regional doctors and/or research experts knowledgeable regarding Bird Flu.
    - They will know how to treat it and how to contain it. You may find that this sort of assistance and expertise may only be available at the Federal level, depending on your locality, and such contact needs to be made as quickly as possible so the proper authorities and such can be dispatched to your location.
- Neighboring Public Health Officials.
    - It is entirely possible, of course, that if a Bird Flu case has been discovered in your jurisdiction, that there may be others waiting in the jurisdictions around you. Word must be spread to their Public Health Officials as quickly as possible to start any possible response there, and/or to help you with your work in your own jurisdiction.

- Your agency's Public Information Officer.
  - Someone is going to have to speak to the public about this incident. The public will need to know about possible symptoms, and where to go to get assistance if they are afraid of possibly having caught the disease. The public will also want to know what precautions to take if they don't have symptoms. Another thing to think about related to this is that in this age of instant information, news will leak about this and the media will converge on your locality, bombarding the Public Health Office with phone calls, requests for more detailed status reports and interviews. The PIO needs to be the person to handle all of this, as you will not have time.
- Police and Local, State Government Officials
  - You will need to work with both these entities to discuss a possible quarantine station if other cases exist, or to remove the current case from the medical center in order to avoid the risk of infecting other patients or caregivers. The public will need to know where this area is so as to avoid it, and the police will be needed to not only help set it up in some cases, but also to provide protection.
- EMS (Local and Regional)
  - It is not unlikely that once word is released of this case, a sort of panic will fall over the population in your jurisdiction, and anyone who feels they are suffering from symptoms similar to those described for Bird Flu may start calling for emergency assistance. The local and regional EMS units have to be put on alert for this possibility, both to quickly respond in the correct fashion, and also to have time to call in reinforcements and volunteers if necessary if the volume of requests for assistance proves to be tremendous.
- Centers for Disease Control

    - Obviously, the CDC will want to know of these developments, and they will be the foremost experts in what steps the PHO and agency should take next both in dealing with the patient, caregivers and the public. They will also quickly dispatch experts into the locality and may well take the lead on that side of things. This will leave the PHO with more of the coordination and support response.

      In addition, experts from the CDC can also advise, based on the situation, if any kind of Personal Protective Equipment (PPE) is necessary and who should have it. You will need to know this so that you understand if PPE is readily available in your jurisdiction, or if you are going to need to call on health agencies in neighboring jurisdictions to provide resources.
- Strategic National Stockpile Personnel
    - While you have received a report that there are medicines and supplies available for the one case that you are aware of, will your locality be ready if you suddenly discover in the next few hours that there are 4 cases? 8? 20? Officials from the SNS must be called on immediately. The SNS can have supplies, medicines, surgical and medical equipment and other such needs delivered to your locality within 12 hours, with the help of state officials.

So, 3 hours have now passed. You have made all the contacts above, because the training you and your staff have gone through in the Public Health agency required opening lines of communications with all these contacts. Because they expected to hear from you in this situation, they aren't getting their news from the TV or radio, but from those involved in the coordinated response effort that is operating efficiently and effectively to this point.

In the next 3 hours, the situation continues to unfold. The original patient has been successfully moved to a different facility and quarantined. The PIO has taken to the TV and radio airwaves with instructions for the population, both those that feel they may have symptoms and want assistance; and those that don't but want to protect themselves. A call for calm has been sounded, so as to not have a panicked population making bad decisions that could harm the emergency response effort. The SNS is sending supplies in case they are needed and a delivery method and location has been secured. Officials from the CDC are in route, and experts in how Bird Flu develops and is transmitted are working with area doctors and staff in your agency to try and track down how this case ended up in your locality.

So what are the PHO's main responsibilities during this time?

- Maintain contact
  - Because of all the communications lines that are opened up, and all the various agents and facets of the response that you must deal with, it is important to be available to continue to receive these communications. You may or may not be near the quarantine site – such an emergency as this may not require direct, on-site involvement. But you will need to be constantly updated on the patient, the reaction, and all the steps that those involved in the response are taking. Constant communication with the Incident Commander – if one is designated for this case – is critical.
- Reassure the public
  - It is very important that the PIO is active in the public during this time. While everyone is obviously worried about the possible spread of the disease – you also must coordinate an effort to soothe and educate the public. Something important to remember in this example is that

much of the population in your jurisdiction will have no idea what they should or shouldn't do in this situation in terms of staying safe. Panic is one of the leading risk factors to an effective emergency response, so information is going to be quick, accurate, and consistently available in multiple formats (and probably, multiple languages) so that everyone in your jurisdiction clearly understands the situation, how to stay safe, and what to do if an evacuation is ordered, etc.

- National Guard assistance?
  - Depending on the response of the public to this situation, or if there is a lack of resources available in your jurisdiction, you may need to work with military authorities to receive National Guard assistance in maintaining order in your jurisdiction. Word spreading about the Bird Flu case in your area may be as dangerous as the spread of the disease itself. The National Guard may be needed to make sure the response area is secured, while also possibly being called in to help bring in people who are suffering symptoms and want to be examined.
- Finalize SNS delivery details
  - At this point, it is too early to tell if you are going to have more than just an isolated case on your hands. While primary caregivers on site have determined that what they need currently is available, that may not remain true should the situation change in the next 6-12 hours, and effectively coordinating the delivery of supplies and medicines with the SNS will leave your jurisdiction ready to handle such an increase in cases in the coming hours and days should they occur.
- Something else to think about … while it may not necessarily be the case with Bird Flu, how will you coordinate the mass

> dispensing of vaccines if the SNS is able to deliver such an item that will keep a large portion of the population in your jurisdiction from being affected? This is where you need to continue to work with local police, government officials, and volunteer organizations to make sure such a large-scale effort to deliver a vaccine can be done in a calm, orderly fashion. Again, the PIO will be called on in this situation, as well, because information will have to be given to the public on where to go to receive such a treatment, as well as any special precautions that they should take.

One thing you will see in the 3- to 6-hour range, depending on the incident, is an increased Federal presence of agencies and responders. But remember, the incident is still a local one. Only you have the first-hand information on what is happening, where it is happening, and who can potentially be affected. Any state or Federal officials that join the response during this time period will need this communicated to them before knowing what next steps they should take. While you may not be the lead in such a response, you will most certainly play an important role and that role doesn't diminish, even when it appears that more of the response is being handled by officials and authorities from outside your jurisdiction.

As you enter the range beyond 6 hours, looking toward the end of the day and beyond, you now will need to consider future issues. You will need to advise local government officials on whether or not there needs to be quarantine or condemning of the building where this case was first discovered. You may think that such an action would only happen in extreme cases, but extreme cases are exactly what you have to plan for in Emergency Management. All other facets of the response that have been discussed in the first hours after you received word of this case are progressing. To this point, you and your staff have followed their training very well.

It's been determined that area utilities, such as the water supply, are safe. There has been no need to call for an evacuation, and no major issues on the roads and with transit. SNS supplies and medicine reinforcements will arrive in the next couple hours, and the public has been made aware of the process for receiving the attention they need, what time that will begin, where to go, and so on.

These times leading out to the 12-hour mark and beyond are also important for another reason. There will be shift changes taking effect and new people will be called into the response who perhaps are not up to speed on what has taken place to this point. You, or someone you designate, will need to cover that with new responders from a Public Health perspective. And at some point, you will also need to designate someone to fill in for you that can handle all of these responsibilities that you have carried out over the last day.

In this Bird Flu scenario, one final task awaits for the PIO, as it will be him/her, or you, that will have to deliver the news either in the next couple hours or in the coming days that the person diagnosed originally to set off this response has passed away. Again, this will be a time to prevent panic among the population in your jurisdiction, and to stress that while this is an extremely unfortunate event; everyone involved in the response is doing their job, and there is no further immediate threat to the public. Through your long-standing communications with a Bird Flu expert in your jurisdiction, he has been able to report back to you that this was, in fact, an isolated case after all, and there is no threat to the population.

Upon this news, again, communication with the public is key. As the response winds down and any necessary clean up and breakdown of equipment and such takes place, the Emergency Management cycle isn't over. Now the Preparedness stage begins all over again. Beyond practice drills and tabletop exercises, the PHO now has a live event to study, learn what went well, what went wrong, and what should be done and how the emergency response should be altered should this situation occur again. In a sense, Emergency Management for the Public Health Officer never really ends, because the PHO is always either involved in a response, or training for the next one. While it may seem overwhelming; this is, in fact, the key to being a successful contributor to the entire emergency response operation.

CHAPTER 15

# Community Surge

• • •

**Robert J. Muller**

SURGE, THE ABILITY TO INCREASE public health and medical systems is a critical component of disaster preparedness and response. Surge is a complex topic, presenting many challenges to effective incident management. The aftermath of Hurricane Katrina and the concern of emerging infectious diseases have focused attention on this issue. The communication and coordination principles, systems and processes that have proved effective for all aspects of disaster response are especially applicable to public health and medical surge. It is extremely challenging to assess, develop strategies, quickly take action and use resources effectively in the early stages of a rapidly evolving incident.

The dimensions of medical surge capacity include healthcare facility-based surge capacity, public health surge capacity, and community-based surge capacity. Healthcare facility-based surge capacity refers to the ability of health care facilities to treat increased numbers of sick, and injured, especially when inpatient care is required. This is in addition to the increased demand anticipated by the worried well. Public health surge capacity refers to the ability to increase core public health functions during a public health emergency. This includes enhanced public health surveillance and epidemiological investigation along with increased and expanded laboratory testing, emergency public information and warning, non-pharmaceutical interventions and if we are fortunate, medical countermeasures distribution and dispensing, such as mass antibiotic prophylaxis or vaccination. Community-based surge capacity encompasses the community's ability to support both healthcare facilities and public health response. Coordination with the community is necessary to avoid over-extending healthcare facilities. Communities assist in the public health response with logistical support activities such as mass prophylaxis or vaccination campaigns. Individuals and communities will be called on to make informed decisions within the shifting context of social media and the mass media industry.

An initial step in exploring this theme is to distinguish surge capacity from surge capability.

Surge *capacity* refers to the ability to evaluate and care for a markedly increased volume, one that challenges or exceeds normal operating capacity. Surge requirements may extend beyond direct patient care or individual intervention to include such tasks as uncommon and intensive laboratory studies or epidemiological investigations. Because of its relation to volume, many initiatives to address surge capacity focus on identifying adequate numbers of hospital beds, personnel, pharmaceuticals, supplies, and equipment. It is necessary to have quantities of each critical asset, but more important for successful surge are the networks, systems and processes that promote:

- Effective communication
- Coordinated assessment of needs with consideration for vulnerabilities
- Development of strategies and identification of resources to address needs in a timely manner

- Evaluation of the efficacy of response during a dynamic, evolving situation

There are concepts and tools to direct risk communication, information sharing, public information and warning and information. Response partners must be able to briefly and clearly summarize what the issue encompasses, at an early stage, in order to engage participants and gather stakeholder input to create a common operational picture. Communication must continue throughout the entire response. Response partner and stakeholder communication is most effective if it begins before an incident, builds on a trusting network and follows established processes.

Planning and training are best built on a coordinated threat and hazard risk assessment by a multi-disciplinary team. Assessment is based on a shared understanding of information to create a common operational picture. Effective and efficient strategy development requires subject matter expertise, with public health and medical systems relying on current scientific principles, medical intelligence and epidemiological investigation. Implementation requires clear roles and responsibilities in coordination with response partners.

Assessment benefits from a multi-disciplinary approach by subject matter experts to identify, quantify, and prioritize needs for response to a specific incident. Experts bring their understanding of current science, guidance, best practices, along with experience and data such as baseline information.

Effective and efficient strategy development for public health and medical systems requires medical intelligence and epidemiological investigation. Threat and hazard identification, pre planning, workforce development and exercises guide strategy and task development. Implementation includes clear roles and responsibilities coordinated with response partners within a system network.

Resources, both personnel and material are limited during initial response to a disaster; that's part of the equation of disaster. The ability to maximize existing resources and expeditiously move these limited resources to locations of need, then manage and support these people, supplies and equipment is necessary to realize their absolute maximum capacity. Moreover, the coordination of resources, whether standby, mutual aid, State or Federal aid is difficult without adequate management systems.

Evaluation continues throughout response in an effort to adequately utilize resources and adjust to evolving situations. Thus, surge capacity is primarily about effective and efficient systems and processes.

Surge *capability* refers to the ability to manage individuals requiring unusual or very specialized evaluation and care. Surge requirements span the range of specialized medical services, including expertise, current information, procedures, equipment, or personnel, that are not normally available at the location where they are needed. Surge capability also includes patient complications that require special intervention to protect medical providers, other patients, organizations and communities.

The U. S. Department of Health and Human Services and the Centers for Disease Control and Prevention offer guidance and cooperative agreement funding for building surge. This guidance is included in the Surge Management Domain are into capabilities for Fatality Management, Mass Care, Medical Surge, and Volunteer Management. Development and these tools increase the ability of the healthcare and public health systems to survive a hazard impact and maintain or rapidly recover operations that were compromised.

Public health and medical systems should anticipate incidents that significantly impact their usual operations, as occurred with Hurricane Katrina, will likely occur in the future. During an incident requiring surge, organizations must be able to transition from a baseline capacity and capability using a systems and processes for response. Once the surge incident is met, then the system can transition back to its baseline capacity and capability.

Strategies and tasks to enhance management systems must recognize that the required emergency interventions are time sensitive and must be based primarily at the local level. This urgency limits the ability of the Federal Government to independently establish, stockpile, own or control resources necessary. States and local jurisdictions must participate in active asset management. In addition, because most medical assets in the United States are privately owned, strategies must bridge the public-private divide, as well as integrate multiple disciplines and levels of government.

A comprehensive effort to address response requirements must include a system description of how the different response components are organized and managed and a concept of operations, how the system components function and interact through successive stages of an event. It must include "all-hazard" processes and procedures, mutual aid, and other validated emergency management concepts.

Public health and medical systems are challenged to prepare for major disasters. Such emergencies will severely challenge the ability of these systems to adequately care for large numbers of patients (surge capacity) and/or victims with unusual or highly specialized medical needs (surge capability).

To address surge and build system resiliency jurisdictions should frame emergency and disaster response on strong day-to-day operational systems that can effectively manage public health and medical response, as well as the develop and maintain preparedness and recovery programs.

The National Incident Management System (NIMS) makes it increasingly important for health systems to adopt response systems based on Incident Command System principles. NIMS establishes core concepts and organizational processes based on ICS to allow diverse disciplines from all levels of government and the private sector to work together in response to domestic hazards. NIMS compliance is required of all Federal departments and agencies, as well as State, Tribal, and jurisdictional organizations that seek Federal preparedness assistance such as grants or contracts. With this basis in ICS, medical and public health organizations develop relationships, strategies, processes, and procedures, and work as partners, fully integrated into the emergency response community. The lessons of the past and threats to the future require nothing less than the ability to suddenly and powerfully move forward and upward, to surge.

(This chapter was written with the collaboration of Staff from the Louisiana Department of Health and Hospitals. This represents personal knowledge and experience and does not represent the views of the agency.)

CHAPTER 16

# Trauma Disaster Planning

● ● ●

**Norman McSwain**

TRAUMA DISASTER PLANNING DEPENDS ON amount of warning that is expected for the 'disaster event" and the amount of resources immediately available when the 'disaster' hits and then the resources that can be available after short delay.

The amount of warning can be divided into Fast Disasters and Slow disasters. An example of a 'slow disaster' is expected big event such as Mardi Gras or a hurricane; a 'fast disaster', is an unexpected event such as a building falling, a terrorist event (Boston Marathon) or local criminal event such as a mass shooting or explosion.

A slow disaster will allow specific planning for a specific event, while a fast disaster requires general planning for a generic event with the local situations in mind.

There are several components that should be included in the planning of both types. The planning for the slow disaster is easier than the fast as specific needs can be addressed and are not as broad, but the following elements should be included in the process:

- Scope of the requirements
- Length of the disaster
- Personnel
    - Access to the medical facility

- Required
  - Administrative
  - Medical
  - Support
  - Security
  - Job descriptions and cross over
- Backup
- When
- Lock down
- Family preparation for required access
- Certification of 'walk-in' volunteer personnel
- Rotation of personnel on strict rules
  - Do not allow the personnel to over work
  - Decisions will be flawed
  - Mistakes will be made

- Facility
  - Size
  - Beds
  - Power supply
  - Water supply
  - Sewerage resources
- Medical supplies
  - Pharmaceutical
  - Surgical
  - resupply
- Food
  - Patients
  - Staff
  - Medical
  - Re-stocking of supplies
- Security
  - protection of facility

    - protection of personnel
    - Lock down
- Evacuation
    - Vehicles
    - Location
    - Acceptance
    - Medical records
        - HIPPA
    - Family notification
- Communication
    - Power supply
    - Access to phone lines without facility network
    - Cellphone
    - Satellite phones
    - Grid overload
    - Band width competition
        - Other users
        - Media
        - Military
- Training
    - Mock disaster
    - Real time drill
    - Table top drills
    - ALL PERSONNEL MUST BE TRAINED

General Eisenhower said that 'planning is everything but plans are worthless'. He said in a few words that it is extremely important to plan for an event or for an unknown disaster but when the event occurs the plans rapidly become obsolete and the managers must be able to 'think on their feet'.

Such is extremely important in the training of the personnel. Unless they are knowledgeable of their job description, are trained, and understand the extent of what to do and what not to do, what resources are available and if and when resupply and evacuation are expected, patients will be lost needlessly.

Personnel must do the jobs that they have the most experience; Untrained elective surgeon must not be placed in a triage position. The floor nurse should not be placed in the ED or the OR.

A physician is not a physician is not a physician. A nurse is not a nurse is not a nurse.

The makers of plans must be experienced planners, and know that when the event happens they must have the experience and understanding of the event to improvise as required.

CHAPTER 17

# The Emergency Department and EMS Surge

• • •

**Joseph DiCorpo**

In the past 20 years we have seen significant changes and improvements in our communities Pre-Hospital Emergency Medical Services Systems (EMS) and local Fire Departments (FD). Due to changes in the Life Safety and Building codes across this country, the incidence of major fires in commercial and residential structures has greatly decreased. FDs have changed in this environment and now almost all FDs in the US now actively participate in their local EMS system. As this change occurred we also saw the maturation and development of sophisticated EMS systems to respond to a marked increase in the number of calls for EMS service and the development of new life saving technologies and first responder/public education programs. The natural amalgamation of these two services was the incorporation of many FD Policies and Procedures into evolving EMS systems. One of these was the Incident Command System (ICS)[2][3], which is a demonstrable, dedicated, organized and expandable communications and command structure for any emergency response which either requires more than one agency or entity, or may have more than a single victim. The purpose of this chapter is to discuss how we can apply the ICS model to the real world problem of the emergent arrival of multiple critical, urgent, and "walking wounded" patients to the hospital Emergency Department (ED), without the luxury or necessity to institute a full-fledged hospital Disaster Plan[1] response.

In the preparation for response to "Mini-Disasters" (single incidents which create 4-20 significantly injured citizens at the same location) Emergency Departments (ED) have had to develop plans and methodologies to handle this "Surge" of patients in the ED.

One may argue that with a good EMS and FD system in place, when these incidents occur, that the victims will be triaged, stabilized accordingly, treated on the scene, and then transported and divided up appropriately between local hospital ED's so that no one facility becomes taxed beyond their capabilities.

We cannot rely on this happening in all cases, and therefore, we should have a plan and methodology for handling this type of "Surge".

## Pre-Surge Planning

It is important not to rely solely on the general JACHO required Hospital Wide Disaster Plan [1]. Case studies have shown over time that this type of plan is not applicable to a situation like the EMS Surge, and this can be handled more efficiently within the confines of the ED and with experienced ED staff. This EMS Surge plan should be a separate ED plan, which should be practiced independently of the Hospital Wide Disaster Plan, and on an annual basis.

## Notification

Before a plan can be effective to handle the Surge is important to have a notification plan in place to make sure the facility is notified before the patients are transported to the facility.

If the facility is not notified before the patients are enrooted, the necessary preparation time factor will be lacking in order to facilitate the arrival of anticipated victims.

The establishment of community 911 and e911 systems throughout the United States are multiple ways to ensure the facility is notified well in advance.

Computer Aided Dispatch (CAD) systems can be programmed to automatically send a message to your ED when the initial call is received based on certain criteria agreed upon with your 911 center. The 911 center can program and electronic update to the ED as to general patient/victim count as it is advised by the field units. EMS/Ambulance Service Radio Traffic is a normal part of ED communications and by pre-planning with your local communications centers you can make sure you are notified in multiple technologies and methodologies as the situation unfolds on the scene.

Ensure time to educate yourself and your staff on understanding the EMS/FD Pre-Hospital Incident Command System (ICS). It is not only important to know what you are hearing, but also who you may be hearing it from.

As in any stressful situation each person on the scene has a different perspective of what is evolving as the scene progresses. Although, ideally, the Incident Commander (IC) has an overall knowledge of what is being done at the scene, the EMS Transportation Officer will be the one directing where each patient is to be transported for definitive care.

In any Multiple Casualty Incident (MCI) there is a plethora of misinformation, more so than accurate information that may be presented t to the ED. Exercise caution, but above everything else, be sure to stay ahead of the information curve and the Surge; always stay thinking about 15 to 30 minutes ahead of where you are right now in the response process. This will help you from being "blindsided" by an unexpected turn of events.

Planning and implementing an ED ICS for the Surge;
The first step in planning for the Surge is to decide at what level of patient influx you need to activate your Surge plan [4].

If the ED is large, then the Surge of 4 patients may not be of any consequence; but if the ED is small and less sophisticated then that same surge may be much more significant and taxing to the facility.

If a level of influx is decided, and also then establish within the notification system(s) with your local 911 center and/or EMS system, it then becomes an organizational drill which would follow the plan.

The Surge plan is a very time sensitive plan because from the time of notification to the actual time of delivery of the first patient it is only a matter of minutes. Therefore the planning document must incorporate an actual time line for the plan's implementation.

Notification is considered Time Zero (T0) and the clock starts immediately.

There are many things that have to be done, but the first 5 minutes is the most critical.

The **first 5 minutes after initial notification** the following tasks should be performed:

1) Establish the ED Incident Command System and activation of the Surge plan by general announcement over ED paging system. This way personnel in the ED know what the Standard Operating Procedure is for the next few hours within the ED, and that as of now policy and procedures have changed.
2) The RN staff can immediately begin to assess their patients and decompression of the ED can begin as soon as possible. This paves the way for the Surge plan participants to clear space for the incoming Surge patients within the next 5 minutes.

3) The Secretarial Staff in ED should notify the departments of Anesthesiology, Operating Room, Pre-Op, Post-Op, Holding Areas, and Post Anesthesia Care Unit. These departments and practitioners should all be asked to place elective surgical operative cases on hold; and no new non emergent operative cases should be started. The reversal of this order can only be issued by the ED Incident Commander in consultation with the hospital Chief of Staff, hospital administration, Anesthesiologist in Charge and Trauma Surgeon in Charge.
4) The Trauma and Orthopedic Surgeon(s) On Call should be notified and requested to respond to ED.
5) Request an Anesthesiologist/Anesthetist to respond to the ED.
6) Request that the RN House Supervisor respond to ED.
7) Notify Administration and Public Relations/Media Relations that the Surge plan has been activated in the ED.
8) The Incident Commander for the Surge plan in the ED should be the pre designated ED MD.
9) The Triage Officer for the Surge plan in the ED should be the on duty ED Charge Nurse or other pre designated individual in the plan.
10) Call Security and have the Security Supervisor become the Transportation Coordination/Traffic Officer. His/her job is essential since he/she must maintain clean egress and exit routes at all times around the ED. He/she should use their fellow Security Officers and request local Police Department assistance for local street clearing, coordination, and assistance as deemed necessary. They must keep all EMS vehicles out of entrance ways and not allow EMS vehicles to back up, stall, be abandoned, and block critical egress and exit pathways for any extended periods of time other than to unload their patients.

11) Assign and plan for an Asst. Security Supervisor as the ED Security Officer. Request that all available Security Officers report to ED within 5 minutes according to the pre plan but do not leave other areas of the hospital without security as may be necessitated by the size and type of event. The ED should be placed on Lock Down-- to secure the area, prevent wanderers, and prohibit unauthorized personnel from coming to the ED and "looking around", especially members of the news media.
12) The senior ED Technician may serve as the Communications Officer and have him/her assigned exclusively to the EMS Radio or communications system. He/she should then issue portable VHF/UHF (hand held) ED radios to Incident Commander, Triage Officer, and Security Supervisor and Assistant Security Supervisor, and other key ED staff, as per the pre plan (these should be numbered, and signed out for tracking purposes). These radios must be acquired before the event and all appropriate staff must be trained in their utilization. These radios are a dedicated, short range, single frequency, handheld radio system. It is essential not to depend on other systems due to system overloading/ congestion, such as cell phones or cellular direct connect systems. The Communications Officer will be responsible for notifying all members of the Surge team, via these common channel radios, of all updates from the scene of the incident and expected delivery of patients, including severity and Estimated Time of Arrival (ETA) to the ED. He/ she also will communicate back to the 911 center or the IC at the scene if the ED becomes saturated and another ED be designated for patient diversion.
13) The Incident Commander, Triage Officer, Transportation Coordinator, Communications Officer, and ED Security

Officer, as well as any other key individuals should be issued bright colored light weight vests designating who they are in the ED Incident Command System. This is not a popular idea but very necessary in the real world Surge. As you have probably noticed by this point the Surge plan is VERY organized. This is why it works. Each member of the Surge response team is trained, oriented, equipped, labeled, identified, and tasked with certain responsibilities. As long as each participant does his/her own individual assignment then the entire system works well. The Incident Commander or Triage Officer have the responsibilities to oversee the entire operation of the Surge plan and make assignment and patient care changes as needed.

14) The Incident Commander MD and Triage Officer/ ED Charge RN should **"Decompress the ED".** This means that they, along with other RN and MD staff assigned to the selected patients, will temporarily or definitively discharge/transfer any stable patient or patients, who are in a Triage/Resuscitation Room, or other ED bed, within **10 minutes** to any available space in ICU, CCU, Holding Area, or Pre or Post-Op Holding areas. Once each of these transfers are completed then the ED staff involved in the transfer will immediately return to ED.

15) A complete bed and capacity assessment should be done and return notification made to the EMS/FD/911 or scene Command Center of the Critical Care Capacity in the ED. An estimate of the capacity for non-critical stretcher cases, and "Walking Wounded" should also be communicated to the EMS/FD/911 Center. Lastly, it is essential to request and confirm casualty estimates from scene.

16) Finally, all participants in the Surge plan should review, agree, and organize a Patient Flow pattern and establish treatment teams and new patient care assignments in ED.
17) It is now approximately **12 minutes** post notification and you should be ready to accept Surge patients.
18) Based on Casualty estimates coming from the EMS/FD/911 Center, and the actual number of patients delivered to the ED as part of the Surge, the ED Incident Commander and Triage Officer will decide whether to call in additional ED MDs, RNs and Technician Staff before normal shift change and/or keep on duty staff on overtime for staffing the Surge. One of the key differentiators of the Surge plan from the general hospital disaster plan is that the Surge plan does not recommend requesting or utilizing non-ED staff respond to ED for Surge staffing.

The Surge plan and the ED Incident Command System described in this chapter are designed and implemented for a single, sudden, fixed number, and influx of patients from a single isolated incident. It is not a hospital disaster or community disaster plan. It is a temporary plan for a specific incident [5]. Most of the time, depending on the severity and number of patients received, the Surge plan will be in effect for about 2 to 6 hours then be deactivated. At that time ED operations will return to normal. Any patient who was temporarily housed outside the ED and not admitted to the hospital may then be returned to the ED for final assessment and appropriate discharge.

The essence of this plan is to create a rapid response organization based on a sudden influx of patients into an already busy ED. As we all know, we hardly ever see the activation of the full hospital disaster plan. But we all know of nights in the ED when we were already full, and the call came in for a six victim motor vehicle accident on the interstate. It is at that moment that we wish that someone would plan for and now be able to activate a Surge plan, to free up critical space and personnel in response to this incident [6].

I know we wish the plan was in place long before the six or eight ambulances lined up outside the ED door and at the same time a helicopter was landing simultaneously on the roof.....?

There is no substitute for specific and dynamic planning --- NONE.

Footnotes:

[1] Joint Commission Accreditation of Healthcare Organizations, Chicago, Illinois, Revised 2012 EC. 4.20 – The organization regularly tests its Community Emergency Operations Plan

[2] National Incident Management System
Department of Homeland Security
December 2008
http://www.fema.gov/pdf/emergency/nims/NIMS_core.pdf

[3] ICS Response to Mass Casualty Scenario with Active Shooter
Department of Homeland Security
December 2013
http://www.usfa.fema.gov/downloads/pdf/publications/active_shooter_guide.pdf

[4] Parkland finds way to handle growing ER volumes
Dallas Morning News
April 28, 2014
http://thescoopblog.dallasnews.com/2014/04/parkland-finds-way-to-handle-growing-er-volumes.html/

[5] Transforming the Emergency Department: Herman Miller's Role in ER One, an Effort to Improve Readiness
http://www.hermanmiller.com/research/solution-essays/transforming-the-emergency-department.html

[6] Hospital Capacity, Patient Flow, and Emergency Department Use in New Jersey
by Derek Delia, Ph.D.
http://www.nj.gov/health/rhc/documents/ed_report.pdf

CHAPTER 18

# Hospital Administrative Planning and Considerations

Robert J. Muller

## Admissions

In the new computerized era most hospitals register patient data via their IT system and give each patient their own unique patient number as well as an admission number that is related to that particular date of their encounter. While their patient number usually remains the same, each encounter number is different, and obviously so, for tracking purposes of that particular admission.

This system is very vulnerable to electrical outage and or collapse of the IT system. Therefore the system should have some redundancies built into it to help mitigate this potential problem.

This may be done by:

A. Ensure that the admit system has adequate backup power from either the internal hospital generator system, or a portable external generator to drive the system.
B. Utilize a battery powered back up laptop computer that has a pre-established emergency program that is capable of providing encounter numbers until the main system is reestablished.

C. Utilize a manual system to issue encounter numbers from a previously established pre designated aliquot of numbers assigned just for these potential emergency situations. These may be pre coded with the letter "E" to indicated their emergency status use so that they are easily identified and may be changed at a later date if necessary (i.e. E-8-735-09)

This indicated an emergency situation (E), -the eight month (8), -and encounter number (735) and the year (09). Additional identification information could be included in this numbering system including the digits of a drivers' license or digits of social security numbers, particularly the last four digits. (E-8-735-09-6288) A relatively simple system may be utilized that can be manually tracked until such time the system can be updated as necessary.

## Census

If there is time to prepare for an impending disaster, i.e. a hurricane, or flood, the hospital should be ***decompressed*** to reduce the census, of all patients that can be *safely* discharged home.

If this is not possible, then patients can be ***transferred*** *to hospitals who have previously executed transfer agreements.

***Evacuation*** of patients differ from transfer, in that the patients are usually evacuated to facilities which have not previously executed agreements for transfer; are further distance, and may or may not be government mediated.

No matter which terminology or methodology is utilized, the MOST important factor is patient safety as well as that of the facility staff and administration.

## Committees

### Bioterrorism Committee

All hospitals should have some form of bioterrorism planning and the size, extent and degree if preparedness should be commensurate with the hospitals ability to serve the community in this aspect.

Many communities have a bioterrorism plan through a conglomerate plan of city or county entities, i.e. fire, police, sheriff department, public works, etc.

If some form of a community plan is not in place then the extent of a hospital plan should be further enhanced, especially decontamination plans.

A hospital bioterrorism planning committee should be composed of the following hospital staff members/representatives:

1. Administrator or administrative representative, i.e. Chief Nursing Officer
2. Physician---Infectious disease or Internal Medicine
3. Physician---Emergency or Critical Care
4. Emergency Department Manager or Supervisor
5. Laboratory Supervisor or Medical Technologist
6. Pharmacy Director
7. Infectious Disease Control Nurse
8. Radiology Supervisor
9. Director of Security
10. Director of Plant Operations

Additional committee members may be added as necessary for the facility size and complexity; however, the committee should be kept to a reasonable size to facilitate adequate discussion and interaction without prolonged discussions that would hamper the accomplishment of the necessary goals. Meetings should be held at time periods commensurate with the time frame necessary to achieve the goals then held in the future to further refine and update the committee objectives.

## Community Disaster Committees

It is a good idea to form a local committee of business leaders for the sole purpose of establishing some form of plans for continuity of business recovery as well as plans for maintaining some form of a supply chain should durable goods be needed during or after an emergency situation.

One community has devised a "CHAT" (Community Hurricane Action Team) committee which serves the purpose of an all disaster planning team to aid in the continuity of supply management. The hospitals even offers embedding of the company personnel in case of a disaster so that there is assurance that he company personnel will be immediately available to open their respective businesses to supply the necessary materials or products post event.

In any events community partners should be established and regular meetings should take place at least every 6 months to keep the mission in sight as well as establish a liaison with the personnel involved and to keep up with new personnel changes especially in the national store chains. Good examples for liaison partnerships would be banks, food stores, big box stores, commercial fuel suppliers, sporting goods stores, and local merchants that have adequate inventory to be of value in a disaster situation. These meeting should include local and county government officials, sheriff, police chief, fire chief, and public works director to name a few.

Plans should be formulated with collaborative agreements to be able to access the necessary supplies available within a community without having to wait for delivery from outside resources if the resources are locally available.

Food, fuel, ice, recovery tools and supplies, only to name a few, may be accessed immediately with previous determined plans. Why allow food to ferment rather than be properly channeled to hospitals or to feed the emergency response workers? Gas/diesel can be accessed from fuel station tanks and serve as a backup fuel plan for emergency generators and vehicles; ice from food marts, and service plazas; clothing from sporting goods stores, etc.

Do not allow local assets to be LOST or wasted due to poor planning.

## Credentialing

The increased need for healthcare personnel during and after a disaster poses the problem of credentialing when utilized from other facilities as well as other cities and other states.

A plan should be determined and adopted by the hospital governing board as under what circumstances and conditions altered credentialing will be utilized and is acceptable.

The MOST difficult problem that needs to be planned for in advance is when there is <u>no communication</u> links to allow for verifications from other facilities, or boards, etc.

Predetermined memorandums of understandings (MOU) can be established among local and county hospitals and within larger hospital systems but becomes problematic when healthcare personnel cross state lines, unless they fall under the terms and stipulations of the EMAC agreement.

Agreements need to be stipulated as to the minimum credential that will be needed and acceptable to allow a healthcare professional to work within your facility; will this be a state license, an ID from a hospital with a previous established MOU, a known central credentialing system as within larger hospital systems, etc. In any event this is BEST established well in advance and a SOG is written and approved through the appropriate channels as well as the legal staff.

Also within these documents, there should be a standard operating guideline (SOG) documents that describes such things as who and how these individuals are to be compensated, travel expenses, volunteer status, illness or injury sustained while in service, etc.

Also many states have enacted a volunteer medical corps program that have been pre-credentialed by the state, have ID cards in their possession, meet and train on a regular basis in disaster preparedness situations and can be activated through state call out procedures.

It likewise would be prudent to see if your state has such a volunteer group of professions, agreement of reciprocity with other states and to become familiar with the contact information necessary to implement when and if needed.

There is NO such thing as too much planning and having the proper MOUs and SOGs in place is essential.

## EMAC - Emergency Management Assistance Compact (EMAC)

The Emergency Management Assistance Compact is a mutual aid agreement and partnership between states and territories. It exists because all states share a common enemy: the constant threat and occurrence of natural and man-made disasters as well as the threat of terrorism.

EMAC offers a responsive and straightforward system for states to send personnel and equipment to help disaster relief efforts in other states. When resources are overwhelmed, EMAC helps to fill the shortfalls. Once the conditions for providing assistance to a requesting state have been set, the terms constitute a legally binding contractual agreement that make affected states responsible for reimbursement. Responding states can rest assured that sending aid will not be a financial or legal burden and personnel sent are protected under workers compensation and liability provisions. EMAC allows states to ask for whatever assistance they need for any type of emergency, from earthquakes to acts of terrorism.

EMAC has been endorsed by the National Governor's Association and the regional Governor's organizations, the National Guard Bureau, the Federal Emergency Management Agency, and the Department of Homeland Security. EMAC has grown to become the nation's system for providing mutual aid through operational procedures and protocols that have been validated during disasters where assistance was provided under the Compact. The Compact facilitates the sharing of resources, personnel and equipment across state lines during times of disaster and emergency. EMAC is formalized into law by member states.

Acting as a complement to the national disaster response system, EMAC provides timely and cost-effective relief to states requesting assistance from compact members who understand the needs of jurisdictions that are struggling to preserve life, the economy, and the environment. EMAC does not replace federal assistance, but can be used alongside federal assistance or when federal is not warranted, thus providing a flow of needed goods and services to an affected state. This ensures the maximum use of all available resources within member states' inventories and acts as another venue for mitigating resource deficiencies. Fifty states, the District of Columbia, Puerto Rico and the U.S. Virgin islands have enacted EMAC legislation. For more information, go to www.emacweb.org and select Mutual Aid Resources, Mission Ready Packages and review the 37-minute Webinar recording.

Prior to Hurricanes Katrina and Rita, which in 2005 struck within a few short weeks of each other in Alabama, Florida, Louisiana, Mississippi, and Texas, many states had enacted emergency management laws to allow for emergency waiver or modifications of licensure standards to facilitate the interstate use of licensed healthcare practitioners. Within the public sector, all 50 states have ratified the provisions of the **Emergency Management Assistance Compact ("EMAC")** which allows for the deployment of licensed healthcare practitioners employed by state and local governments to other jurisdictions to provide emergency services without having to be licensed in the affected jurisdictions. Today, all states have ratified EMAC.

The entire EMAC document is approximately 50 pages in length.

Copies of this Act may be obtained from:

NATIONAL CONFERENCE OF COMMISSIONERS
ON UNIFORM STATE LAWS
211 E. Ontario Street, Suite 1300
Chicago, Illinois 60611
www.nccusl.org

CHAPTER 19

# Decontamination Team/Protocol

• • •

**Robert J. Muller**

EACH HOSPITAL SHOULD HAVE SOME type of decontamination plan in association with their community they serve and the risks and hazards of their particular service area. Each hospital does not need to have a full decontamination set up and team BUT should have some sort of Decon plan no matter how small their risks and vulnerability.

In many small communities with volunteer fire departments the hospital may be the primary Decon facility; whereas in other communities with larger departments and full professional training the primary role for Decon will be at the scene rather than the hospital. In this case the hospital may have total confidence on the primary Decon process or may desire to have a secondary Decon protocol.

In any event, mitigation and planning for this scenario should generate some type of protocol appropriate for the situations that may present themselves.

Unless there are well trained personnel, level 3 suits should be sufficient for hospital decontamination. Personnel should be trained as well as drilled on a regular basis in the use of suits as well as the techniques of decontamination. If this is not feasible due to any reason, then this job should be turned over to another group within the public service or military community.

**Improper training and lack of exercising can lead to breaches resulting in the safety of hospital personnel.**

The hospital also should have an adequate budget to provide for the necessary equipment as well as maintenance of the equipment. This can be expensive on an annual basis, but necessary to maintain competence and safety.

Members chosen from hospital personnel for a Decon team should not include any professionals (M.D., R.N., Respiratory, etc.) as these people will be needed for triage and treatment; the use of ancillary personnel best serves this function. A good section to recruit from would be engineering, business office personnel, housekeeping and food services. These people may likewise enjoy being part of a somewhat "clinical" experience that is beyond their normal routines.

CHAPTER 20

# Disaster Code Standardization

• • •

**Robert J. Muller**

Hospital disaster codes should be standardized according to some form of pre agreed protocol with local, county and if possible state hospital agencies.

Today, with nursing pools being available, nurses may rotate to several different hospitals in a single month. Code standardization makes sense so there is uniformity which avoids any confusion when codes may be called.

Also there are large hospital groups which may share staff on a regular basis and particularly in an emergency situation and may have codes which vary from hospital to hospital.

We see a few codes as being universally acceptable such as code blue, red and code pink but other codes have various meanings depending on the locale: code white, code black, etc.

All codes should have a universally recognized meaning and this can be easily accomplished by mutual agreements and may someday be a Joint Commission standard.

## Code Recommendations:

CODE BLUE - Medical Emergency – Cardiac/Respiratory Arrest

| | | |
|---|---|---|
| CODE RED | - | Fire |
| CODE GREY | - | Severe Weather |
| CODE BLACK | - | Bomb threat |
| CODE PINK | - | Infant/Child Abduction |
| CODE YELLOW | - | Disaster – Mass Casualty |
| CODE ORANGE | - | Hazardous Materials |
| CODE WHITE | - | Security Alert – Violence/Hostage |
| CODE SILVER | - | Active Shooter |

Note that while the above main colors remain constant, there is flexibility built into the system for individual hospital needs. Emergency code colors not stated may be used by individual organizations to address specific facility or geographic concerns. The goal is to have a common set of base colors and for hospitals to customize them to meet their needs albeit a response to these events is very similar hospital to hospital.

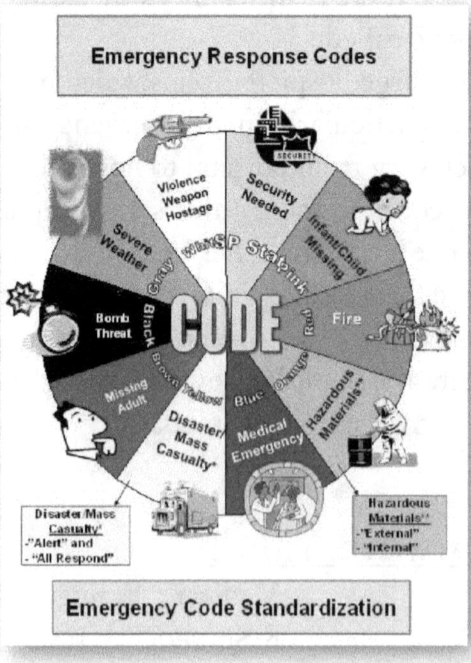

CHAPTER 21

# Evacuation

● ● ●

**Robert J. Muller**

NOW THE TIME IS HERE to make a decision, stay in place or evacuate the facility?

When the situation becomes such that a decision has to be made to evacuate the facility then where do we go from here? What does it take to evacuate a facility? How many patients --- adults, ICU, OB, children and neonates do we have in house to evacuate? Where and how do we begin to evacuate them-these are the questions that have to be answered and should be answered in advance of a critical situation.

The number of patients should have been reduced by decompression so the remaining patients are those that definitely cannot be discharged to home or for family to independently take the responsibility for their safe evacuation.

How do we begin to evacuate 50 or say 100 patients of all different types of acuity? Finding 50 or more local ambulances may prove to be an impossible task, so we must plan and think out of the box.

Ambulance transportation contracts must be formulated with numerous providers depending on the possible anticipated census that may be in-house at the time of an impending and somewhat anticipated disaster, such as a hurricane. But then, what about a tornado that provides no warning or an earthquake or flood from a breach or overtopping of river banks.

Look NOW for providers and services for several hundred miles circumferentially where ambulance can be brought in to aid in facility evacuation as it is likely the local providers will be inundated with requests for service on an acute basis as well as a transfer basis from other facilities as well.

Think about the use of busses: large tour carriers, school busses within the community, assisted living commuter buses, etc. Consider also the off route use of busses from the local transit company. The problem that you will have is usually not the bus but obtaining the services of a sufficient number of bus drivers. Remember they have families likewise and will also want to evacuate.

Think about vans from whatever source you may be able to make an agreement for utilization in an emergency situation; Auto dealerships, company employee transport vans, and any and all other that you may start to seek out in advance and form contractual agreements for their utilization and service. Think about staff, gas, insurance and damages just to name a few of the item that need to be addressed in agreements.

The last resort is to make some agreement with the local or state military organizations, such as the national guard, and, while they will be more than busy with other tasks, if they know in advance that this will be one of their assignments, they likewise will start to pre-plan to assist in hospital evacuation.

They usually are part of the state plan for air-vac evacuation of patients and neonate transport in some areas, such as the coastlines and the Florida Keys, etc.

When an evacuation is determined by the administrative staff in conjunction with local officials then the state department of health and hospitals needs to be notified and a cursory plan sent to them so that they are aware that the hospital will be evacuated and closed for the duration of the event and where the patients will be transported.

It is likewise essential that the facility have agreements in place with several local hospitals in case a local evacuation may be needed due to an internal disaster such as a fire, as well as several distant facilities that are in opposite directions from the threat and not lateral to the threat so as to achieve a "one time only" evacuation. Hence a hospital on the coast of Mississippi should not evacuate to a facility on the coast of Louisiana but should have arrangement with facilities to their North that will be out of harm's way for the threat or the threat will be greatly diminished when it gets to that location. Usually the recommended area would be 30 miles or greater as a minimum to begin to plan for evacuation as well as being at a higher elevation and decreased threat level. Therefore the evacuation of a hospital in Key West to a facility in Marathon, Florida, while is greater than 30 miles to the North, the threat level remains the same and thus evacuation has to be planned further to central or Northern Florida, etc.

Arrangement for the evacuation of neonates and ICU patients requires a facility that has the same services to offer and not only must have the physical space, but likewise must be prepared for up-staffing.

In the contractual agreement for transfer, it must also be addresses who will provide the increased staffing as well as all the cost factors associated with the transfer.

If the sending facility agrees to send staffing with the patients, then new problems and cost may be encountered with the food and lodging for the staff as well as the point of credentialing of the professional level personnel.

ALL of these factors MUST be taken into consideration in ADVANCE and planned for before the situation presents itself on an emergent basis and with critical decision making necessitated without fore-thought.

IF a hospital facility and staff are inadequate or unable to provide for all the necessary needs of their patients then a decision to evacuate must be made. One hospital in New Orleans following Hurricane Katrina was flooded and had no electrical power to sustain hospital operations including air conditioning in August. The ambient temperature of the facility rose to 100 degrees and THEN a decision was made to evacuate the remaining critical and very elderly patients in the worst possible conditions------needless to say many died in the transfer attempt as well as the hospital being tied up in litigations for next eight years for failure to plan and provide. No matter how well prepared in advance, it is likely there will be some patient attrition but the numbers will probably be much lower based on proper planning.

Also the proper pre-planning can be a significant factor in the determination and defense in litigation that may arise from numerous reasons within the facility from staff stating they were not advised they would be sent to another facility to patient deaths. Again---always play the devil's advocate in planning and it is not IF an event will happen but what to do WHEN it happens.

CHAPTER 22

# Hospital Cyber Security

● ● ●

**Willard Hatcher**

A HOSPITALS PRIMARY FOCUS IS, understandably, on patient treatment and care, perhaps an overlooked aspect in the preparation of a hospital complex is the vulnerabilities of its Electronic Medical Record (EMR) system and the supporting medical data systems. The recent rapid deployment of EMR systems across the nation in order claim federal grant funding has led to increased reliance and vulnerabilities of critical health care systems. The federal grant monies were rewarded for implementation of systems and not necessarily the security or hardening of the systems.

These EMR systems replaced reliable paper and film systems with vulnerable digital systems, which if not properly implemented, can crash when needed most during a crisis. Also, an EMR system exposes health care institutions to increased data breach risk. In this chapter we are going to illustrate the risks of EMR systems and related digital medical care systems as well as some tried and true solutions.

## Financial Incentive To Rush Into Emr And Phi Data Breach Risk

On February 17, 2009, President Barack Obama signed the American Recovery and Reinvestment Act (ARRA). Title XIII of ARRA, called the Health Information Technology for Economic and Clinical Health Act (HITECH), allocated $19.2 Billion toward the development of healthcare IT (Information Technology). This act seeks to bolster health IT to improve the delivery of healthcare in the U.S. by incentivizing the implementation of EHRs and meaningful use of them. With various provisions and regulations, the Act provides assistance, tools, and resources to providers to allow for implementation and utilization of electronic health records.

The Medicare and Medicaid EHR Incentive Programs provide financial incentives for the "meaningful use" of certified EHR technology. To receive an EHR incentive payment, providers have to show that they are "meaningfully using" their certified EHR technology by meeting certain measurement thresholds that range from recording patient information as structured data to exchanging summary care records. The US Department of Health and Human Services (HHS) has established these thresholds for eligible professionals, eligible hospitals, and critical access hospitals (CAHs).

The Medicare and Medicaid EHR Incentive Programs include three stages with increasing requirements for participation. All providers begin participating by meeting the Stage 1 requirements for a 90-day period in their first year of meaningful use and a full year in their second year of meaningful use. After meeting the Stage 1 requirements, providers will then have to meet Stage 2 requirements for two full years. Eligible professionals participate in the program on the calendar years, while eligible hospitals and CAHs participate according to the Federal fiscal year.

Many providers implemented EHR systems to meet these standards and receive thousands (small providers) and millions of grant dollars. For some this was an economic decision and not a service decision. Many of these providers did not in turn increase their IT (Information Technology) staffing or IT security systems to properly administer or secure these systems.

This movement of patient identity and medical data from paper file records to a stored digital record has led to a bonanza of PII (Personal Identifiable Information) and PHI (Protected Health Information) more vulnerable to theft than traditional financial institution systems. These systems many times have not budgeted to include professional level of IT security staff, security systems nor security or risk assessments.

Further exasperating this risk are the regulations requiring EHRs to be shared across state health exchange networks. These underfunded/under staffed IT professionals are being asked to store PII/PHI records while making them readily available to local medical staff as well as making them available to other regional providers. At the same time these woeful IT professionals are being asked to make this data readily available to payers (government-insurance companies) while maintaining the data privacy from skilled organized crime hackers.

After rewarding handsomely with federal dollars the implementation of EHRs, HHS is following up with audits of recipients of these dollars for proper security threatening to fine those institutions that have not properly implemented HIPAA (Health Insurance Portability and Accountability Act) and HITECH security standards. These audits intend to punish those who have not properly implemented EHR to the federal standards. These same audits and fines hopes to incentivize the implementation of proper IT security standards.

EMR records are increasingly being targeted by sophisticated organized Cyber-criminal enterprises. The FBI issued a rare PIN (Private Industry Notification) #140408-009 in April of 2014 warning the health care industry "Cyber actors will likely increase cyber intrusions against health care systems..." The highly regarded non-profit IT security group, SANS, issued a report in February of 2014 indicating health care security strategies and practices are poorly protected and ill-equipped to handle new cyber threats exposing patient medical records. SANS stated its real world analysis of Cyber activities indicated that multiple devices (e.g. radiology imaging software, digital video systems, faxes, printers) and security application systems (e.g. VPNs, Firewalls and Routers) of health care institutions were found to be compromised.

According to the Ponemon Institute report of March 2013, sixty-three percent of the health care organizations surveyed reported a data breach in the past two years with an average monetary loss of $2.4 million per data breach. Forty five percent of these organizations had not implemented proper security measures to protect PHI.

Global data security experts, Crowdstrike, in 2014 reported that there were around fifty core active Cybercriminal groups. Some of these groups included Russian and Chinese threat actors. Information Week magazine reported in 2013 that on the black market PII records were worth anywhere from ten to twenty-eight dollars per record, yet when coupled with PHI records the value jumped to fifty dollars.

A scary trend is recent Eastern European CryptoWall or CryptoLocker Cyber ransom virus attacks have rendered some health care organizations temporarily inoperable. These recent viruses infect an employee's laptop or workstation through Phishing Email solicitation or drive by web surfing of malicious site where it loads its malicious software. This software systematically starts going through computer drives alphabetically (a, b, c,) and encrypts all data files with some sophisticated encryption algorithm that is nearly impossible to break. If a hospital machine is on a network with shared network drives, then those network drives get encrypted as well which can make EMR records inaccessible. The virus leaves a ransom note with instructions where to wire the money in order to get the decryption key to release the data. It is about a fifty-fifty chance that the criminals will give a proper key when paid.

Normally the only recovery from a Crypto-Ransom attack is to wipe the drive of infected machines and restore drives from backup copies. Of course this at least temporarily makes systems unavailable and can result in lost PHI. The bottom line is HIPAA compliance does not equal security.

Another significant risk is the risk of HHS fines for not meeting HIPAA/HITECH security standards and the risk of PHI being compromised during a data breach. HHS requires reporting of PHI data breaches and makes public those over 500 records. Typically HHS fines an institution up to $1,500 per PHI record exposed during a breach or unauthorized release. There is also the loss of reputation risk when a PHI data breach is made public and the cost can be higher than the fines. In order to help avoid some of these audit and penalty risk I would recommend the following actions at a minimum:

1. Use Strong Passwords and Change them regularly – Passwords should be at least eight characters in length and include at least one special character or number or capital letter. These passwords should be changed at least every ninety days.
2. Install and Maintain Anti-Virus Software – Anti-Virus software needs to be installed on every computer and kept up to date.
3. Use a Firewall – Install a network hardware firewall that can filter in and out bound digital traffic. This firewall should be configured to block all traffic and opened up only to the absolute minimum EHR and other medical traffic absolutely necessary.
4. Control Access to PHI Data and Systems – Require username and passwords to all EHR/PHI systems including medical

devices such as EKG and Imaging machines. Require a time out screen saver that locks and requires re-authentication.

5. Control Physical Access – Have adequate physical security to all PHI/EMR devices and supporting network equipment, especially, portable devices like laptops, USB media, Ipads, etc. Use cable locks when necessary. Be also aware of dangers of fire, water, HVAC and sprinkler systems to electronic systems. These systems tend not to fare well in damp or hot environments. Don't forget the network switches stored in the communications closets.
6. Limit Network Access – Peer to peer networking tools like Google Drive, Dropbox and Skydrive are appealing to workers yet open PHI/EMR networks open to remote unauthorized access. Have policies and training forbidding staff to loading such software or using it at work.
7. Prepare and Plan for Disasters – Fire, flood, hurricanes, tornados, pipe/roof leaks, black outs, power surges, backhoes, etc. can cripple a PHI/EMR network. Have a plan to operate for at least 48 hours without outside utilities or resupply or shift change. Have a plan to operate offsite and/or off of backup systems. Backup tapes, UPS, HVAC and generator power systems are a minimum. Don't forget to secure these backup systems as well.
8. Good IT Security Habits - Medical workers are familiar with healthy habits like hand washing. The same culture or awareness needs to be implemented for IT security. Have a standard secure configuration for workstations that does not allow unessential applications like games, messaging clients, etc. Find out if EHR/Medical vendors maintain an open back door connection for maintenance, if so, then it must be blocked at the Firewall and only opened

when necessary. Disable remote file sharing, remote desktop access (RDP, PC Anywhere, etc.) except to system administrators.

9. Protect Mobile Devices – If access via IPad or Smartphone or other mobile devices is required then have a standard configuration requirement (pin code, screen lock, etc.) and secure with a mobile device security application.
10. Promote an IT Security Culture - Conduct employee "awareness" (not training to educate about IT security) threats such as Phishing Emails and remote data programs like BitTorrent, Google, Yahoo, Dropbox, etc. The weakest link in any computer system is the user.

## Controls Tend To Be Bypassed During A Crisis

A natural disaster (Hurricane, Tornado, Earthquake, Wild Fire, or other utility/personnel disruption) can cause the few existing Cyber controls to be turned off or bypassed in order to maintain access to EMRs. Being the primary mission of providers is to provide care, when a conflict between controlled access to EMR and the providing care occurs, the providing of care wins.

For example, a power outage or surge can cause many electronic systems default to open to allow access (doors, Firewalls, etc.). The default to close could lock out users. So an attacker may cause an outage to gain access to a network or building.

Backup IT systems tend to be configured without IT security due to budget constraints. Many of these backup systems will not be updated or patched or are the latest release, thus vulnerable to outside attack and/or may not be compatible with the current EMR/PHI systems.

Many of the backup systems do not have Anti-Virus or protected by a Firewall or have up to date access controls (usernames/passwords) due to duplicate cost of implementation. Thus, during a crisis, an intruder or employee may have unfettered access to EMR/PHI records and/or data.

Many times these backup systems are running in an offsite with the proper security architecture. Thus, even in normal times these systems are vulnerable to attack 24/7.

The somewhat expensive but necessary solution to this problem is to properly maintain backup IT systems with duplicate systems. This risk verses cost benefit analysis needs to be conducted via a BIA (Business Impact Analysis) that can highlight the most critical systems. The BIA will **be utilized to build a proper disaster recovery plan.**

## Reliance Of Emrs Makes Staffs Vulnerable A Crisis

The resulting over reliance of EMRs makes staffs vulnerable to diversion due to system unavailability resulting from natural and manmade disasters (power spikes, Cyber attacks, etc.). Now that health care systems have gone electronic and everyday new healthcare workers only know these electronic systems, what happens when these systems fail? How is patient care going to be delivered?

Some EMR systems, like Epic, have system plans to operate in standalone mode when network connectivity to the servers is not possible. These systems allow for local input and caching of EMR data to be loaded and correlated later when the master EMR server becomes available.

Yet many EMR systems do not have this standalone connectivity. For example, one small hospital in a rural area in 2014 suffered a power spike and brown out one hot summer day. This power surge reset all the network switches on the floors to default settings due to the fact the communications closets on each floor did not have UPS (battery) backup to protect the local switches. Therefore, the entire hospital computer network was down for the entire day till administrators could get back in and reconfigure the network settings. Since the workers were using an EMR system that no longer operated, the hospital had to go on diversion the entire day sending patients out of town.

Sometimes your disaster can be your own doing. A larger hospital had to close one day due to fact a plumber was working on pressure pipe system when it broke and started flooding from an upper floor. Normally this would shut a hospital down but the flooding was pouring down the vertical shaft of the electrical/communications closets of the hospital, thus knocking out the IT and telephone switching equipment for most of the hospital.

One major hospital IT department in a notorious hurricane zone had thought of everything. They had backup systems with weeks' worth of backup generators and fuel, hardened concrete building on upper floor data center so impervious from wind/rain/flooding, they had food, water and shelter for personnel and yet after about 24 hours of a category four hurricane they had to shut down. Why? The local city water supply had cut off due to pipe breaks. How does this affect a data center? The HVAC chillers relied on a clean water supply to operate so once the water pressure went down so did the air conditioning and being August in the south the temperatures of the data center quickly rose to intolerable temperatures.

## What Can We Do To Mitigate These Risks

As you may know there are ways to address risk: Mitigate, Accept or Insure, but one cannot not eliminate risk. To address the above enumerated risk I would recommend a health care institution undertake a full risk assessment looking at the IT/EMR/PHI/PCI (Payment Card Industry), physical, environmental and regulatory risk. Then conduct a BIA to classify those systems and processes that are most essential to the institution. Follow that up with a comprehensive DR plan managed by a full time DR or emergency manager who can update and exercise the DR plan.

CHAPTER 23

# Hospital and Medical Facilities as Soft Targets

● ● ●

Robert J. Muller

HOSPITALS AND HEALTHCARE FACILITIES ARE prone to being soft targets to terrorist groups or lone individuals with a personal or political agenda.

These facilities focus on healthcare for the sick and injured as well as preventable maintenance programs for patient wellness. This is their **main** focus --- not tight security--- as that is a low priority in providing patient care.

As a result, there are many areas of vulnerability in hospitals, clinics, laboratories, surgery centers and attaches as well as free-standing office complexes --- all that meet the full definition of a soft target.

Some areas of vulnerability to evaluate can be done by playing the "What If" scenario for discussion to harden out the thought process.

The physical plant of most facilities offers a point of major vulnerability in that there is no real security areas and those that are protected can be easily penetrated by anyone who may have some serious intensions on disruption, distraction or destruction.

A good example for starters is facility entrances. There are usually many --- other than those common ones for patient and visitor admittance.

Many times a soft area is the loading dock where items are received on a daily continuous basis, and people have access into the facility and go virtually unnoticed. These include delivery people, UPS, Fed Ex and the like, and if not included in this group, then all it would take are a few hours of observation from a distant point in real time or by recording, as to what the protocol may be for access via this portal of entry.

How many entrances are there into the facility? Where do they enter into and what access do they provide once inside the facility? What if I gained easy access into a facility that allowed me to get into the men's or women's locker room and access to uniforms or ID cards that maybe in that room What if there is a stack of scrub suits and lab coats on hangers from others who have changed and have identification of these coats with a name or designation? Where could I go if I donned one of these coats or scrub suits --- what access would that allow me to other areas of the facility such as electrical panels, generators, air handlers, duct work, laboratory, medical supplied or general stores only to name a few.

What if I had access to the restrooms and changed out the air fresheners to aerosolized containers with virus particles or chemical vapors to sicken the staff over a period of time?

What if I had access to the sewer system that could be blocked and cause a backup within the facility as a diversionary measure? What if I brought in timed explosives and dirty bombs in packages on the loading dock allowing time for them to filter though the normal supply chain lines?

What if I was able to get to the food supply and contaminate it, resulting in distribution to facility personnel and patients?

The normal daily flow of patients and personnel thru the hospital make it very difficult if not impossible to provide complete security unless very sophisticated systems would be put in place at great initial expense plus continuous monitoring and maintenance expenses. In addition, this would also hinder patient flow and cause serious delays within the system resulting in internal as well as external patient anarchy.

A current flow in a normal day in medical facilities sees hospital personnel, patients, visitors, law enforcement and fire personnel and sales and service representatives from all areas and walks of life. Anyone of these would be very easy to impersonate with little to no effort, and to gain further facility access virtually undetected, especially within the larger and more vulnerable facilities.

All staff hospital personnel should have some form of a **picture identification card**, including administrative staff, physicians and board members; frequent hospital contractors may likewise be given a different color ID with or without a picture but redeemable upon demand as well as a predetermined expiration date. After the expiration date on ID cards, a different color card should be used. The "RepTrack" type system may also be effectively utilized if in place within the hospital that can be used to track business representatives and contractors.

If it is not hospital policy for ID cards to be returned upon completion or termination of employment, then a 6 month revalidation process must take place. This can easily be done by placing a validation sticker on the front of the ID card with a different color (that can be easily recognized from a distance of 6-10 feet) with an expiration date printed on it. This keeps all ID cards current without the expense of remaking new ID cards for all employees.

The use of some form of **uniforms** is extremely important to the security of a hospital, no matter what size the hospital, they allow easy identification of personnel from a patient perspective, as well as other employees in larger facilities. But they must be protected and treated as an important item that by its very nature allows a certain security clearance.

Today scrub suits are readily purchased in every type of store from uniform stores to grocery stores, and this allows unlimited access to the general public.

Today many hospitals allow the wearing of scrub suits from their nursing staff to their janitorial staff. Unless some form of parameter is set up within the hospital, this can be a serious breach of security and safety for the hospital as well as the patient.

Security may be established with types of uniforms required of certain department personnel, like engineering, housekeeping, janitorial, etc.; while professional staffing may wear the traditional white nursing apparel or if scrub suits are permitted for these people, then a color should be established. This may be based on departments, i.e. nurses-white, physical therapist-blue, and respiratory therapist-green, laboratory-black, etc. Likewise, colors may be differentiated by floors or units, such as nurses in different color pants and shirts, i.e. ICU white pants, blue tops; OB pink, etc.

During times of high level security this uniformity can be a great help in identifying potential breaches within the hospital system, and is an easy as well as a very cost effective system to implement.

If a person is wearing a white top and red pants that is assigned to a coronary care unit is seen in the physical plant area then a red flag maybe raised as a possible breech of security for the area and should be reported and investigated.

Also a floor that houses critical or technical equipment such as the computer server should have special security access to that area such as double doors, scan ID access either fingerprint or eye retinal scan, or access by a coded elevator with special key access, etc.; not to mention once again special uniforms that identify employees of that floor.

Visitor wrist banding works very well is efficient, easily recognizable and cost efficient.

One color may be utilized or multiple colors to signify different areas for security purposes. For example a patient may be banded at the security check point with a blue wrist band to indicate they are going for a radiology procedure. If they are seen wondering around the third floor patient area by a staff member or security person, then they immediately know this person should not be in that area.

Hospital access is of the utmost importance and depending on the locale and physical setup, pre-determined access routes could be determined and marked by property signage for the general public, employees and emergencies presenting to the hospital.

A vulnerability analysis of the facilities' water supply should be conducted and a plan formulated to maintain continuity in any way that is feasible to achieve this goal.

The hospital facility **water supply** should be assessed as to the possibility for loss of continuity due to any means of disruption. This may be in the form of loss of a main pump, pipeline disruption due to explosion, earthquake, or flooding of the primary service electrical supply.

Alternatives must be identified to sustain the facility ---from hours to days due to the loss; this includes having an alternate water supply, a stored water supply in tanks, bottles, bladders, tank trucks or the ability to manufacturer or purifies water from a local stream, river or lake. The use of commercial purification systems that are uniformly available may solve the emergent need of a facility and may be contracted through various vendors.

The loss of facility water supply, electrical and or communications can result in internal disastrous consequences.

Alternate water sources, or the main water supply system that has possibly been damaged and comes back on line, **should be tested** in the laboratory, and this should be anticipated in advance as most hospital laboratories are not prepared for water testing.

**Fire Systems** should be analyzed as to vulnerability as false alarms as well as water shedding from sprinklers could cause a very significant diversion and distraction.

**Roof top access** should be limited as this likewise can provide a possible target to air handlers and vent systems as well a communication lines and radio antennas and elevator/lift equipment.

**Parking Lots and Garages** --- those facilities that have parking in lots and/or garage facilities should have some form of security in terms of either manned security or automated gated security to both enter and exit the facility.

Entry points into the hospital or clinic facilities should have some form of planned security with special cards or tokens and should be monitored by surveillance cameras, to prevent unauthorized or undetected entry.

## Computer Systems

Today, since the advent of computerization, multiple hospital systems from air conditioning to patient records are on some type of computer platform. Most of these go through some type of central server and or stored in clouds; many may be on an individual computer network or individual system without networking.

In order to help avoid hacking into these systems remember the following points:

Use Strong Passwords and Change Them Regularly – Passwords should be at least eight characters in length and include at least one special character or number or capital letter. These passwords should be changed at least every ninety days.

Install and Maintain Anti-Virus Software – Anti-Virus software needs to be installed on every computer and kept up to date.

Use a Firewall – Install a network hardware firewall that can filter in and out bound digital traffic. This firewall should be configured to block all traffic and opened up only to the absolute minimum and other medical traffic absolutely necessary.

Control Access to Data and Systems – Require username and passwords to all systems including medical devices such as EKG and Imaging machines. Require a time out screen saver that locks and requires re-authentication.

Control Physical Access – Have adequate physical security to all devices and supporting network equipment, especially, portable devices like laptops, USB media, IPad, etc. Use cable locks when necessary. Be also aware of dangers of fire, water, HVAC and sprinkler systems to electronic systems.

Limit Network Access – Peer to peer networking tools like Google Drive, Dropbox and Skydrive are appealing to workers yet open networks unauthorized access. Have policies and training forbidding staff to loading such software or using it at work.

**Prepare and Plan For Disasters** – Fire, flood, hurricanes, tornados, pipe/roof leaks, black outs, power surges, backhoes, etc. can cripple a network. Have a plan to operate for at least 48 hours without outside utilities or resupply or shift change. Have a plan to operate offsite and/or off of backup systems. Backup tapes, UPS, HVAC and generator power systems are a minimum. Don't forget to secure these backup systems as well.

**Good IT Security Habits** - Medical workers are familiar with healthy habits like hand washing. The same culture or awareness needs to be implemented for IT security. Have a standard secure configuration for workstations that does not allow unessential applications like games, messaging clients, etc. Find out if vendors maintain an open back door connection for maintenance, if so, then it must be blocked at the Firewall and only opened when necessary. Disable remote file sharing, remote desktop access except to system administrators.

**Protect Mobile Devices** – If access via IPad or Smartphone or other mobile devices is required then have a standard configuration requirement (pin code, screen lock, etc.) and secure with a mobile device security application.

**Promote an IT Security Culture** - Conduct employee "awareness" not training to educate about IT security threats such as Phishing Emails and remote data programs like BitTorrent, Google, Yahoo, Dropbox, etc. The weakest link in any computer system is the user not to mention even worse --- the hacker.

There are so many ways of using hospitals and medical facilities as soft target due to the numerous reasons previously elaborated, and many that I have not touched upon. In order to case harden medical facilities this would mean to restrict and limit access or delay access to those that maybe in dire emergency need for medical care.

There would be ways of personal altruistic attacks within medical facilities from explosives to viral and bacterial releases that could be devastating in both a short term and long term scenarios or at the very least cause havoc and another means of possible distraction for something far reaching taking place.

The day may come, as it is now with critical triage at accident scenes, that potential patients may have to be screened before entry into a facility, i.e. scanners or the like and outpatient visits limited to certain facilities away from a main structure, and visitors going through a screening process much like that within the current airline industry.

There is **NO perfect system** and all security systems have their flaws as we have seen by various instances in the past, BUT the day may come when what we know of today is no longer, and we enter into a new generation of life which we have been totally unaccustomed in seeking and receiving medical care.

CHAPTER 24

# Federal Grants

• • •

**Robert J. Muller**

Hospitals are eligible for federal grant funding, depending on the type of grant, and the eligibility requirements of the grant.

Grants may be individually applied for in the name of the institution, or generally disbursed through a central grant application for various facilities. States may receive grant funds and then disburse the funds to various hospitals based on needs or various formulas they may choose.

The **MOST** important fact to remember about applications for federal grants is that they MUST be very specific and if the grant is received the funding must be spent EXACTLY on what was specified in the original grant application; thus if a laptop computer was specified in a federal grant, then a desktop cannot later be the item that is purchased; if a Nikon digital camera Model XY was specified, then a Cannon model ZX cannot be later purchased.

All items purchased with federal grants should be kept in a separate inventory listing, individually labeled and MUST be stored on site at the facility and not be stored at an offsite location, or loaned out to other facilities or locations of the same facility. Remember --- the grant must be followed according to the letter of the grant as far as specificity and location of the grant application. If an item is to be used in a roaming manner, this must be specified at the time of the grant application; Following these simple rules will keep you out of trouble with the feds when there is a facility audit.

A suggestion: if applying for a federal grant, train or employ someone with experience at writing grants; while not difficult, they can be tricky and very technical. Small mistakes can make the difference of whether a grant request is approved or rejected.

CHAPTER 25

# Releasing Protected Health Information

• • •

**Kenneth Rhea**

## A Short History

On Wednesday, August 21, 1996, President Clinton signed into law and Act that was to have a massive impact on health care in the US and in particular the privacy and security of individually identifiable health information. The Act was extensive and required in part that the Secretary of Health and Human Services (HHS) proposes standards for the protection of health information by health care providers throughout the US. The Act was named the "Health Information Portability and Accountability Act of 1996" better known by the acronym "HIPAA".

The first of several rules was known as the "Privacy Rule" published in the Federal Register Thursday, December 28, 2000. In general terms the Privacy Rule introduced standards to "... address the use and disclosure of individuals' health information..." The intent was to "...assure that individuals' health information is properly protected while allowing the flow of health information needed to provide and promote high quality health care and to protect the public's health and well-being." The Rule was modified August 14, 2002 with a date of compliance required by April 14, 2003. This Rule set the standards for protections of health information that was individually identifiable related to "covered entities" such as health plans, health care clearinghouses, and health care providers. The individually identifiable health information becomes "protected health information" according to the Rule when it is (i) Transmitted by electronic media; (ii) Maintained in electronic media; or (iii) Transmitted or maintained in any other form or medium. There were more rules to come.

A second Rule was published February 20, 2003 known as the "Security Rule". This Rule primarily protected the "...confidentiality, integrity, and availability..." of electronic protected health information (ePHI). Compliance with the Security Rule was required by April 20, 2005 for most health care providers.

A third related regulation was a part of the American Recovery and Reinvestment Act of 2009 and was actually a separate Act known as "The Health Information Technology for Economic and Clinical Health Act" better known as the "HITECH" Act. This Act became law February 18, 2009 with the stated intent to "...promote the adoption and meaningful use of health information technology" The Subtitle D of this Act specifically increased civil and criminal enforcement of HIPAA Rules related to electronic health information. Section 13410(d) revised section 1176(a) of the Social Security Act and established four (4) classes of violations with four (4) corresponding levels of penalty for each violation. It also set the maximum penalties for violations of identical provisions.

Some of these rules were enacted as "interim" rules which became final on January 13, 2013 which corresponded to the publication of most recent Rule on Friday, January 25, 2013 in the Federal Register. This Rule with a compliance date of September 23, 2013, included significant modifications to parts of earlier rules, in other cases adoption of interim rules already in place, and some new additions. This new Rule had a long name:

> *"Modifications to the HIPAA Privacy, Security, Enforcement, and Breach Notification Rules Under the Health Information Technology for Economic and Clinical Health Act and the Genetic Information Nondiscrimination Act; Other Modifications to the HIPAA Rules"*

It is known with the shorter name of the Omnibus Final Rule (OFR) or Megarule and was in itself composed of four rules one of which was to finalize modifications issued as a proposed rule on July 14, 2010. The stated Rule general purpose was to "...make certain other modifications to the HIPAA Privacy, Security, Breach Notification, and Enforcement Rules (the HIPAA Rules), to improve their workability and effectiveness, and to increase flexibility for and decrease burden on the regulated entities." While the intent is usually acknowledged there has been considerable discussion on how much the "burden" to medical institutions, physicians, and other health care providers has actually been decreased.

## Privacy and a Public Health Event

Since the dates for covered entity (CE) compliance with the various rules, i.e. compliance by medical institutions, physicians, and other health care providers, the Office for Civil Rights (OCR) has had "...responsibility for implementing and enforcing..." the HIPAA regulations. This enforcement which has increased through 2014 has had the effect of emphasizing the need for regulatory compliance by health care providers.

However, in the fall of 2014 an event occurred on Saturday, August 2, 2014 which brought into prominent public concern the relation of HIPAA regulations and handling of protected health information.

The following news report from Fox News and the AP appeared August 1, 2014:

> *"Plans are underway to bring back the two American aid workers sick with Ebola from Africa. A small private jet based in Atlanta has been dispatched to Liberia where the two Americans work for missionary groups. At least one of the Americans is expected to be treated in the U.S. at Atlanta's Emory University Hospital, which has a special isolation unit.* ***The hospital declined to identify the patient, citing privacy laws.*** *The private jet can only accommodate one patient at a time. In a press conference Friday afternoon, Emory's Dr. Bruce Ribner, said the facility had been informed that two patients were coming to the facility; one in a few days, the next a few days after that.."* [Edited with highlight]

It was assumed that the "privacy laws" referenced were the HIPAA regulations related to the privacy and security of individually identifiable health information that was protected health information (PHI). Clearly the decision to refuse identification was made, but was such a decision actually required?

Since the two missionary physicians were treated we have also seen the first diagnosis of Ebola infection in the US at Texas Health Presbyterian Hospital, Dallas, Texas on September 26, 2014. Thomas Eric Duncan, a Liberian man who traveled from Monrovia to Dallas was evaluated at the hospital on September 24, 2014, was released, and was later readmitted with eventual death October 8, 2014. On October 12, 2014 it was announced that a hospital employee working with Mr. Duncan had contracted the first transmitted case of Ebola infection. Once again the hospital elected not to identify the new patient in this situation stating wishes of the family. The patients survived the infection, but the actions and the stance of the hospital and government were widely discussed in the media with extensive commentary and speculation on medical actions taken, i.e. actions of covered entities (CEs) under the HIPAA regulations and the eventual effects of the Ebola virus in the US. Most authorities feel that this threat while not receiving as much media attention in the remainder of 2014 has not by any means ended, e.g. limited control in several African nations with Sierra Leone at the end of 2014 being in a "state of emergency" and declaring a "lockdown" of public activities in an attempt to gain control of the continuing loss of life. Of little comfort was the statement by an individual without medical background or training appointed by President Obama as an "Ebola Czar" who said that "...Americans should expect more domestic cases...".

While the eventual course of this virus in the US is of considerable concern and is unknown there are several things that can be stated with certainty. One is that the HIPAA regulations on the privacy and security of protected health information are in place, regulations have not changed due to the Ebola concerns, and regulations apply to situations of patients having or who are suspected of having Ebola infection as well as other medical conditions. Another is that requests for patient status, types of treatment, and other information involving protected health information (PHI) will frequently be requested by third parties such as relatives and media. The allowed disclosure of protected health information (PHI) under the HIPAA regulations must be understood by every medical institution, physician, or other covered entity (CE) in order to make appropriate decisions for protection of health information and regulation compliance.

## Relevant Regulations

The action of allowing disclosure of protected health information (PHI) has been addressed since the Privacy Rule which as noted was the first of HIPAA privacy and security regulations with required compliance by April 14, 2003. The most recent modifications and additions to regulations occurring with the Omnibus Final Rule in 2013. Patients have always had a right under these regulations to request their protected health information (PHI) as stated in 45 CFR §164.524 (1) that a right of patient access to PHI maintained in a designated record set exists "… as long as the information is retained in the designated record set..." However there are some exceptions such as whether or not the PHI involves "(i) Psychotherapy notes; (ii) Information compiled in reasonable anticipation of, or for use in, a civil, criminal, or administrative action or proceeding; and (iii) Protected health information maintained by a covered entity" that is subject to the Clinical Laboratory Improvement Amendments 1988 with access prohibited or is exempt from the these amendments. Also access to PHI may be denied to patients in a number of situations of patient request some of which allow review of the decision to deny access and some which do not. In certain situations use or disclosure of protected health information requires an opportunity for the patient to agree or object, e.g. facility directories, involvement in a person's care, and for notification purposes. However, there are many other situations in which release of protected health information (PHI) may be done without patient permission.

In the Omnibus Final Rule it was stated that the Privacy Rule "… recognizes that covered entities must balance protecting the privacy of health information with sharing health information with those responsible for ensuring public health and safety, and permits covered entities to disclose the minimum necessary protected health information to public health authorities or other designated persons or entities without an authorization for public health purposes specified by the Rule." Release of protected health information (PHI) prominently associated with high profile medical treatment such as possible Ebola virus cases may involve release to third parties either related or unrelated to the patient and in situations where such release has not been requested or authorized by the patient. In respect to patient permission to release information HIPAA regulations specifically allow for the "uses and disclosures for which an authorization or opportunity to agree or object is not required". Stated in another way the physician does not need permission from the patient to use or disclose the protected health information (PHI) in certain situations. These include 1) victims of abuse, neglect, or domestic violence, 2) health oversight activities, 3) judicial and administrative proceedings, 4) release related to decedents, 5) cadaveric donation purposes, 6) research purposes, 7) specialized government functions, and 8) workers' compensation.

Of particular interest are four additional categories which may be particularly relevant to medical care of patients with threatening diseases such as Ebola virus infection. These are 1) law enforcement purposes, 2) uses and disclosures required by law and to the limited extent required by law 3) "use or disclosure to avert a serious threat to health or safety" and 4) "uses and disclosures for public health activities".

In relation to the first two involving law enforcement and disclosures required by law the information may be disclosed, but within limits, i.e. the "...use and disclosure complies with and is limited to the relevant requirements of such law". This may include judicial and administrative proceedings mentioned above and may require "satisfactory assurance". This would include assurance such as written statements and necessary documentation of necessary actions for a "protective order", i.e. "an order of a court or administrative tribunal" or a "stipulation" by the requesting party limiting the use of the PHI and return or destruction of the PHI after the intended use. Release is also possible by the covered entity (CE) if "reasonable efforts" have been made to obtain a qualified protective order. Disclosure for other law enforcement purposes might include those "pursuant to process" such as a court order, a court-ordered warrant, a subpoena, or summons "issued by a judicial officer". Also included are administrative requests, administrative subpoenas, administrative summons, a civil demand, or an "authorized investigative demand." Limited disclosures to law enforcement authorities may also be done for requests involving identification and location of a person, for victims of a crime, decedents, crimes on the premises of the covered entity (CE), and reporting crime in emergencies. In any case the PHI requests cannot be total and must be "relevant and material" to the law enforcement enquiry and be "...specific and limited in scope to the extent reasonably practicable...", e.g. in situations of identification and location purposes the covered entity (CE) may disclose to the requesting law enforcement official only certain information including name and address, date and place of birth, SS number, blood type and Rh factor, type of injury if any, date and time of treatment or death, and a description of "...distinguishing characteristics...". A "law enforcement enquiry" demanding without reason the total medical records of an individual would not be acceptable.

While law enforcement has been and in the future might well be involved in activities related to infectious disease problems such as Ebola infection with a need for understanding of HIPAA regulations by health care providers, the most prominent regulatory areas will be those of public health activities and averting serious threats to health and safety.

Of prominent note is the allowance of use and disclosure of protected health information (PHI) in situations of "...public health surveillance, public health investigations, and public health interventions..." when such activities are for the "...purpose of preventing or controlling disease, injury, or disability, including, but not limited to, the reporting of disease..." to "A public health authority that is authorized by law to collect or receive such information…". These situations, as many others, require appropriate identification of the requesting person, documentation of authorizations, and complete record documentation by the health care provider.

Equally in force, but not as closely related to problems of infectious disease are uses and disclosures of PHI for public health activities "… for the purpose of activities related to the quality, safety or effectiveness…" of "…an FDA regulated product or activity…". This applies if the requesting person is "subject to the jurisdiction of the Food and Drug Administration (FDA) with respect to an FDA-regulated product or activity for which that person has responsibility…." This would include in some situations a medical device company or its identified representative. A covered health care provider, i.e. covered entity (CE) may provide protected health information (PHI) to a medical device company representative if the disclosure is for the provider's own treatment, payment, or health care operation (TPO) purposes. Also PHI may be disclosed to a device company representative without patient consent when the device company is actually a "health care provider" under HIPAA regulations, i.e. "…furnishes, bills, or is paid for "health care" in the normal course of business." The various scenarios can become complicated, but must be closely evaluated by the covered entity (CE) health care provider before the release of PHI.

Also PHI may be released to a "…public health authority or other appropriate government authority authorized by law…" to receive information about child abuse or neglect. A school may also receive PHI under defined criteria.

With considerations of "…applicable law and standards of ethical conduct…" PHI may be released under the second major category of averting a "…serious threat to health or safety…" such as might be the case with Ebola infection. These kinds of PHI releases by a health care provider can be done if the covered entity believes "…in good faith…" that such a release will in his/her best judgment "…lessen a serious and imminent threat to the health or safety of a person or the public;" and that the person to whom the PHI is provided is someone who is "reasonable able to prevent or lessen the threat…"

In other situations relating to violent crime such releases can be made by a covered entity allowing law enforcement to "identify or apprehend" an individual unless the information obtained by the covered entity has been obtained in the course of treatment, counseling, therapy or the request for such. In these situations there is a restriction of the amount of PHI released to only the "statement" by the person about a violent crime. In all of the situations relating to the aversion of a threat to health and safety there is a "presumption of good faith belief" by the covered entity (CE) releasing the protected health information (PHI) meaning that the covered entity (CE) has relied on his/her actual knowledge or the "…credible representation by a person with apparent knowledge or authority."

As these regulations indicate the specific protected health information (PHI) disclosure allowances without patient consent in many instances provide for health care provider medical decisions which will be in the best interest of privacy and security of PHI, but which will also serve the public health and safety. In the earlier situation the hospital was not specifically constrained by the regulations to refuse patient identification. Instead, as shown in the discussion above, the regulations allowed a choice. In the case of the 1st Ebola diagnosis in the US and the later 1st proven transmission of Ebola at the same hospital the decision not to identify was allowable, though PHI could have been released if the health care provider felt that one of the above criteria applied.

In all situations the general prime interest is the best protection of health information consistent with federal law requirements. It is important to understand that in some cases situations of individually identifiable health information are also addressed by state law. In these situations if a provision of federal law is "...contrary to a provision of state law..." federal law preempts state law unless the Secretary of HHS might for several reasons determine otherwise or the state law " ...is more stringent..." The determination of whether some provision is "contrary" is based on whether a "...covered entity or business associate would find it impossible to comply with both the state and federal requirements" or "...The provision of state law stands as an obstacle to the accomplishment and execution of the full purposes and objectives..." of the federal law.

## Summary

The short summary is that in the described situation, as well as many other medical situations, choices in handling of protected health information (PHI) are available to medical institutions, physicians, and other health care providers, but knowledge of what HIPAA regulations and other laws allow is necessary. Every health care professional should therefore be aware of these allowed uses and disclosures not only for the purpose of covered entity (CE) compliance with regulations and avoidance of potential civil or criminal penalties, but for provision of appropriate medical care and assistance with public health. Given regulatory allowances the final institution and physician informed decisions must then be made based on good medical judgment.

## Disclaimer

Information provided by MER Consulting LLC is risk management opinion and should not be construed as legal advice. Legal advice should be obtained from licensed legal representation. No contained information is intended to take the place of either the written law or regulations. Readers are always encouraged to review any specific statutes, regulations, and other interpretive materials for a full and accurate understanding of their contents.

CHAPTER 26

# Financial

• • •

**Robert J. Muller**

It is recommended for follow up and documentation that all paperwork be documented with signatures and the event, date and time, so that they can be easily followed up and retrieved at a later date if necessary. An example would be KATR0829051710RJM—indicating Katrina event on August 29, 2005 at 5:10 P.M. by RJM.

A follow up initial and or signature is imperative especially for purchase orders, requisitions, etc. that have a present, as well as a future financial impact and may be utilized for submission for FEMA reimbursement.

It is imperative that it be conveyed to all the employees the importance of obtaining CASH prior to an planned disaster events as many retail outlets will not be able to accept credit or debit cards due to absence of electricity or computer connections.

The hospital likewise may need to have cash on hand, unless pre agreements have been made within the community for credit should recovery materials and supplies need be purchased.

Cash on hand to supplement or provide payday loans to employees can be a very nice BUT very dangerous as well as a laborious process. If large amount of cash are held on premise, strict confidence must be kept until the last moment when this service is announced to the staff, and significant security must be provided due to the nature of this situation and the vulnerability it presents.

CHAPTER 27

# Hospital Emergency Incident Command System (HEICS)

• • •

**Robert J. Muller**

HEICS IS AN EMERGENCY MANAGEMENT system made up of positions based on an organizational chart. Each position has a specific mission to be address in an emergency situation. Each position represented has an individual checklist designed to direct the assigned individual in disaster operations and recovery tasks. The HEICS plan includes job description forms to enhance this overall system and promote accountability.

The HEICS plan is flexible. Only those positions, or functions, which are needed, should be activated. The HEICS plan allows for the addition of necessitated positions, as well as the deactivation of positions as needed at any time. This equates to promoting efficiency and cost effectiveness. Full activation may take hours or even days. The majority of disasters or emergencies will require the activation of a limited number of positions.

More than one position function may be performed by an individual. Situations of a critical nature may require an individual to perform multiple tasks until additional support personnel can be activated and this can be aided by the use of the position checklists. See appendix.

HEICS is required by Federal Law (Title 29 CFR OSHA 1910.120) for events involving any type of hazardous materials situations and accurate record keeping of the events is a necessity for FEMA reimbursement.

The more complex the event and the longer the duration of an event, the MORE experienced and knowledgeable the personnel should be in the command system and should be trained above the ICS 100 level.

## NIMS

The *National Incident Management System* (NIMS) provides a systematic, proactive approach to guide departments and agencies at all levels of government, nongovernmental organizations, and the private sector to work seamlessly to prevent, protect against, respond to, recover from, and mitigate the effects of incidents, regardless of cause, size, location, or complexity, in order to reduce the loss of life and property and harm to the environment. NIMS self-study course IS 700 is available through the FEMA Emergency Management Institute.

NIMS works hand in hand with the *National Response Framework* (NRF). NIMS provides the template for the management of incidents, while the NRF provides the structure and mechanisms for national-level policy for incident management. The NRF self-study course is IS 800 and is likewise available through the FEMA Emergency Management Institute (see link above).

CHAPTER 28

# The Role of the Hospital Safety Officer

• • •

**Michael J. Fagel**

IN EVERYDAY OPERATIONS, SAFETY & health planning and processes are usually routine operations that we have all become accustomed to in our day to day work.

During a crisis, we may be asked to do different tasks other than our "normal" daily routines.

In this light, we must NOT take safety for granted, and think that it is SOMEONE ELSES JOB.

In fact, safety is OUR responsibility --- to us, our families, our co-workers and our customers, the patients we care for.

During the heightened time of escalating operations, the safety officer is often times disregarded as an important resource during extended or immediate operations. Regardless of the type of incident or event, SAFETY must be paramount.

Each state or territory is covered by Federal OSHA regulations or by equivalent state equal regulations.

Upon notification of an event, the safety officer needs to be engaged quickly with the officials involved in the ongoing operation. The Safety officer's roles should be that of a consultative participant in the decision making of the team leading the response, investigation or the daily work.

Being consultative at the outset will help to set parameters of the EXPECTATIONS of the roles, as well as the proper outcome of the events.

The safety officer needs to also understand that many elements of the standard require testing, selection and fit testing according to the standard. The various states (about 50%) have adopted their own standards that must be as protective as the Federal Standards.

A good program of ensuring safety and health is a continuous process that requires an adequate knowledge of the hazards that the employees may or will likely come into contact.

Procedures may vary, and it always better to have a more comprehensive PPE (personal Protective Equipment) program in place before the event occurs.

Selection of the proper personal protective equipment for various roles should be done BEFORE the events, following established protocols.

The top 5 causes of injuries to hospital workers (From BLS data 2011)

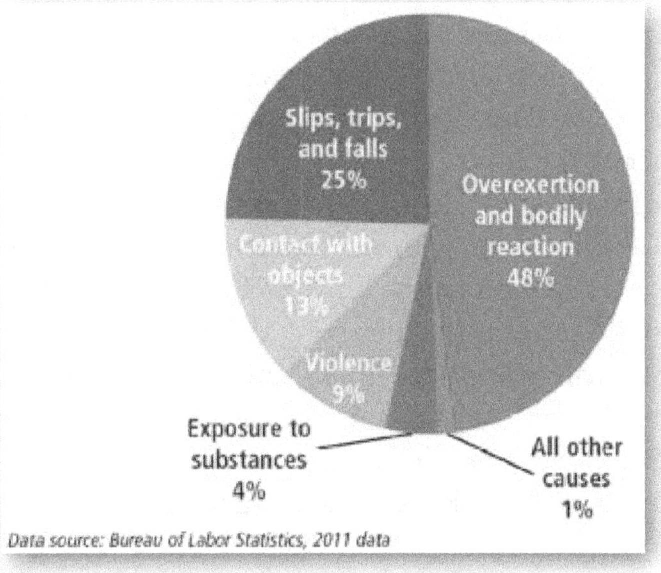

With the above data in mind, let's cover a few important points.

Lifting and moving patients can easily be one of the biggest risk factors in the above data.

If it requires more help, then let's do our best to make sure we can do so safely. It might require a 2 person lift or carry, and or a mechanical assist.

BUT, we know that during a crisis, we may not have the ability to use the tools and techniques as we would like to.

Once we get injured; we are of little value to the rest of the team.

Slips trips and falls are the next highest category.

Walking and working surfaces, change in elevations, are some causes of these events.

Contact with objects could be lacerations, burns, punctures or other elements that we MAY HAVE the ability to control.

Situational awareness, PPE and overall safety guidance may help to prevent injuries in this category.

The next pervasive category is Violence in general. It could be from a combative patient or family, or other external factors as well. Make sure that YOU are not placed between the assailant and the door, and keep yourself acutely aware of your surroundings.

During any crisis situation, tempers flare, and desperate people do desperate things.

Our facilities are chock full of tools and instruments that may be used against us at any time. Situational awareness is the key.

The next element on the list is EXPOSURE to substances.

It could be from Blood or body fluids (OPM) other potential infectious materials gloves, masks, eye protection are a front line of defense, along with the appropriate mask or respirator that is designed for that type of exposure.

When in doubt, GEAR UP at all times, until it has been proven safe.

Following OSHA 1910.32d (which is required) will help to establish the appropriate personal and protective equipment necessary for the task at hand.

OSHA has guidelines that are under continuous updating that can be a useful tool for preparations for emergency response.

(https://www.osha.gov/SLTC/emergencypreparedness/gettingstarted.html)

Each local OSHA office (or their state equivalent) has a research library available as well as the OSHA.gov website that has numerous resources available for enhancing the PPE and response process.

Several standards come into the forefront of emergency response.

The General Duty Clause (5(a) 1) is a standard that states:
SEC. 5. Duties
(a) Each employer --
(1) shall furnish to each of his employees employment and a place of employment which are free from recognized hazards that are causing or are likely to cause death or serious physical harm to his employees;
(2) shall comply with occupational safety and health standards promulgated under this Act.
29 USC 654
(b) Each employee shall comply with occupational safety and health standards and all rules, regulations, and orders issued pursuant to this Act which are applicable to his own actions and conduct.
https://www.osha.gov/pls/oshaweb/owadisp.show_document?p_table=OSHACT&p_id=3359
The rule as stated above clearly indicates that the EMPLOYER has a duty to follow appropriate procedures and training as required.

Other standards that may come into play would be:
Personal Protective Equipment

U.S. Department of Labor
Occupational Safety and Health Administration
OSHA 3151-12R
2003

This informational booklet provides a general overview of a particular topic related to OSHA standards. It does not alter or determine compliance responsibilities in OSHA standards or the Occupational Safety and Health Act of 1970. Because interpretations and enforcement policy may change over time, you should consult current OSHA administrative interpretations and decisions by the Occupational Safety and Health Review Commission and the Courts for additional guidance on OSHA compliance requirements.

One of the most common overlooked standards is the RESPIRATORY protection standard, 1910.134 (https://www.osha.gov/SLTC/respiratoryprotection/standards.html)

Respiratory Protection1910.134 (a) (1)

In the control of those occupational diseases caused by breathing air contaminated with harmful dusts, fogs, fumes, mists, gases, smokes, sprays, or vapors, the primary objective shall be to prevent atmospheric contamination. This shall be accomplished as far as feasible by accepted engineering control measures (for example, enclosure or confinement of the operation, general and local ventilation, and substitution of less toxic materials). When effective engineering controls are not feasible, or while they are being instituted, appropriate respirators shall be used pursuant to this section.

1910.134(a) (2)

A respirator shall be provided to each employee when such equipment is necessary to protect the health of such employee.

The employer shall provide the respirators which are applicable and suitable for the purpose intended. The employer shall be responsible for the establishment and maintenance of a respiratory protection program, which shall include the requirements outlined in paragraph (c) of this section. The program shall cover each employee required by this section to use a respirator.

The responsibility of the safety officer is to become familiar and conversant with all of the applicable standards as promulgated by the regulatory authority having appropriate jurisdictions over the laboratory or of the response/investigation site.

The absence of a Federal or state official DOES NOT NEGATE the safety officer from following appropriate standards and programs.

Policies and procedures that FOLLOW appropriate guidelines are critical for the success of your safety and health PROCESS. Note that I have used the term process as well as program, as a PROCESS is continuous cycle that begins with:

Identifying the hazards

Selecting the APPROPRIATE Personal Protective Equipment for the SPECIFIC Hazard (PPE)

Identifying those jobs, procedures or operations that require PPE

Identifying what TRAINING is required

Identifying what EDUCATION is required (it is NOT THE SAME AS TRAINING)

Establishing appropriate safeguards for approval and utilization of safety equipment

Providing adequate time for identification, training and retraining is critical.

If you take the time now to accurately identify what the employees will or may be exposed to, the time to prepare is now.

CHAPTER 29

# Role of the Chaplain in a Disaster

● ● ●

**Rev. Rodney Bourg**

## Introduction

In time of a disaster the chaplain as well as all first responders and civil leadership is faced with ultimate chaos and turmoil. Everyone is working basically off of adrenalin. The Chaplains role is to attempt to bring calm and peace to this very difficult situation and time. That is the ideal, however, human nature being what it is – a best attempt is all we can ask.

The chaplain needs to be present to and work with not only the victims but the first responders, medical personnel and team leadership to any situation. His/her primary role is one of communications and discernment of the situation at all levels. The chaplain must greet people where they are and attempt to calm and comfort them, no matter the trauma they may have faced or be facing. The chaplain must bring God's presence and re-assurance to these times.

The only way that this can happen is if the chaplain himself/herself has a strong personal and intimate relationship with the Lord and understands God's unconditional love for him/her and all others.

## Victims

One of the chief concerns for the Chaplain should be to never blame the victim for their own circumstances, whether the disaster is natural or man-made or the result of the victims on actions. The primary role of the chaplain is to be present to the victim and to seek to find ways to facilitate responses for them in meeting their needs.

## First Responders

Another group that the Chaplain must be present to is the first responders. These men and women are on the front lines responding to any and all needs of the victims, usually at a great cost to themselves (emotionally, physically and spiritually) and their families. During major natural disasters many times they may or may not know if their own families are safe.

Another concern is the duration of deployment during a disaster adrenaline will only take them so far. They must take downtime even it is for a short time, so that they can continue to serve affectively. After the disaster it is essential that all responders be de-briefed and assessed for post disaster stress and given the appropriate counseling.

## Medical Personnel

Another group the chaplain needs to minister to is the medical personnel. Like First Responders they have similar situations and challenges. However, unlike First Responders their expertise demand a constant presence and many times in extremely difficult and trying times. There work even in good times is stressful and demanding, but is compounded during a disaster.

The chaplain again needs to be present to and creative in finding ways to be able to encourage them to take breaks on a regular basis with some extended down-time.

## Prolonged Stress

During any disaster regardless whether man-made or natural all responders – Chaplains included, have to come to grips with their own human limitations. The operative word among all responders needs to be balance. Once the immediate threat subsides, some kind of schedule for all responders needs to be developed and followed, giving all parties some down-time so that they can more effectively serve for the long haul.

## De-Briefing

It is essential for all responders to participate in some form of review of the disaster. This is an opportunity for all parties involved to review, evaluate and be better prepared for the next disaster. It is also a chance to surface any physical, emotional or spiritual challenges the individual has faced and can be offered the appropriate help they need to re-gain their balance in life.

## Communications & Discernment

The chaplain is in a unique situation to be able to discern what he/she is hearing from the victims and responders and convey this information to the leadership team in a disaster. This information coming from all levels of the disaster operation can be extremely beneficial to those who must make difficult decisions in times of crisis.

CHAPTER 30

# Human Resource Attrition

• • •

**Robert J. Muller**

IT IS IMPORTANT TO BE cognizant of the fact that depending on the type of disaster, the facility will experience some type of absenteeism. It is important to have pre-planned agreements or understandings with the staff in place prior to an event, but numerous circumstances arise in individuals lives that prevent even the best planned staffing from becoming a reality.

During weather related emergencies, staff may not be able to find child care, husbands or significant other may be away; pets may not have been properly pre planned for care, and may not be left alone; access ways may not be accessible due to debris or rising water; modes of transportation may fail, etc.

During a public health emergency such as a pandemic, personal or family sickness or contamination may prevent employees from being able to get to work, as well as official advice for self or a mandatory quarantine. The fear of "bringing home" disease or sickness is a very real reality.

Bio terrorist, nuclear or chemical events may be limited for access depending on the nature of the event, the proximity of the events and the procedures that have been pre-established for access credentialing of essential personnel.

The point is that the facility must plan on functioning with loss of few, or many of the scheduled personnel and alternative protocols must be in place to provide service in the event that this becomes reality.

## Personnel Pool

Create a plan and a location for a personnel pool. During and after a disaster there are many volunteers that show up at the hospital facility, i.e. staff families, friends, relatives, and outsiders from the community as well as those that come to your aide from out of state including movie stars and celebrities (John Travolta, Nick Lachey, Brad Pitt, Matthew McConaughey----to name a few).

Make advanced assignments where anticipated staffing needs may require additional personnel.

Good examples may be *security* (internal and external) and may utilize those with previous law enforcement or military experience, or federal agents who may volunteer; *traffic and parking* direction, helicopter landing zone security (use those with prior military experience preferably in aviation)-a *heliops manager*; outside *animal control*; outside *logistics* (to procure barricades, tents, etc.); staff *babysitting* (teenage family members are excellent for this function); if there is only one or two access roads into the facility --staff a *checkpoint* to help alleviate unnecessary traffic and movement around the facility and secure the area that may be utilized a landing zones (LZ) for helicopters; others may include *PBX operators, food preparation/disbursing assistants; receiving and supplies, etc.*

Post disaster donations in the form of food and clothing can rapidly become problematic; think about assigning at least one person to be in charge of *donation management*. There is also an excellent FEMA EMI course on the subject.

A *Pet Manager is essential. This person needs to be responsible to register and keep track of all pets within the facility area.

A Hotel Manager is necessary to assign rooms to those that will be embedded within the facility. This position is best served by a hospital employee rather than a volunteer. This position requires someone that is not only totally familiar with all the areas of the facility that can be utilized for embedding, but also the personnel that require embedding. Designated areas also may be defined as to staff, volunteers, etc.

Identify and list potential needs in the facility disaster plan where personnel can be easily referenced and assignments made rapidly as qualified volunteers become available.

All volunteer personnel should have some form of ID. Generic IDs' can be made and kept for pool use or the use of color wrist banding will likewise serve the same function. Whichever the case maybe some form of identification is a requirement within the hospital facility and surrounding grounds, parking, clinic, office buildings, etc.

# Section Two

• • •

# Policies and Procedures

CHAPTER 31

# Active Shooter

• • •

## Robert J. Muller

An active shooter is an unpredictable individual(s) activity engaged in killing or attempting to kill people in a confined area, typically through the use of firearms, but knives and explosives may also be instruments of implementation.

Victims are usually selected at random or at least until a specific targeted victim is found or identified.

The event is unpredictable and evolves quickly, although some well-planned events have been known to take place in the past and do occupy longer spaces of time.

Having a policy and knowing what to do can save lives.

Denial of such an event within a facility can be a major mistake and failure to plan and exercise can prove to be a monumental mistake.

While no facility ever hopes to see such an event evolve, it is plausible within the realms of today's society that such an event has a real possibility of taking place within the facility. This is likely to occur within facilities as disgruntled employees, depressed patients, irate families or just a great place for a high profile random event.

Have a plan and have organized meeting with the staff and employees to advise of the plan and the need for planned action within the various areas and departments within the hospital bases on the accepted guideline. Utilize local law enforcement to actively participate in the creation of the plan and to know in advance how your facility plan to deal with such situation should the need arise--- BEFORE it happened --- not a "we should have...", after it happens.

## Active Shooter and Emergency Operations

Health Care Facilities, hence known as **HCF,** face many challenges in emergency planning in terms of their environment, geography, governance and their population served.

HCF's are complex, multifaceted enterprises that incorporate many roles. In their primary role as a health care provider, they often serve as community centers as well as emergency care facilities.

Security personnel may or may not be present which can vary the levels of protection available to the employees and staff as well as those visitors and patients forever present and any one time.

Often HCF's include many different buildings and locations within the same campus physical locale, including such as clinic and office buildings, ancillary facilities. i.e., ambulatory surgery centers and parking facilities either as lots or garages. This increases the vulnerability potential as well as necessitating increased staffing to deal with the potential for an organized or random violent assault.

Many of the facilities are research oriented and may contain sensitive information, radioactive materials, storage of deadly pathogens, and other dangerous pharmaceuticals such as narcotics are just one example.

These are individual or combined resources can attract individuals or radical groups with opposing beliefs to the goals and directions upon which the HCF may be oriented. Depending on the national significance of facility, the importance of adequate safeguard from terrorist and potential criminal threats becomes paramount.

Emergency Management and preparation often times becomes a facility step-child due to the fact that there are more pressing needs in competition for shrinking budgets. The inclusion of such line items as patient care, equipment purchases and upgrades, facility management and salaries, just to mention a few, require the brunt of administrative attention on a daily basis.

The potential versus the possibility become essential in the thinking process of dealing with strict budgetary constraints. While all are important, usually the squeaky wheel gets the grease and thus many times the security budget takes a back seat in the planning process. When an emergency situation arises then and only then does its' importance and significance get emphasis.

When an emergency does occur within a facility, the HCF personnel should be adequately pre trained and exercised to react immediately, being able to activate the plan; notify responsible agencies and being able to provide direction through actionable information in accessible formats before first responders even begin to arrive.

HCF officials should include pre-designated incident commanders, should be engaged in a coordinated effort with local, state and federal partners without compromise of ANYONES safety and only adequate pre planning can determine the roles to be played by employees and personnel.

Active shooter incidents are defined as those where an individual is "actively engaged in killing or attempting to kill people in a confined and populated area."

Many times incidents occur within buildings, other times outside in spaces such as parking lots, and entrance ways. In each incidence, law enforcement response to the scene should follow a preset of protocols that require them to find and end the threat as soon as possible, and then to evaluate and make sure everyone is safe and accounted for within the area confines.

Other gun related incidents that may occur within the HCF environment, i.e. domestic situations, are not defined as active shooter incidents are they are usually isolated events and not with the original intent of loss of life to multiple victims. While these do not fit the criterion, the plans should likewise account for these types of events.

The natural human reaction of such events, even for highly trained individuals, is startled, fear and anxiety, disbelief and many times even denial.

Training for personnel must focus on the mantra of "RUN, HIDE, FIGHT", and should be viewed on a continuum. Everyone should be trained to run away from the shooter and encourage others to follow without hesitation. If that is not possible, they should seek a secure place to hide and learn the technique of barricading themselves within confines. As a very last result a decision may be made to fight and obviously this should always be a last resort decision when all else have failed or is impossible. The more the better, as it becomes virtually impossible for one assailant to deal with multiple persons fighting back unless he/she has the advantage of an automatic weapon. Also remember the element of surprise is a powerful one especially when combined with joint forces.

Healthcare personnel may also be faced with the added dilemma of the safety of patients and visitors within the facility who may not be able to perform any of the above three recommendations due to the condition, age, injury, disabilities, or engaged within medical procedures such as X rays, and surgery.

## Planning

A HCF planning team should be established with goals, objectives and courses of action to be taken and like this book, be placed in a plan annex.

The plans will be impacted by the assessments conducted at the outset of the planning process and require updating as ongoing assessments occur, especially through vigorous and extensive plan exercises.

The plan should be created with the external partners from the local, state and federal levels, including the local police and sheriff office, state police, FBI, EMS, fire and office of emergency management.

The internal partners should include the administrative leadership who MUST find the time to participate, clinical care providers, security, facility management, human resources, chaplains and risk management.

The plan should include:

1. Proactive steps that can be taken by employees to identify individuals who may be prone to commit violent acts due to their current like situations, depression and despair. This should become a part of a planned seminar or training program of some type that is best formulated for the facility's' needs.
2. A system for reporting an active shooter incident such as an announced code to help prevent others from entering into the situation either internal or external.
3. Emergency escape procedures and routes --- familiarity with the floor plans and potential safe areas internally as well in some cases maybe external to the facility.
4. Lockdown procedures for floors, sections (ER, X ray, OR, etc.), office buildings and facilities on campus, etc.
5. Cooperation and integration of the facility incident commanders and the external incident commanders and a planned communication system as well as multiple alternate backup systems.
6. A communication system both written and in digital form on computers or thumb drives of all the responding agencies

direct numbers that are planned on being used during an emergency.

7. Preferable secure internal command center when evacuation is not possible with multiple door or steel door access only, etc. An attempt to activate and run an internal command center should only be under taken in certain situations and under the advisement and approval of the external partners.
8. How to lock evacuate, shelter in place and lock down patients, visitors and staff.
9. How to and where to evacuate when the primary evacuation routes are unusable.
10. How to select and pre select effective shelter in-place locations, i.e. locations with thick walls, brick, mortar, cinder blocks, solid doors, no interior windows, etc. These areas can likewise be used for natural hazards such as tornados, hurricanes and earthquakes and should be stocked with some vital supplies to stop hemorrhage, facilitate communications and sound alarms, such as a monitored fire alarm.
11. Train staff in psychological first aid to reduce the initial stress caused by traumatic events and to foster long-term adaptive functioning and coping.
12. An adaptive internal security plan based on what is available within the HCF, time of day, day of week, etc.

Research shows that perpetrators of targeted acts of violence engage in both covert and overt behavior preceding their attacks. They consider, plan, prepare, share and in some case move to action. One of the most useful tools for HCF to develop is to identify, evaluate, and address the troubling signs through the formation of a multidisciplinary threat assessment team---TAT.

A TAT with diverse representation will operate more efficiently and effectively and should include HCF administrators, human resources, counselors, current employees, medical and mental health professionals, chaplain, public safety and law enforcement personnel.

The TAT should serve as the central body to ensure the warning signs observed by multiple people are not considered isolated events and that they do not slip through the cracks as they may represent escalating behavior that is a serious condition and can become a fatal event.

The HCF TAT should only rely on factual information and avoid unfair labeling or stereotyping to remain in compliance with civil rights, privacy and other applicable Federal and state laws. The TAT protocol should probably be established with the HCF legal counsel in agreement and accepted compliance before augmented.

The TAT may review the threatening behavior of current or former patients, family members, visitors, staff and any other persons brought to the attention of the TAT. The TAT considers a complete evaluation of the potentially threatening person's life, more than focusing on warning signs and threats alone. The TAT may also identify any potential victim(s) with whom the individual may interact. Once the TAT identifies an individual who may pose a threat, the team then must address an appropriate course of action to address the situation through the various entities that comprise the TAT; whether this is counseling or possible law enforcement involvement and intervention or any continuum in between.

Law enforcement can be of help to assess reported or troubling behavior quickly and privately and have the ability to reach out to available Federal resources such as the Federal Bureau of Investigation behavioral experts in the National Center for Analysis of Violent Crime at Quantico, Virginia, are available 24/7 to help develop threat mitigation strategies for persons of concern.

The TAT should consult with its HCF administration and develop a process to seek these additional resources.

This chapter written with information provided by: United States Department of Health and Human Services, Office of the Assistant Secretary for Preparedness and Response, "Incorporating Active Shooter Incident Planning into Healthcare Facility Emergency Operations Plans", Washington, DC, 2014

## Active Shooter Events

When there is an active shooter in the vicinity, there must be preparation both mentally and physically to deal with the situation. There are three options:

Run
Hide
Fight

If you choose to RUN:

- have an escape route plan in mind
- leave your belongings behind
- evacuate regardless of whether others agree to follow
- help others escape
- do NOT attempt to move the wounded
- prevent others from entering an area where the active shooter may be
- keep your hands VISIBLE
- call 911 when you are safe:
  a. give location of active shooter
  b. number of shooters
  c. physical description of the shooter(s)

d. number and type of weapons (if known)
e. number of potential victims

If you choose to HIDE:

- hide in an area out of shooter's view
- lock doors and block entry to your hiding place
- silence your cell phone including the vibrate mode, remain quiet as possible

If you choose to FIGHT:

- fight as a LAST resort and only when your life is in imminent danger
- improvise weapons, i.e. scissors, broken glass, light bulbs fire extinguishers,, door hinge pins, etc.
- attempt to incapacitate the shooter, i.e., gouge eyes, etc. Remember your life depends upon your actions. You are fighting for YOUR life. Act with as much physical aggression as possible.
- Commit to your actions----YOUR LIFE DEPENDS UPON IT.

When law enforcement arrives, remain calm and follow their instructions.

Drop items in your hands, i.e., bags, jackets, etc. ANYTHING in your hands DROP it - remember tensions will be running high and flight of thought and assessment rapid.

Raise hands and spread your fingers

Keep your hands visible at all times

Avoid quick movements to officers such as holding onto them for safety

Avoid pointing, screaming or yelling
Do NOT ask questions when evacuating

## REMEMBER

The first officers on the scene will not stop to help the injured. Expect expert trained rescue teams to follow the initial officers. These rescue teams will treat and remove the injured. Do not attempt to assist them to do their jobs unless you have been specially trained for such an event in which case identify yourself to the responding officers and your qualifications. Remember they still make ask you to leave or escort you out as they do not know until final assessment is made as to who the active shooter may be or might have been --- comply and do not be offended.

Once you have reached a safe location, you will likely be held by law enforcement until the situation is under control and all witnesses have been identified and questioned. DO NOT leave the area until cleared by law enforcement authorities.

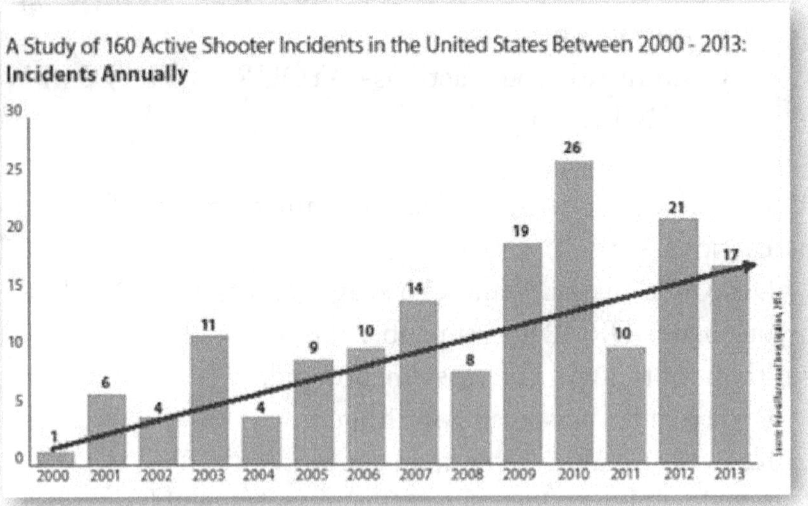


Ref. FBI Headquarters National Press

CHAPTER 32

# Bomb Threats

• • •

**Robert J. Muller**

Hospitals are often a favorite target of potential bomb threats, often as pranks from a disgruntled employee, kids out of school, or mentally deranged persons seeking self-gratification, etc.

**ALL** bomb threats should be taken **SERIOUSLY**. Do **NOT** ignore them as being some type of prank.

The usual threat is received via the PBX by a hospital operator that customarily answers calls for referral to patient rooms, departments or administrative services. These operators are not trained in dealing with this type of call and its importance and significance are somewhat underplayed.

It is imperative that all hospital operators be adequately trained in answering this type of call and training may be obtained by requesting local law enforcement, the FBI or ATF, to conduct a training session. While as in most training session, not all can attend at one time, and therefore a video should be made of the session and converted to a DVD that can be distributed to those who were absent. Training should be MANDATORY and records should be kept of all of those who have attended the session or have viewed the video.

Take all phone calls of a bomb threat seriously. DO NOT take as a hoax.

1. SPEAK slowly and gather as much detail as possible: ASK
   A. Location
   B. Time of detonation
   C. Type of device
2. OBSERVE:
   A. Background noise, i.e. train whistle, paging, auto noise, etc.
   B. Accent
   C. Tone of voice, i.e. serious, straight forward, slurred, playful, nervous
3. NOTIFY:
   A. House Supervisor
   B. Administration
   C. Security
   D. Local Police
   E. Local Sheriff Office.
   F. FBI Field Office or local Resident Agent
   G. Call code as directed by administration
   H. Begin evacuation as directed.

CHAPTER 33

# Facility Policies

● ● ●

**Robert J. Muller**

## Cafeteria Policy

A policy should be established as to how the cafeteria will handle the feeding of the hospital personnel in a disaster situation, with the possibility in a reduction of cafeteria staffing as well as the possibility of rationing of the supplies on hand.

A system may be pre-arranged with the staff and be known well in advance of situations developing whereby an alphabetical system, a departmental system or a floor by floor system may be utilized to prevent a disorganized rush on the cafeteria at any one time. A "what-ever" works system that is best for your facility should be the one that is chosen to be adopted for your facility---but adopted well in advance of need.

## Embedding

A policy should be in place in preparation for embedding of those essential personnel of the hospital and it ancillary staffing personnel essential to the operations and well- being of the hospital in preparation, operations and recovery of the event.

This may include outside ancillary personnel essential to the operations of the facility, i.e. IT or electrical engineers, mechanics, etc. who are not normal daily hospital staff but yet essential to operations and their physical presence becomes a necessity in anticipation of an event.

## Facility Plan

An emergency management facility plan may be written in many ways --- use the format that works best for your facility and staff structure.

The plans may be written addressing each of The Joint Commission (TJC) sections that require addressing; somewhat a question and answer as to how the facility addressed and plans for that particular section.

The plan may be written to comply with the ICS system --- addressing each of the operational areas of the HEICS, i.e. Operations, Logistics, Financial and Planning.

The plan may be written addressing each department responsibilities, i.e. administration, nursing, ancillary services, etc.

The plan that I feel is the most comprehensive is the plan that address the issues and solves the problems and addresses who will ultimately be the person or persons responsible to solve them. Then divide this plan into sections using whatever system that works best for the facility, i.e.

Security issues related to parking and building entry and integrity --- who, numbers of persons needed to facilitate resolution of the problem and how will resolution take place --- what is the plan?

Then place this plan under a) operations b) administrator responsible for security c) plan book section "security" d) alphabetical placement, etc.

The MOST import thing is to **PLAN** and do so in advance and to exercise and revise the plan on at least an annual basis or as needed.

There are numerous consulting hospital consulting companies that are available that can help with plan preparations if needed that can range in cost from $ to $$$$$ depending on the company used and what is expected from them. Be specific as to what services you are expecting to receive before signing any contracts as well as a deliverable in the contract for copies of the plan, how they will be presented i.e. binders, hardback copies, etc. and most important the expected date of completion which past a reasonable time make the contract null and void.

## Facility Relocation Plan

In hospital facilities that may be prone to flooding on the first floor, a plan should be implemented for alternate sites, either within the facility or at nearby surrounding facilities, to continue operations of that particular service. What about if an internal fire temporarily shuts down an area?

Many hospitals have their laboratory located on the first floor. Where could it be located in order to continue operation if flooding facilitated its relocation??? What about the food preparation facility??? Are there any schools in the area where contractual agreements may be made to utilize their facility to continue food preparation?? Preplan and anticipate possible needs.

Many other areas may be in similar situations. Identify the critical service areas and facilitate a plan for relocation to ensure continuous operation before a crisis might take place.

## Firearms Policy

All facilities should have some type of written firearms policy, regarding employees working as well as guests visiting the facility. The nature and extent of this policy should be totally dependent upon the locale of the facility as well as the community standards and situational status in the surrounding area.

All **law enforcement officers** are required to retain their firearms in all situations but should be easily identifiable by uniform or in plain clothes by wearing an easily recognizable badge on their belt facing forward and visible from a reasonable distance. Do NOT allow any type of armed security service to provide services to the facility unless they are **uniformed**. (In a critical disaster or national emergency they may be mistaken as looters or terrorists by local or federal law enforcement officers if not readily identifiable). Notify local law enforcement agencies as to the presence of contracted security at your facility.

Firearms removed or confiscated from patients or victims brought into the hospital in emergency situations should be tagged with identifying information and secured in the hospital safe until such time they can be **signed** over to a family member or law enforcement official. If possible allow the firearm to only be handled by security or someone totally familiar with various types of firearms. They are usually loaded and must be considered very dangerous. DO NOT allow a weapon to sit on a counter---they must be handled with care and taken immediately to a secure location. The same policy should be for knives, stun guns, Tasers, pepper sprays, etc.

If a weapon is turned over to a law enforcement office make sure the event is properly documented with a basic description of the weapon, time/date, officer's name, badge number, agency and have him/her sign for the weapon.

In an emergency situation where family members or employees may be utilized for security purposes, unless they are bona fide commissioned law enforcement or retired law enforcement officials, they should not be allowed to be armed by written policy.

## Food Preparation

Hospital facilities should have alternate plans for the preparation of food as well as alternate food supply sources.

In the event of loss of power or gas, alternate preparation sites should be pre identified. The utilization of local school cafeterias, restaurants, or local catering companies that have adequate facilities may be alternatives. On a limited basis, the use of such things as propane tank grills and or barbecue pits can be utilized. However, this is not feasible for the large scale preparation of foods.

Additional food sources should be identified within the community, especially areas that may be evacuated and or abandoned including large grocery stores, Wal-Mart, Sam's Club and restaurants than may store large supplies of meat and food stores, i.e. Outback, Applebee's, etc.

Preplanning within the community should involve these potential suppliers and their general manager as well as their store managers. Complete listings of these persons contact numbers and alternate means of communication should be established, i.e. text messaging, contact via a headquarters phone number or email address, etc. A good community activist program is essential for all the local sources that maybe beneficial to the hospital facility.

## Pet Policy

A survey taken of hospital employees shows that in anticipated disaster preparation (i.e. weather related), many of the staff responded by stating their intention to work and or stay at the hospital facility **only IF** they could bring their pets. Many parents today are single, one parent families, and have made arrangements with other for the care and evacuation of their children----but not their pets. Pet boarding may be difficult if not impossible to find in view of an impending disaster.

Pet policies should allow a place that is protected for the staff's pets. This may be on a loading dock, in a secure warehouse area or a provided containerized area such as a garbage dumpster turned over on its side. The hospital facility should be evaluated for possible secure site(s) that could be utilized to secure pets during a disaster.

Pets should be registered, secured in an airline approved (owner provided) type carrier with doors secured by plastic zip ties, and all care should be provided by the owner. At the time of registration, the owner should supply a picture of their pet to be placed in a plastic sleeve with the registration information. The owner should provide bedding, food and toys for their pets.

The staff should be allowed adequate time from their duties to care for their pets several times a shift. This also provides a period of relief for them from their very stressful situation of working during the disaster away from the family unit.

This policy should be announced well in advance or even at the time of employment and the requirements for pet registration taken care well in advance or any disaster situations.

Following a disaster, many victims bring pets with them to the hospital as they have no place else for them to be taken care. This can pose a secondary problem as many of the pets are frightened from having gone through the disaster, and may be disoriented or injured.

The hospital should have some portable plastic fencing available to rapidly create an outdoor kennel area for containment of these animals. The facility should also have some form of large netting to throw over any unruly or wild pets/animals and should have some heavy pairs of gauntlet-type gloves available to handle pets should this become necessary. The facility should also have a pre -arranged agreement with a local veterinarian for care of injured animals post disaster as well as an arrangement for bulk food from local stores. (Following Hurricane Katrina, one hospital handled over 300 animals that had been brought to the facility through evacuation)

XYZ Regional Medical Center
Disaster Pet Policy

We're aware that 63% of the population are single pet owners, and that 45% of that group actually own more than one pet.

We strongly encourage you to make advanced arrangements for the long term care of your pet outside of the hospital, with relatives, friends or your local veterinarian clinic for boarding --- should disaster preparation become eminent.

Pets will thrive much better with the constant attention they receive in a secure environment and the loving hands of those they are most familiar.

In the event that this is totally impossible and it becomes a necessity to bring your pet to the hospital, we are happy to accommodate your pet. We will provide a place for sheltering only --- YOU MUST provide care to your animal(s) as outlined in the following rules before placement will be facilitated.

1. You must check-in and register your pet upon entering the hospital.
2. You must have a 3" X 4" color picture of you and your pet, taken and printed prior to arrival, to be turned in at the time of your pet registration.
3. You must complete and sign the consent form agreement (to which your picture will be attached).
4. You must bring your pet in a secure airline type approved cage so your pet can stand, sit and turn around.

5. You must bring proof of inoculations or current veterinarian issued tags.
6. You must provide all food, water (a supply may not be available depending on the type of emergency condition), blankets/toys and clean- up supplies.
7. You must bring a collar and leash
8. You must bring a supply of 30 zip ties with a box cutter, side cutting pliers or large scissors to cut them free from securing of the cage door when removing your pet for personal attention. The door must be re secured with zip ties each time your pet is removed.
9. You must be responsible for pet visitation, feeding, walking, relief and cleaning of your pet, cage and area, if applicable.
10. PREPARE NOW --- **do not wait until the last moment** --- secure all necessary papers, supplies, cage, etc.

## Pet Registration Protocol

1. Request Form Completion
2. Attach Picture of Pet
3. Verify Inoculation
4. Verify Supplies – cage, collar, leash, etc.
5. Signed Verification Form
6. Place Registration Form including picture in clear sheet protector...place on cage with wire tie
7. Secure Pet carrier door with wire tie
8. Assign location to pet carrier

**Pet Manager:** ______________________________

**Date:** _______________________

# Pet Registration Form

**Name: ____________________________________________**
**Address: __________________________________________**
**Phone No. ______________ Cell No.________________**
**Hospital Work Location___________________________**
**Floor Work Location 1st 2nd 3rd 4th**
**MOB Other_________________**

**Type Pet:**
**Dog Name_________________________________________**
**Cat Name_________________________________________**
**Other____________________________________________**
**Vet Name:________________________________________**
**Telephone:_______________________________________**
**Inoculation Date:__________________________________**
**Checked In and Verified By:__________________________**
**Date:____________________________________________**

***Attach photo of pet below***

## Volunteer Plan

Have a plan as well as a person identified to be the facility volunteer coordinator in place well before the need arises.

With all disaster situations there will be numerous volunteers that present to the facility and it should be planned well in advance as to where you may need to fill in with volunteer positions to new positions that you may need during the situation for which you would ordinarily not have a person needed to handle that need. You should also think about how and who will credential people in these situations and people will show you telling you stories about what they can do from surgery to cooking and someone has to be assigned to determine not only the need but the correct person for the job.

You may need physicians, nurses, techs, security personnel, babysitters, cafeteria servers, cooks, runners, helicopter landing zone security and heliops managers, etc. The list can go on and on, but what is important is to identify these possible positions in advance and make a list of criteria to identify persons to possibly fill these positions. A good example is the husbands of in-hospital personnel who may have prior military experience and can help out with security (unarmed), heliops management; teenage siblings that may be great runners or baby sitters, etc.

Again the most important aspect is to pre-plan and to mitigate wherever possible --- in advance --- and the operation will run very smooth because it has already been planned.

## Seasonal Flu Plan

Seasonal flu (influenza) is a respiratory illness caused by a virus either the "A" or "B" type strains, resulting in severe and sometimes fatal illness.

During a characteristic flu season approximately 5-20% of the United States population comes down with the flu.

## Symptoms

Symptoms of the flu range from high fever, headaches, fatigue, muscle aches and sometimes vomiting and diarrhea.

The flu can be complicated by dehydration, ear and sinus infections, pneumonia, and exacerbation of chronic medical conditions such as asthma, chronic pulmonary disease, diabetes and congestive heart failure as well as others.

Influenza is a small virus and therefore can be spread easily thru droplet contamination as well as aersolization via coughing, sneezing and objects that have likewise been contaminated—enhancing its spread and distribution, i.e. computer key boards, telephones, door handles and countertops to only name a few.

While flu is best prevented by annual vaccinations, many people are complaisant and don't get their immunization, OR are afraid to receive the vaccine as they believe they actually come down with the flu OR the vaccine may pose present or future medical problems such as Guilliane Barre syndrome.

Whatever the type or strain of the flu virus, IF there is any chance for contamination, the health and well-being of patients as well as the hospital staff become eminent in our planning efforts.

During community influenza outbreaks, admitting patients infected with the virus can lead to nosocomial transmission of the disease. Unimmunized healthcare workers and visitors can likewise contribute to nosocomial dissemination.

Transmission of influenza among hospital employees and staff leads to absenteeism and disruption of the healthcare process.

In order to best prepare the facility and control influenza a set of strategies MUST be implemented, starting with a review of the state and national pandemic plans.

The basics that must be adhered to are:

1. Daily routine infection control practices utilizing appropriate barrier precautions during patient care.
2. Early recognition of symptoms and surveillance of suspected cases within the facility.
3. Isolation of suspected or known patients to private rooms and utilization of the limited visitor policy.
4. Vaccination of all healthcare personnel willing to take the vaccine is recommended.
5. Utilization of anti-viral to treat ill persons as well consideration of the efficacy for use in prophylactic treatment.
6. Staff and patient education regarding the nature of the virus, the symptoms and the prevention of spread of the disease.

## Elements of Routine Infection Control

## Hand Washing

Decreasing the risk of transmission of microorganisms in health care settings, accomplished primarily by hand washing is a major component of infection control. Hands should be washed or disinfected with a hand sanitizer immediately before and after touching a patient. Hands should be washed after touching blood, body fluids, secretions, excretions, and contaminated items, even when gloves are worn. Hand washing with plain soap or detergent for at least 10-15 seconds under running water is an effective method of removing soil and transient microorganisms. If sinks for hand washing are not readily available, alcohol-based agents can be used and are allowed by DHH/OPH policy.

## Gloves

Clean, non-sterile, disposable gloves should be worn when touching blood, body fluids, secretions, excretions and contaminated items. Gloves should be removed after use and before touching any non-contaminated items or touching another patient, and hands should be washed immediately with soap and water or an antiseptic hand rub.

Due to the significant number of health care workers with latex hypersensitivity, other strategies should be available such as non-latex products alone or in combination with latex gloves, powder-free latex gloves, "low protein" latex gloves, and vinyl gloves.

If gloves are in short supply (i.e., the demand during a pandemic could exceed the supply), priorities for glove use might need to be established. In this circumstance, reserve gloves for situations where there is a likelihood of extensive patient or environmental contact with blood or body fluids, including during suctioning.

Use other barriers (e.g., disposable paper towels, paper napkins) when there is only limited contact with a patient's respiratory secretions (e.g., to handle used tissues). Hand hygiene should be strongly reinforced in this situation.

## Masks

To be consistent with droplet precautions, health care workers and visitors should wear masks when they are within 3 feet of an infected patient or a patient suspected of being infected with influenza virus. Infected patients or patients suspected of being infected should wear a mask when being transported.

Wear a mask when entering a patient's room. A mask should be worn once and then discarded. If pandemic influenza patients are cohorted in a common area or in several rooms on a nursing unit, and multiple patients must be visited over a short time, it may be practical to wear one mask for the duration of the activity; however, other PPE (e.g., gloves, gown) must be removed between patients and hand hygiene performed.

- Change masks when they become moist.
- Do not leave masks dangling around the neck.
- Upon touching or discarding a used mask, perform hand hygiene.

## Gowns

Wear an isolation gown, if soiling of personal clothes or uniform with a patient's blood or body fluids, including respiratory secretions, is anticipated. Most patient interactions do not necessitate the use of gowns. However, procedures such as intubation and activities that involve holding the patient close (e.g., in pediatric settings) are examples of when a gown may be needed when caring for pandemic influenza patients.

A disposable gown made of synthetic fiber or a washable cloth gown may be used. Ensure that gowns are of the appropriate size to fully cover the area to be protected. Gowns should be worn only once and then placed in a waste or laundry receptacle, as appropriate, and hand hygiene performed.

If gowns are in short supply (i.e., the demand during a pandemic could exceed the supply) priorities for their use may need to be established. In this circumstance, reinforcing the situations in which they are needed can reduce the volume used. Alternatively, other coverings (e.g., patient gowns) could be used. It is doubtful that disposable aprons would provide the desired protection in the circumstances where gowns are needed to prevent contact with influenza virus, and therefore should be avoided. There are no data upon which to base a recommendation for reusing an isolation gown on the same patient. To avoid possible contamination, it is prudent to limit this practice.

## Goggles and face shields

In general, wearing goggles or a face shield for routine contact with patients with pandemic influenza is not necessary. If sprays or splatter of infectious material is likely, goggles or a face shield should be worn as recommended for standard precautions.

## Personal Protective Equipment (PPE) for special circumstances

PPE for aerosol-generating procedures

During procedures that may generate increased small-particle aerosols of respiratory secretions (e.g., endotracheal intubation, nebulizer treatment, bronchoscopy, suctioning), healthcare personnel should wear gloves, gown, face/eye protection, and a N95 respirator or other appropriate particulate respirator. Respirators should be used within the context of a respiratory protection program that includes fit-testing, medical clearance, and training. If possible and when practical, use of an airborne isolation room may be considered when conducting aerosol-generating procedures.

PPE for managing pandemic influenza with increased transmissibility. The addition of airborne precautions, including respiratory protection (an N95 filtering face piece respirator or other appropriate particulate respirator), may be considered for strains of influenza exhibiting increased transmissibility, during initial stages of an outbreak of an emerging or novel strain of influenza, and as determined by other factors such as vaccination/immune status of personnel and availability of antivirals. As the epidemiologic characteristics of the pandemic virus are more clearly defined, CDC will provide updated infection control guidance, as needed.

Precautions for early stages of a pandemic

Early in a pandemic, it may not be clear that a patient with severe respiratory illness has pandemic influenza. Therefore precautions consistent with all possible etiologies, including a newly emerging infectious agent, should be implemented. This may involve the combined use of airborne and contact precautions, in addition to standard precautions, until a diagnosis is established.

Know what is clean, know what is contaminated, keep them apart. Healthcare personnel should be particularly vigilant to avoid cross contamination. Some of the mistakes commonly observed are:

1. Touching eyes, nose or mouth with contaminated hands (gloved or ungloved).
2. Making adjustments to the PPE during patient care or removal. Careful placement of PPE before patient contact will help avoid the need to and risk.
3. Touching contaminating environmental surfaces that are not directly related to patient care (e.g., door knobs, light switches).
4. Touching pen, glasses and other personal items during patient care.

Patient placement

Isolation plans for use during a pandemic should be developed in advance. Under ideal circumstances, patients with suspected or diagnosed influenza should be in a private room. However, during a pandemic this may not be practical as it is currently impractical during seasonal epidemics. During a pandemic, private rooms are unlikely to be available and containment of infection is likely to be difficult. Consideration should be given to cohorting patients with active confirmed or suspected influenza infection.

Isolation procedures for other pathogens, including use of a private room, should continue to be utilized. Use of dedicated staff that has been immunized should be considered for care of those with suspected or confirmed influenza infection.

Patient movement

Movement and transport of infected patients should be limited as much as possible. If a patient must be transported, he or she should wear a surgical mask to decrease the risk of virus transmission to other patients and health care workers. Congregation of patients should be minimized. This will prevent spreading of illness by non-symptomatic or undiagnosed persons. Patients should also be educated about personal hygiene measures that decrease virus transmission (i.e. covering their mouth and nose when coughing or sneezing, hand washing, discarding tissues, using disposable eating and drinking utensils, etc).

Linen and laundry

Standard precautions are recommended for linen and laundry that might be contaminated with respiratory secretions from patients with pandemic influenza:

Place soiled linen directly into a laundry bag in the patient's room. Contain linen in a manner that prevents the linen bag from opening or bursting during transport and while in the soiled linen holding area.

Wear gloves and gown when directly handling soiled linen and laundry (e.g., bedding, towels, personal clothing) as per standard precautions. Do not shake or otherwise handle soiled linen and laundry in a manner that might create an opportunity for disease transmission or contamination of the environment.

Wear gloves for transporting bagged linen and laundry.

Perform hand hygiene after removing gloves that have been in contact with soiled linen and laundry.

Wash and dry linen according to routine standards and procedures

Dishes and eating utensils

Standard precautions are recommended for handling dishes and eating utensils used by a patient with known or possible pandemic influenza:

Wash reusable dishes and utensils in a dishwasher with recommended water temperature.

Disposable dishes and utensils (e.g., used in an alternative care site set-up for large numbers of patients) should be discarded with other general waste.

Wear gloves when handling patient trays, dishes, and utensils.

Patient Care Equipment

Follow standard practices for handling and reprocessing used patient-care equipment, including medical devices:

Wear gloves when handling and transporting used patient-care equipment.

Wipe heavily soiled equipment with an EPA-approved hospital disinfectant before removing it from the patient's room.

Follow current recommendations for cleaning and disinfection or sterilization of reusable patient-care equipment.

Wipe external surfaces of portable equipment for performing x-rays and other procedures in the patient's room with an EPA-approved hospital disinfectant upon removal from the patient's room.

Environmental Cleaning, Disinfection

Cleaning and disinfection of environmental surfaces are important components of routine infection control in healthcare facilities. Environmental cleaning and disinfection for pandemic influenza follow the same general principles used in healthcare settings.

Cleaning and disinfection of patient-occupied rooms

Wear gloves in accordance with facility policies for environmental cleaning and wear a surgical or procedure mask in accordance with droplet precautions. Gowns are not necessary for routine cleaning of an influenza patient's room.

Keep areas around the patient free of unnecessary supplies and equipment to facilitate daily cleaning.

Use any EPA-registered hospital detergent-disinfectant. Follow manufacturer's recommendations for use-dilution (i.e., concentration), contact time, and care in handling.

Follow facility procedures for regular cleaning of patient-occupied rooms. Give special attention to frequently touched surfaces (e.g., bedrails, bedside and over-bed tables, TV controls, call buttons, telephones, lavatory surfaces including safety/pull-up bars, doorknobs, commodes, ventilator surfaces) in addition to floors and other horizontal surfaces. Clean and disinfect spills of blood and body fluids in accordance with current recommendations for Isolation Precautions

Cleaning and disinfection after patient discharge or transfer

Follow standard facility procedures for post-discharge cleaning of an isolation room. Clean and disinfect all surfaces that were in contact with the patient or might have become contaminated during patient care. No special treatment is necessary for window curtains, ceilings, and walls unless there is evidence of visible soiling.

Do not spray (i.e., fog) occupied or unoccupied rooms with disinfectant. This is a potentially dangerous practice that has no proven disease control benefit.

Postmortem care

Follow standard facility practices for care of the deceased. Practices should include standard precautions for contact with blood and body fluids.

Laboratory specimens and practices

Follow standard facility and laboratory practices for the collection, handling, and processing of laboratory specimens.

Targeted Influenza Control Measures: Respiratory hygiene/ Cough etiquette

Respiratory hygiene/cough etiquette has been promoted as a strategy to contain respiratory viruses at the source and to limit their spread in areas where infectious patients might be awaiting medical care (e.g., physician offices, emergency departments).

The impact of covering sneezes and coughs and/or placing a mask on a coughing patient on the containment of respiratory secretions or on the transmission of respiratory infections has not been systematically studied. In theory, however, any measure that limits the dispersal of respiratory droplets should reduce the opportunity for transmission. Masking may be difficult in some settings, e.g., pediatrics, in which case the emphasis will be on cough hygiene. The elements of respiratory hygiene/cough etiquette include:

Education of healthcare facility staff, patients, and visitors on the importance of containing respiratory secretions to help prevent the transmission of influenza and other respiratory viruses

Posted signs in languages appropriate to the populations served with instructions to patients and accompanying family members or friends to immediately report symptoms of a respiratory infection as directed

Source control measures (e.g., covering the mouth/nose with a tissue when coughing and disposing of used tissues; using masks on the coughing person when they can be tolerated and are appropriate)

Hand hygiene after contact with respiratory secretions, and Spatial separation, ideally >3 feet, of persons with respiratory infections in common waiting areas when possible.

### Health Care specific guidance: Hospitals - Detection of persons entering the facility who may have pandemic influenza

Post visual alerts (in appropriate languages) at the entrance to hospital outpatient facilities (e.g., emergency departments, outpatient clinics) instructing persons with respiratory symptoms (e.g., patients, persons who accompany them) to:

- Inform reception and healthcare personnel when they first register for care, and
- Practice respiratory hygiene/cough etiquette

As the scope of the pandemic escalates locally, consider setting up a separate triage area for persons presenting with symptoms of respiratory infection. Because not every patient presenting with symptoms will have pandemic influenza, infection control measures will be important in preventing further spread.

During the peak of a pandemic, emergency departments and outpatient offices may be overwhelmed with patients seeking care. A "triage officer" may be useful for managing patient flow, including deferral of patients who do not require emergency care.

Designate separate waiting areas for patients with influenza-like symptoms. If this is not feasible, the waiting area should be set up to enable patients with respiratory symptoms to sit as far away as possible (at least 3 feet) from other patients.

Post signs that promote respiratory hygiene/cough etiquette in common areas (e.g., elevators, waiting areas, cafeterias, lavatories) where they can serve as reminders to all persons in the healthcare facility. Signs should instruct persons to:

- Cover the nose/mouth when coughing or sneezing.
- Use tissues to contain respiratory secretions.
- Dispose of tissues in the nearest waste receptacle after use.
- Perform hand hygiene after contact with respiratory secretions.
- Facilitate adherence to respiratory hygiene/cough etiquette by ensuring the availability of materials in waiting areas for patients and visitors.

**Provide** tissues and no-touch receptacles (e.g., waste containers with pedal-operated lid or waste container) for used tissue disposal.

**Provide** conveniently located dispensers of alcohol-based hand rub.

**Provide** soap and disposable towels for handwashing where sinks are available.

Promote the use of masks and spatial separation by persons with symptoms of influenza.

Offer and encourage the use of either procedure masks (i.e., with ear loops) or surgical masks (i.e., with ties or elastic) by symptomatic persons to limit dispersal of respiratory droplets.

Encourage coughing persons to sit as far away as possible (at least three feet) from other persons in common waiting areas.

## Hospitalization of Pandemic Influenza Patients

### Patient placement

Limit admission of influenza patients to those with severe complications of influenza who cannot be cared for outside the hospital setting.

Admit patients to either a single-patient room or an area designated for cohorting of patients with influenza.

### Cohorting

Designated units or areas of a facility should be used for cohorting patients with pandemic influenza. During a pandemic, other respiratory viruses (e.g., non-pandemic influenza, respiratory syncytial virus, parainfluenza virus) may be circulating concurrently in a community. Therefore, to prevent cross-transmission of respiratory viruses, whenever possible assign only patients with confirmed pandemic influenza to the same room. At the height of a pandemic, laboratory testing to confirm pandemic influenza is likely to be limited, in which case cohorting should be based on having symptoms consistent with pandemic influenza.

Personnel (clinical and non-clinical) assigned to cohorted patient care units for pandemic influenza patients should not "float" or otherwise be assigned to other patient care areas. The number of personnel entering the cohorted area should be limited to those necessary for patient care and support.

Personnel assigned to cohorted patient care units should be aware that patients with pandemic influenza may be concurrently infected or colonized with other pathogenic organisms (e.g.,

*Staphylococcus aureus*, *Clostridium difficile*) and should adhere to infection control practices (e.g., hand hygiene, changing gloves between patient contact) used routinely, and as part of standard precautions, to prevent nosocomial transmission.

Because of the high patient volume anticipated during a pandemic, cohorting should be implemented early in the course of a local outbreak.

**Patient transport**

Limit patient movement and transport outside the isolation area to medically necessary purposes.

Consider having portable x-ray equipment available in areas designated for cohorting influenza patients.

If transport or movement is necessary, ensure that the patient wears a surgical or procedure mask. If a mask cannot be tolerated (e.g., due to the patient's age or deteriorating respiratory status), apply the most practical measures to contain respiratory secretions. Patients should perform hand hygiene before leaving the room.

**Visitors**

Screen visitors for signs and symptoms of influenza before entry into the facility and exclude persons who are symptomatic.

Family members who accompany patients with influenza-like illness to the hospital are assumed to have been exposed to influenza and should wear masks.

Limit visitors to persons who are necessary for the patient's emotional well-being and care.

Instruct visitors to wear surgical or procedure masks while in the patient's room.

Instruct visitors on hand-hygiene practices.

**<u>Control of nosocomial pandemic influenza transmission</u>**

Once patients with pandemic influenza are admitted to the hospital, nosocomial surveillance should be heightened for evidence of transmission to other patients and healthcare personnel. (Once pandemic influenza is firmly established in a community this may not be feasible or necessary.)

If limited nosocomial transmission is detected (e.g., has occurred on one or two patient care units), appropriate control measures should be implemented. These may include:

- Cohorting of patients and staff on affected units
- Restriction of new admissions (except for other pandemic influenza patients) to the affected unit(s)
- Restriction of visitors to the affected unit(s) to those who are essential for patient care and support

If widespread nosocomial transmission occurs, controls may need to be implemented hospital wide and might include:

- Restricting all nonessential persons
- Stopping admissions not related to pandemic influenza and stopping elective surgeries

# Section Three

• • •

# Operations

CHAPTER 34

# Par Values

• • •

## Robert J. Muller

Par values should be established for the operation and internal sustainment of the facility for a minimum of 96 hours; longer if the facility is located in an environmentally vulnerable zone with high probabilities of occurring events (i.e. a hospital located along coastal areas, earthquake areas, etc.)

The values should likewise take into account the patient *volume* of the hospital as well as its *service area* and *support* from other surrounding facilities in the community and or region, (i.e. the only hospital in a coastal community versus a hospital 30 miles inland with 2 other hospitals in the service area; a hospital in a community that is totally evacuated versus one in a community of a sustainable population of 20,000, etc.).

All critical supplies should be maintained by computerized inventory as well as manual inventory and should be assessed preceding seasonal environmental events as well as National Security Alert elevations to higher levels.

Each hospital's supply par value will be dependent on its locale, accessibility, supply chain, and physical facility limitations on storage.

Par values should include all critical areas of the hospital from dietary to pharmacy.

ALWAYS plan for the worse and do not assume that your supply chain will always be easily accessible.

Multiple contracts should be in place to establish a redundancy of the supply chain, in case of failure for whatever reason, of one or more of the primary suppliers.

One value level to keep in mind for the recovery phase is the need for tetanus toxoid and snake bite venom as the need for these items often escalates depending on the type of disaster, as well as the locale.

CHAPTER 35

# Dialysis Management

• • •

**Robert J. Muller**

During a prolonged local or regional disaster, dialysis patients become problematic, especially in facilities that have been seriously compromised by limited water supply and electrical power, not to mention limited specialized staffing.

There is no easy way to mitigate against this possibility.

Probably the best mitigation is to have the staff physicians who have dialysis patients, made aware of this scenario and to have their patient look into alternate plans for additional sites outside of the area that may be able to handle their dialysis treatments, intrastate as well as interstate, should regional evacuation become necessary. It is imperative for the well-being of these patients that alternate treatment programs be emphasized and the patients be educated through hospital sponsored community seminars or other modes such as informational literature, etc. This is an excellent project to be assigned to the command staff Liaison and PIO officers for execution and familiarization.

Pre, during and post disasters, chronic renal failure patients requiring dialysis need and REQUIRE special attentions as well as preparation.

As of 2004 statistics, there were 355,000 patients in the United States requiring dialysis; Four percent of the population has diabetes and by 2010 that number is expected to rise to seven percent.

It is imperative that chronic renal failure (CRF) patients be properly educated on what, when and where of dialysis planning. This is something that should be encouraged by the physicians, diabetic educators and dialysis facilities.

The requirements for dialysis are:

1. Electrical Power --- one dialysis machine requires approximately 1.0-1.7KW of power alone.
2. Potable water for use in the treatment. Each treatment requires a minimum of 60 gallons of treated water and the water must have sufficient water pressure to drive the dialyzer. The exception is the Continuous Renal Replacement Therapy (CRRP) units which are waterless.
3. Personnel qualified to perform dialysis.
4. Physician order for dialysis and medical records to support the treatment.
5. Facility to perform the procedure must be set up appropriately. Therefore it is imperative to seek, well in advance, possible alternate areas or facilities to be able to meet these requirements --- not at the last minute when planning choices may be limited.

CHAPTER 36

# Infant Abduction Protocol

• • •

**Robert J. Muller**

1. Notification of abduction by staff.
2. Call Code Pink
3. Notify Security
4. Notify House Supervisor
5. Begin in house search
6. Notify Local Police Dept.
7. Notify Administrator On Call
8. If necessary-------Notify FBI ask for agent of the day.
9. Ask appropriate agency to call AMBER Alert
10. Notify News Media if ok with lead law enforcement agency or have protocol in place as to who will notify news media, i.e. hospital administration PIO, local law enforcement or FBI. This should be established beforehand in agreement with all agencies involved so that improper information or release of information timing is inappropriate.

CHAPTER 37

# Mass Casuality Events

● ● ●

**Robert J. Muller**

- By definition, mass casualty incidents overwhelm the resources of individual hospitals. Equally important, a mass casualty incident is likely to impose a sustained demand for health services rather than the short, intense peak customary with many smaller scale disasters. This adds a new dimension and many new issues to preparedness planning for hospitals.
- Hospitals, because of their emergency services and 24 hour a day operation, will be seen by the public as a vital resource for diagnosis, treatment, and follow up for both physical and psychological care.
- Hospital preparedness for disasters has focused historically on a narrow range of potential incidents. To increase their preparedness for mass casualties, hospitals have to expand their focus to include both internal and community-level planning.
- Traditional planning has not included the scenario in which the hospital is the victim of a disaster and may not be able to continue to provide care. Hospital planners should consider the possibility that a hospital might need to evacuate, quarantine, or divert incoming patients.

- Hospital preparedness can be increased if state licensure bodies, working through the Federation of State Medical Boards, develop procedures allowing physicians licensed in one jurisdiction to practice in another under defined emergency conditions. (See under EMAC.)
- Hospital preparedness can be increased if the medical staff Credentials Committees develops a policy on the recognition of temporary privileges in emergency or disaster situations and if hospitals in a community regularly share lists of the medical staffs and their privileges.

If the disaster is a mass casualty event, such as a major earthquake or biological terrorism, the patient load may overwhelm all of the hospitals, the offices of physicians, and the general resources of the community. A disaster plan limited to an individual facility is inadequate. A single facility's plan may address part of the spectrum of disasters appropriately, but its weakness is that it may ignore larger scale incidents. Therefore, hospital preparedness should expand from planning within the context of a single hospital organization to planning by the hospital to become part of a community-wide initiative to address mass casualties. This would necessitate participation in community-wide preparedness drills.

While the majority of hospitals are accredited by the JCAHO and work to comply with its standards, some hospitals are not JCAHO accredited. Many of the unaccredited hospitals are in small rural communities, which may not perceive themselves as likely to experience a mass casualty incident. Nevertheless, all hospitals should include responding to the basic elements of mass casualty incidents in their preparedness plan. When hospitals are not JCAHO accredited, it was suggested that the state licensing body or a similar entity have the responsibility for assuring that the hospital's disaster plan addresses both incidents of limited and mass casualties.

In a disaster, especially one for mass casualties, the hospital may receive more patients than it can handle. Or, if the incident results from chemical or biological exposure, the community may need to protect its self by designating some hospitals as open to victims and others as open only to patients who have not been exposed to the chemical or biological contaminants.

The implementing regulations for the Emergency Medical Treatment and Labor Act (EMTALA) state:

If any individual (whether or not eligible for Medicare benefits and regardless of ability to pay) comes by him or herself or with another person to the emergency department and a request is made on the individual's behalf for examination or treatment of a medical condition by qualified medical personnel (as determined by the hospital in its rules and regulations), the hospital must provide for an appropriate Medical Screening Examination within the capability of the hospital's emergency department, including ancillary services routinely available to the emergency department."

The EMTALA interpretive guidelines provided by HCFA state:

A hospital may deny access to patients when it is in 'diversionary' status because it does not have the staff or facilities to accept any additional emergency patients at that time. However, if the ambulance disregards the hospital's instructions and brings the individual on to hospital grounds, the individual has come to the hospital and the hospital cannot deny the individual access to hospital services.

Individuals coming to the emergency department must be provided a medical screening examination beyond initial triaging. Triage is not equivalent to a medical screening examination. Triage merely determines the 'order' in which patients will be seen, not the presence or absence of an emergency medical condition.

A hospital, regardless of size or patient mix, must provide screening and stabilizing treatment within the scope of its abilities as needed, to the individuals with emergency medical conditions who come to the hospital for examination and treatment.

- Mass casualty incidents that result from infectious causes are different from all other types of incidents for many reasons, including:

  (1) the onset of the incident may remain unknown for several days before symptoms appear,
  (2) even when symptoms appear, they may be distributed throughout the community's health system and not be recognized immediately by any one provider or practitioner,
  (3) once identified, the initial symptoms are likely to mirror those of the flu or the common cold so that the health system will have to care for both those infected and the "worried well,"
  (4) having gone undetected for several days or a week, some infectious agents may already be in their "second wave" before the first wave of casualties is identified,
  (5) public confidence in government officials and health care authorities may be undermined by the initial uncertainty about the cause of and treatment for the outbreak,
  (6) health care authorities and hospitals may want to restrict those infected to a limited number of hospitals but the public may seek care from a wide range of practitioners and institutions, and

(7) health care workers may be reluctant to place themselves or family members at increased risk by reporting to work.

- Biological incidents will be the most difficult for the community to understand and effectively coordinate its response. Valuable time is lost if public health officials are unable to rapidly identify and communicate the threat represented by what appears to be a series of unrelated illnesses. The federal government should continue to provide support for epidemiological programs which allow hospitals to submit information rapidly on atypical patients so that community-wide patterns can be identified as soon as possible.
- The traditional separation between the medical care community (e.g., hospitals, physicians, and nursing homes) and the public health community needs to be bridged in preparation for mass casualty incidents. Mass casualties will provide more work than any organization itself can address. Coordination is key, and the historic separation is a genuine disadvantage.

CHAPTER 38

# Mass Fatality Planning

• • •

**Capt. Ronald Frey (Ret.)**

THERE IS A NECESSITY FOR the pre-planning for mass fatality events with the various scenarios that may be part of the vulnerability data assessment plan. Depending upon the locale and situational status of the facility and locational proximity some various scenarios may necessitate planning; i.e. location near a large airport, truck stops, chemical and other Haz Mat handling facilities, interstate highways, rail lines to name a few. It is also important to plan for mass fatalities in the event of pandemics as well as other possible weather related catastrophic events, i.e. tornados, floods, mudslides, earthquakes, and hurricanes.

The primary objectives for the mass fatality plan are:

- To ready the county and region for managing a mass fatality.
- To identify decedent operational areas, the stakeholders and organizations responsible for these operational areas, and develop a plan for providing and for coordinating operational activities.
- To specify the command and control structure, who will activate the plan, and criteria for levels of activation?
- To present information on and guidelines for the decedent operational areas.

- To provide logistics information that enables readiness and scalability.
  - Supplies and equipment
  - Staffing requirements
  - Facility requirements
- To provide information on infection and other health and safety threats; mass fatality information systems, pandemic influenza considerations, security requirements; family, cultural and religious considerations; and staff and volunteer management.
- To describe how the plan will be exercised, updated and maintained.

Hospitals should pre plan with the local medical examiner/coroner, funeral homes and the state mass fatality task force as well as local emergency management officials.

Plans should be formulated as to body storage, including a very detailed labeling and identification process to avoid losing, switching or improperly identifying corpses; capacity and handling as well as the timely transport of remains to predetermined locations for future interment.

A hospital morgue manager or other staff person should be chosen to be the point of contact and introduced to the system well before an event may occur. This person should likewise be incorporated into the Hospital incident Command System under the operations section and under the medical care director as a unit leader; and some forms of training should be provided from the numerous state and federal courses that are available.

In case of a mass fatality incident there should be a known, and planned for format in place to deal with, now that the deceased person and all on their valuables and clothing have been collected and secured with the excess intake of human remains. Most people ask, "What is a Mass Fatality Incident?" It is an incident where there are more fatalities than you can normally handle, i.e. if you can handle up to ten bodies in your hospital morgue and an incident happens that produces 25 fatalities at your hospital, than that is a Mass Fatality Incident.

Where could a Mass Fatality Incident occur?

| | |
|---|---|
| Airports | Truck Stops |
| Rails Lines | Refineries |
| Highways | Floods |
| Hurricanes | Snow Storms |
| Mudslides | Tornados |
| Fires/Explosions | |

When planning for a Mass Fatality Incident, the administration of a hospital should make arrangements to furnish unlimited, unmarked 40 foot refrigerated trailers to be delivered within two hours of request by a previously established contractual agreement. The hospital should have a pre- determined area set to place these trailers on a solid cement or asphalt pad. Electrical access to this area will be required in order to power the refrigeration unit and should be pre-established of adequate volts and amperage so the parent power supply is able to handle the increase demand upon the system. Likewise, sufficient electrical cords should be available and if utilized only for this purpose, should then be stored with the disaster supplies.

## Body Storage

The evidence custodian should have the ability, if available either directly or remotely, to go to a computer utilizing barcode software and print a barcode for each deceased person. She/he should print enough labels for placing one label on each piece of evidence collected from the person they are dealing with. Once the labels are completed for labeling of all the evidence, a label should be placed, on a "toe tag' and placed on the victim's right toe with all the vital information necessary for proper identification and organization. Next, a barcode tag should be placed on the right wrist of the victim. Lastly, the victim is placed with in the body bag. When the body is in the body bag, seal the bag by placing a tag through the holes of both zippers; and again write all the vital information on the evidence tag on the outside of the bag and put a barcode tag on the evidence tag. For completion of the process place a barcode tag on each side of the body bag at the level of the victims head for orientation purpose.

When removing the victims from inside the facility to the storage trailer outside this will be the first time the press or the general public will get to see any signs of the victims. Always remember you are being watched and your actions could be recorded. So act professional at all times. If possible utilize barrier screens to limit the areas exposed to the public.

If you are not authorized to speak to the press, **DO NOT**.

As you enter the trailer, to load the body bags remember this is a person and always treat them with the utmost reverence and respect, as if they were part of your family. Do not load them one side to the other side. Always leave a pathway to walk and make a diagram of the internal placement of the bodies to facilitate easy location when the bodies begin to be released to other agencies or funeral homes. Do not stack bodies on top of each other out of respect. If space becomes a problem then an additional truck should be utilized. If autopsies are to be conducted on some of the victims, then the bodies should be placed in a different trailer, marking the trailers as so.

During the time of a massive incident, i.e. an airline disaster, bodies may initially be placed in various states with and without clothing and missing body parts, etc. In this case the above noted process may not be handled in such an orderly manner until after the event come to fruition and in this case the body bags should be appropriately labeled as to the content or partial contents and properly documented on the body inventory sheet, before you initial completion of the event.

If body parts cannot be definitely identified as belong to a victim, then these parts should be placed collectively in a separate body bag for sorting and definite identifications at a later date by more qualified individuals.

Before returning the 40 foot trailers to the vendor, the trailer should be completely sanitized from top to bottom and front to back.

The remediation of the trailers upon completion and return should be performed by a licensed service that is familiar with the process, has the proper chemicals and equipment and is able to certify the process.

Again—do not wait until the last minute to PLAN.

## Pandemic Preparedness

There is an excellent reference on this subject, that I refer you to the text by Dr. Michael Fagel, "Crisis Management and Emergency Planning" (CRC Press, 2014), Chapter 15 written by Douglas Himberger which is relatively all inclusive and beyond the scope of this text.

CHAPTER 39

# Reentry

● ● ●

**Robert J. Muller**

It is essential to address the situation of disaster reentry into the area where the hospital is located as well as the generalized locale, county and even the state.

It is imperative that reentry plans be made with the local, county and state emergency management offices as to what is necessary for reentry to the hospital following a disaster and what are their criteria for reentry.

There are special ID cards that are issued, placards for automobiles, hospital ID cards, stickers to be placed on ID cards, uniforms, logos, marked vehicles, etc. There are all types of criteria upon which the local, county, and state agencies make the final determination which they feel work best for their locale.

In most instances these criteria are usually the acceptable norm:

1. Proof of employment of the facility as staff, i.e. uniform, ID, etc.
2. A state driver's license or picture ID
3. A single person in a vehicle or each person in the vehicle show proof of employment—no "piggybacking" with others or families.
4. The area has been cleared as safe for reentry

5. The person(s) bring their own "Go Bag" with all of their own self-sustaining supplies, food, clothing, and medication, etc.

It is also important that arrangements be made for contractors, who are not direct hospital employees, but yet are vital to the facility operations, i.e., electricians, IT personnel, communications specialists, etc. They must have some form of identification or letter from the facility introducing them as such to the proper authorities to allow for their reentry.

While there a numerous scenarios, it is very important to know these criteria and be able to disseminate these criteria to the staff before a disaster incident occurs and the staff is unable to gain access back to the facility to provide much needed assistance in the anticipated world of chaos.

CHAPTER 40

# Infection Control and Emergency Preparedness

• • •

**John Curtis Brady**

**Natural disasters**: Hurricane
Floods
Tornados

**Biologic disasters**: Pandemics-- i.e. SARS, Influenza
Bioterrorism-- i.e. Anthrax, imported biologics, i.e. Ebola.

**Diseases**: Pandemic Influenza
Severe Adult Respiratory Syndrome
Imported Tropical diseases
Natural Disaster associated:
- Hepatitis A
- Tetanus
- Staph
- Gastrointestinal
- Contaminated environment

**Natural disasters:**

Tornados, hurricanes, floods and earthquakes

**<u>Biologic disasters</u>**:

- Pandemics, such as SARS, Influenza, or imported biologics like Ebola fever.
- Bioterrorism i.e. Anthrax

**<u>Common factors of disasters:</u>**

Every disaster is different with dynamic challenges before, during and after their occurrence. Some "givens" should be assumed when planning responses, developing emergency preparedness plans and most importantly during drills. These include:

- Loss of essential services, including electricity, water or supply chain.
- Loss of infrastructure, including facilities or electronic information.
- Shortage of workers due to transportation loss, worker or worker family illness/injury or unwillingness to report to work.
- Sudden increase in patients likely beyond care capacity often with serious injury and/or severe conditions.
- Relocation of severely ill patients to another facility may not be possible.
- Inability to resupply quickly and readily.
- Critical decisions regarding use of resources should fall to the hospital incident command system with input from the Infection Control Practitioner (ICP) and well as caregivers caring for patients.

**<u>Planning for the worst and hoping for the best</u>:**

Infection transmission or out-breaks may happen following any disaster. The most likely infection related disasters will occur related to a pandemic (worldwide/continent wide) outbreak of influenza; and imported infectious disease like Ebola fever or a bioterrorism attack outbreak. Plans and protocols for these outbreaks should be individualized rather than a group approach; based upon type or most likely organism's to be encountered.

For outbreaks of an emerging imported infectious disease like Ebola fever, SARS (Severe Respiratory Syndrome) or pandemic Influenza it is recommended plans and precautions should adhere to guidelines advocated by sources such as the Centers for Disease and Prevention (CDC) and or the World Health Organizations (WHO) and some organisms may require their own separate plan and protocols relative to the nature of the disease and levels of precautions. Materials to develop bioterrorism disease plans are available from the same sources.

Diseases associated with overcrowding (i.e. shelters) such as Staphylococcal skin infections and loss of sanitary systems (i.e. flooding) and gastrointestinal illnesses such as Salmonella, and food associated illness should be considered in both planning and patient screening.

Preparations should also include having psychological counseling available for staff and patients. Natural disasters can significantly affect the physical and mental health of survivors and individuals displaced from their homes.

**Role of ICP**: Preparation of policies, guidelines protocols
Active involvement on drills involving natural and biologic disasters
Assess, adopt and train staff on specific issues/diseases
Advise decision makers on needed supplies, equipment, training needs and mitigation issues.
Active member of Incident Command Team

ICPs need to be involved in assessing mass casualty event readiness, including being involved in the facility hazard vulnerability assessment. Health care facilities need to assess all components of their all-hazards emergency management plan. Infection prevention-related aspects of the emergency management plan are only a small piece of the overall plan. ICP's should provide input to guide decision making, Emergency Preparedness planning, protocol development, drills and critiques.

If the ICP of the facility is a solo practitioner it is a good idea to designate an alternate infection prevention person. This person should be given pre-disaster basic infection control training in infection control/prevention principles and practice. It is of course crucial that the primary ICP is involved in the planning of all infection prevention aspects of the emergency preparedness program to validate required standards are being met in a disaster. It is also important to have the ICP as the designed communicator with local, state and federal public health agencies relative to communicable diseases as they will be both knowledgeable as consultants, available resources and medications.

Emphasize with all employees to assume a disaster will occur. It is a matter of when; not if a disaster will happen. To be prepared for it, all staff should know and understand the incident command system, be aware of and know what policies and protocols are in place and how to adapt and overcome obstacles in any disaster.

**Emergency Planning and Exercises**

Emergency Preparedness is an ongoing process based on current and emerging related information. For the ICP it means continuous preparation in the form of:

1. Ongoing review of pertinent literature from national and local health authorities.

2. Mitigation by anticipating how to minimize impact by use of plans, supply allocation and storage of adequate supplies.
3. Control by making certain staff receive critical information on all infection control and prevention methods for various scenarios.

## Emergency Planning and Exercises

Prevention of diseases for which vaccines are available, including Hepatitis A and B, Influenza, Diphtheria, Pertussis and Tetanus. Encourage pre-disaster immunization programs.

Preparation mechanisms should include individualized plans addressing possible scenarios which are likely to be faced, include cohorting of similar infections.

On a regular basis have "live" Emergency Drills conducted which include infection related aspects and include potential for transmission to healthcare workers. Make it real.

## Monitoring

The facility should be aware of and actively monitor for any emerging crisis to be ready for developing crises and use the advance warning, when available, to begin implementing steps to address a disaster.

Invest in a radio system which has unified radio capability for contact with state, local and other officials on agreed upon frequencies; communication with various entities outside the facility will be crucial.

Medical countermeasures including adequate supply of vaccines and antibiotics with periodic rotation of stocks.

Acquire an internal radio capability with handsets for all ICS members.

Have surge capacity of medical supplies, storage and allocation.

**Preventive and ongoing education by the ICP**:

Transmission concepts.
Basic aseptic technique.
Hand sanitation under disaster conditions
Standard and Isolation Precautions including cohorting.
Extraordinary Precautions for unusual diseases like Ebola.
Decontamination of equipment, environment and people.
Use of PPE observers who monitor and live time critique donning and removing PPE.

**Preventive and ongoing education by the ICP**:
**Issues requiring input by the ICP for Emergency Preparedness Plans**

- Having around the clock infection control coverage with back-up.
- Facility assessment/hazard vulnerability assessment
- Participation in all disaster drills even when a biologic agent is not in the plan.
- Strategies for receiving and posting health alert messages within the facility.
- Negative-pressure surge capacity using portable negative air machines.
- Safe patient specimen collection procedures.
- Patient screening/triage protocols for communicable diseases.
- Food safety and storage capability issues.
- Water management.

- Trash/waste control planning.
- Pet management.
- Environmental decontamination.
- Develop and implement emergency standards of care that reduce infection risk.
- Prioritization for limited supplies of anti-infective therapy
- Employee health/safety procedures
- Outbreak investigation protocols and coordination of any suspected internal infections.

**Education topics ICPs should address with all staff**

- Triage procedures relating to communicable disease.
- Patient decontamination.
- Patient management (patient discharge instructions, when to isolate, and others).
- Disease specific information on bioterrorism agents, emerging infections, and pandemic influenza.
- Self-screening and reporting of symptoms.
- Personal Protective Equipment use and reuse for isolation procedures.
- Procedures for obtaining and handling patient specimens safely.
- Hand hygiene.
- Cleaning and disinfection and use of alternative disinfectants.
- Trash management.
- Emergency management procedures and policies that affect infection transmission.
- How to safely reuse respiratory protection when resources are insufficient or short.
- Postmortem care.

Education of all hospital personnel on infection control preparedness need be in multiple forms in a three part phased plan:

**Part One**

The adult learner accepts new information best when it directly relates to them.

Use well publicized disasters and explain how they impacted the healthcare facilities, focus on the job tasks specific to each group, i.e. Nurses, nursing assistants, Emergency staff, Laboratory, Radiology, Dietary, Material Management, Pharmacy, etc. Provide documentation demonstrating the critical nature of being prepared to operate under sub-optimal conditions and deliver good care. Explain the functioning concepts of the Incident Command System.

**Part Two**

The role of educator is of utmost importance. Training the staff before a crisis, ongoing reinforcement, and "live" drills/exercise will not only prepare them but also build their confidence for the day when they must function in a disaster mode. When they can go through an exercise, learn from errors, make mistakes and corrections and have the instructor explain why the protocol is to be followed in a certain way is tremendously beneficial.

During drills a good practice is to "lose" support which could be affected in a real disaster. Examples include not allowing use of utilities like electricity unless you actually have emergency power capability such as diesel generators and an adequate supply of diesel fuel. If local water service could be lost do not permit use of tap water. If sewerage would be impacted such as with a flood determine how to address loss of toilet facilities. **Hint**: A large stock of kitty litter and plastic five gallon buckets can be a great thing to have on hand in a disaster. Losing the support of things we take for granted in our facilities, like utilities, can help staff to really get a grasp of what to expect and how to overcome these challenges.

**Part Three**

A useful tool I have found is to provide staff with small laminated cards with specific information appropriate to different groups. For example with nursing the card lists diseases and what type of isolation; another card demonstrating PPE donning and removal; for Housekeeping the card shows isolation signs and Information on disinfectants in use, all cards include the ICP's office and cell phone number as well as how to contact me by internal radio. Each card is the same size as the hospital photo ID worn by all and has a hole punched to allow attachment to the back of the ID card providing ready access.

These are examples but you should use your own ideas for what will be helpful in your facility.

**The ICP during the disaster**

When dealing with a disaster; make multiple daily rounds of all active care areas but in particularly the emergency room and intake areas. Maintain a high visibility and engage staff to encourage communication, questions and opportunities for "learning moments".

Communication with staff can assist the ICP in knowing conditions on the care unit, supply concerns, any infectious disease cases present, and other staff concerns.

One useful tool for the ICP is either a tablet or small laptop computer loaded with the facility Emergency Plans, protocols and other information such as CDC guidelines which can be readily accessed during "curbside consults" and answering various questions.

From my own experience in Hurricane Katrina in 2005 the ICP should consider a personal disaster kit to be kept in their office as a means of being self-prepared:

> My kit consists of a full size multi-cell flashlight (like the metal five cell flashlight carried by law enforcement officers), a small one for the pocket (the LED type produces a great deal of light) and are very efficient so the batteries don't require replacement quite so often. A smart cell phone can be a great lifeline to communicate with family. During Hurricane Katrina my voice cellular service was not working but I was able to send and receive text messages. The cell phone is also very useful for recording important notes and photos. Most smart phones can also pick up AM or FM radio stations which facilitate knowing the status of the surrounding area if conditions (i.e. flooding/civil disorder) prevent leaving the hospital.
>
> I also maintain a supply of different sized batteries for personal devices and of course a charger for my cell phone. In this way your office can be a quiet place to retire even if emergency power is not available. Keep a personal supply of hand sanitizer, several packages of baby wipes (which can give you an opportunity for what I called a disaster bath. Also a few rolls of toilet paper and a case of bottled water. A sleeping bag in your office also can be a welcome site at the end of a long day. Also consider a small supply of snack foods such as prepackaged crackers and peanut butter or

cookies, A few creature comforts can boost your spirits and make poor conditions a bit more bearable.

If the hospital has an internal radio system one portable radio should be assigned to the ICP for internal communication.

The ICP is responsible for communicating modifications and/or revisions to Infection prevention policy/protocols related to PPE use or protective measures to personnel when they occur during a disaster.

## The ICP after the disaster

The ICP will need to communicate between the facility and outside agencies like public health authorities. The IP's role in external communication and coordination will depend on the health care facility emergency management plan and radio capabilities.

As your institution begins to recover from the disaster and return to normal talk to the staff and get their ideas and feedback. Their experience can be very useful in post disaster critiques to help improve as well as change things that were not helpful.

## Recovery

When the disaster is over there should be a meeting of the Incident Command Team to do a post-disaster review and critique of all elements; what worked, what did not, and how to enhance the disaster plans. The ICP should contribute the positive aspects as well as that which needs improvement.

During recovery from the disaster and return to normal the ICPs should consider compiling their experiences and sharing their findings with colleagues to help others in their disaster planning.

Learn from our past mistakes to avoid making the same mistakes in the future.

CHAPTER 41

# Pharmacy

• • •

**Robert J. Muller**

THE PHARMACY SHOULD BE WELL stocked for potential anticipated disasters. In most states following 9/11 federal grants, called HRSA, have been allocated to hospitals via the state departments of health and hospitals, for the purpose of stockpiling for disasters. A percentage of each of the grants over the past years has been for stockpiling in the pharmacy.

In anticipation of seasonal events such as hurricane season (June 1 – November 30) or other weather related events, increased inventories of such drugs as tetanus and snake bite anti venom should be visited; depending on the hazard vulnerability of the facility as well as the surrounding locale.

Agreements by memorandums of understanding (MOU) should be executed with other hospital pharmacies in the community as well as the regional area for mutual aide exchange of supplies.

While in most disaster scenarios, pharmaceuticals may be readily available through pharmaceutical warehousing and delivery services; they may be precluded in environmental disasters such as earthquakes, tornadoes and hurricanes due to inability to communicate or access the facility.

The National Stockpile is a cache of drugs that is housed in secret locations strategically located around the United States for delivery to requesting areas within 12 hours. This should be requested through the state regional coordinators of the department of health and hospitals or directly through the county/parish Emergency Operations Command Center; (should additional drugs, vaccines or supplies become critically necessary and unavailable from the contracted supply sources or previous MOU facilities.)

If not already established by the healthcare facility, the name and contact information of the regional coordinator or state contact should be made and recorded as a vital part of the facility emergency management plan.

See Appendix for contents of National Stockpile.

Some states have special disaster laws that take effect upon orders of the Governor during declared disasters. Some of these laws allow hospital pharmacies to dispense quantities of medications to patients either via a clinic attached to the hospital or to hospital patients being discharged. (Many hospitals do not have a license to dispense medications on an outpatient basis).

Check with your local state pharmacy board regarding prescriptive authority associated with disasters so that you may be well informed as well as properly inventoried.

Several of the chain pharmacies now have agreements with hospitals to provide medications to be directly delivered to the hospital for patients take home prescriptions at the time of their discharge. Check with your community pharmacies to see if such a plan can be initiated in times of an impending disaster situation as well as on a regular basis for patient convenience as well as to enhance their satisfaction level with the hospital services offered to their patients.

Some of the laws also allow for community pharmacies to dispense/refill patient medications without physician authorization for a period of one month based on the situation and patient need.

CHAPTER 42

# Hospital Emergency Food Preparation and Applied Food Safety Concepts

• • •

**Alfred Trappey**


## Abstract

*"The Hospital Emergency Food Preparation and Applied Food Safety Concepts chapter was developed as a resource guide written to provide an overview of food preparation and safety standards; regulatory standards necessary to support its Hospital Dietary Department food managers, supervisory personnel, volunteers as well as food service vendors, all working collectively in a hospital food service environment during all levels of emergency meal preparation."*

However, "*It is the responsibility of the Hospital Nutrition and Dietary Department's food managers and shift supervisors, to monitor and maintain all mandated regulatory guidelines of local, county and state health departments in both food safety and sanitary compliance of their establishments during meal preparation; not limited to holding, serving and meal delivery to ambulatory and non-ambulatory clients (volunteers and family members) as well as hospital staff.*"

## Introduction

The intent of this chapter is to offer applied food safety standards along with practical reference guidance to assist hospital dietary food service managers, staff and volunteers on essential food safety protocols. Prior knowledge or understanding acquired through the introduction and use of staff training exercises will reinforce the basic principles of applied food safety when used by hospital dietary department in meal preparation during a catastrophic event.

An accredited hospital nutrition and dietary department must address its key role or contribution in support of its hospital's mitigation plan. The hospital's nutrition and dietary department mitigation plan should not only outline emergency census feeding basics on how to keep predetermined quantities of "in-house" food supplies on hand but also how to organize daily delivery of food staples.

For example, activation of a contractually negotiated future delivery of food staples can be pre-approved by the Hospital Administrative staff' as part of its nutrition and dietary department Continuity of Operations-food service vendor agreements (Memorandums of Understanding/MOU).

"Pre-approve/negotiated" dietary emergency feeding support with the use of Vendor MOU's are now an essential resource function within a Hospital's Emergency Operation Center (EOC) and should be annually reviewed and Administratively recognized as an essential financial obligation on behalf of its Hospital's Emergency Operations Guidelines.

The application of the Dietary Department's operational nutritional feeding, food safety preparation and established serving guidelines must be flexible in order to achieve manageable meal preparation decisions.

A hospital's nutrition and dietary mitigation and response feeding guidelines should address not only catastrophic emergency feeding menus but also recognize local nutritional and dietary support due to the potential for "in-house" shelter in-place mandates.

Remember---it is the responsibility of the "Hospital Dietary department's" food managers to monitor and maintain food safety compliance in their establishments during meal preparation, holding, serving and delivery to ambulatory and non-ambulatory clients as well as hospital staff!

Most hospital food managers will, at some point encounter the challenges presented by natural disasters and the subsequent emergencies they can cause extensive power outages, wind damage from tornadoes, and flooding to name a few. Food service operations should immediately be discontinued and re-evaluated whenever food safety is compromised by an emergency incident.

The likelyhood of accidental chemical releases from nearby industrial corridors and urban transportation routes should also be anticipated. Today, the potential threats of biological, radiological and chemical terrorism exist. Therefore, without exception, each hospital mitigation plan must address the probability of a catastrophic event with resulting in mass casualties; triage of patients and survivors all requiring shelter-in-place protocols.

Therefore, food safety feeding programs at all levels (in-house; shelter in place) by the hospital's Nutrition and Dietary Department must be given serious consideration.

*(State Health Department and Federal Health Codes and Hospital Certification Requirements)*

Offers ongoing food security and emergency preparedness advice.

Serving food safely and efficiently "in-house" to both ambulatory and non-ambulatory patients as well as staff and first responders will require a financial commitment by Hospital Administrators. This commitment specifically directs the hospital dietary food service department to have a State approved mitigation strategy for keeping an adequate food storage inventory on-site (72 hrs) and the necessary security measures to ensure a basic and usable safe food supply.

## Food service operations: Staff

When activated, food handlers must employ "Hospital Emergency Food Safety and Sanitation Operational Guidelines", written specifically by the Nutrition and Dietary Department and formally adopted by Hospital management. Remember, the risk of food contamination increases in emergency situations!

Food handlers must:

- wash hands before and during food preparation;
- work on a clean surface;
- use clean utensils;
- wear a hairnet or a net for beards; and
- stay home when sick.

Food handlers, servers and volunteers are typically cross-utilized from other hospital departments, often over-worked and are operating under both unfamiliar and unsatisfactory conditions (i.e. working weekend shift, night shift).

"*Supervisory oversight*" is essential to ensure safe food handling!

For example:

- availability of a continuous safe water supply;
- food-storage methods;
- workers' personal hygiene;
- food preparation and service;
- waste disposal;
- dishwashing and rinsing procedures; and
- overall kitchen sanitation.

## Food workers and Volunteers

All food workers must practice strict hand washing, maintain good hygiene and be without rashes, sores, cuts, or any communicable disease.

Maintain employee and volunteer illness logs.

Report customer illness complaints to the health department.

Train employees on any changes in serving procedures which may be due to the emergency or by a symptomatic communicable disease; necessary to ensure public health protection.

## Food and storage

Carefully examine all sealed food containers and utensils before using. If perishable foods become warm - do not use.

If canned foods are damaged, puffed or leaking - do not use.

Do not accept food or water from unapproved (i.e., home prepared) or unknown sources where quality control cannot be assured by the County/State Health Department Sanitation Section. Use water only from a safe and approved source.

Inspect all incoming items to detect spoilage, outdated packages or contamination and rodent filth.

Store fruits, vegetables, cooked foods, prepared foods and "ready-to-eat" items above raw meat to prevent cross contamination.

Store all items at least six inches off the ground in insect and rodent-proof containers.

Keep all chemicals away from food and utensils. Label all chemical containers.

## Food preparation

Provide hand washing stations with soap, paper towels, and nail brush.

Eliminate bare-hand contact with ready-to-eat food items (provide gloves, tongs, scoops).

Separate areas should be set up for hand washing, food preparation, and washing and sanitizing utensils.

Prepare quantities sufficient for immediate use. Leftovers must be avoided if refrigeration is inadequate.

Use single-service eating and drinking utensils when possible. Avoid customer self-service.

## Temperature controls

Cook all foods thoroughly; meat, fish, poultry should be well done.

Keep hot foods hot at 140°F or above. Quickly reheat all foods to 165°F or hotter.

Keep cold foods cold at 41°F or below.

Limit food items being cooled. Follow the food code closely for fast and safe cooling.

## Cleaning and sanitation

All food preparation and serving areas should be cleaned and sanitized.

Properly wash (clean water & detergent), rinse, and sanitize (sanitizing solution) all utensils and equipment.

Wash and sanitize cutting boards, knives, and other utensils after each use to prevent cross contamination.

Properly dispose of all solid and liquid waste - frequently.

Control insects and rodents in all food-related areas. Use only approved pesticides and control measures.

Maintain sanitation and regularly clean inside and outside the establishment.

## Regulatory Basics for Handling Food Safely

**Storage**

Always refrigerate perishable food within 2 hours—1 hour when the temperature is above 90 °F (32.2 °C).

Check the temperature of your refrigerator and freezer with an appliance thermometer. The refrigerator should be at 40 °F (4.4 °C) or below and the freezer at 0 °F (-17.7 °C) or below.

Cook or freeze fresh poultry, fish, ground meats, and variety meats within 2 days; other beef, veal, lamb, or pork, within 3 to 5 days.

Perishable food such as meat and poultry should be wrapped securely to maintain quality and to prevent meat juices from getting onto other food.

To maintain quality when freezing meat and poultry in its original package, wrap the package again with foil or plastic wrap that is recommended for the freezer.

Canned foods are safe indefinitely as long as they are not exposed to freezing temperatures, or temperatures above 90 °F. If the cans look ok, they are safe to use. Discard cans that are dented, rusted, or swollen. High-acid canned food (tomatoes, fruits) will keep their best quality for 12 to 18 months; low-acid canned food (meats, vegetables) for 2 to 5 years.

## Meal Preparation

Always wash hands with warm water and soap for 20 seconds before and after handling food.

Don't cross-contaminate. Keep raw meat, poultry, fish, and their juices away from other food.

After cutting raw meats, wash cutting board, utensils, and countertops with hot, soapy water.

Cutting boards, utensils, and countertops can be sanitized by using a solution of 1 tablespoon of unscented, liquid chlorine bleach in 1 gallon of water.

## Frozen Product Thawing

The refrigerator allows slow, safe thawing. Make sure thawing meat and poultry juices do not drip onto other food.

Cold Water: For faster thawing, place food in a leak-proof plastic bag. Submerge in cold tap water. Change the water every 30 minutes. Cook immediately after thawing.

Microwave: Cook meat and poultry immediately after microwave thawing.

## Cooking

Cook all raw beef, pork, lamb and veal steaks, chops, and roasts to a minimum internal temperature of 145 °F (62.8 °C) as measured with a food thermometer before removing meat from the heat source. For safety and quality, allow meat to rest for at least three minutes before carving or consuming. For reasons of personal preference, consumers may choose to cook meat to higher temperatures.

Ground meats: Cook all raw ground beef, pork, lamb, and veal to an internal temperature of 160 °F (71.1 °C) as measured with a food thermometer.

Poultry: Cook all poultry to an internal temperature of 165 °F (73.9 °C) as measured with a food thermometer.

## Serving

Hot food should be held at 140 °F (60 °C) or warmer.

Cold food should be held at 40 °F (4.4 °C) or colder.

When serving food at a buffet, keep food hot with chafing dishes, slow cookers, and warming trays. Keep food cold by nesting dishes in bowls of ice or use small serving trays and replace them often.

Perishable food should not be left out more than 2 hours at room temperature—1 hour when the temperature is above 90 °F (32.2 °C).

## Leftovers

Discard any food left out at room temperature for more than 2 hours—1 hour if the temperature was above 90 °F (32.2 °C).

Place food into shallow containers and immediately put in the refrigerator or freezer for rapid cooling.

**Use cooked leftovers within 4 days.**
**Reheat leftovers to 165 °F (73.9 °C).**

## Refreezing

Meat and poultry defrosted in the refrigerator may be refrozen before or after cooking. If thawed by other methods, cook before refreezing.

## Disposal of food

- Remove to a designated condemned food storage area away from food preparation and equipment storage, and secured in covered refuse containers or other isolated areas to prevent either service to the public, or accidental contamination of the facility and other food.

- If the food must be retained until the distributor can credit the facility, it must be clearly labeled as "not for sale" and kept in a refrigerated location separate from other food.

## Conclusion

Hospital Emergency Food Safety and Sanitation Operation Guidelines are based upon a "risk assessment" and should define catastrophic activation levels; when to institute hospital emergency feeding practices to be followed by its Food Service and Nutrition Department specific to employee/patient safety by appropriately applied food sanitation protocols.

Hospital Emergency Operation Food Safety and Sanitation Guidelines should also be annually reviewed by its Hospital Administrative staff and submitted for final review and approval by the appropriate County/State Health Departments.

The Nutrition and Dietary Department's "Hospital Emergency Operation's Food Safety and Sanitation Guidelines" must be understood, employed and strictly enforced during activation of emergency meal preparations!

## Precautions against Food Contamination

Food-borne illnesses can be avoided by following good food-handling practices. Strict sanitary rules must be implemented to ensure that carefully selected, uncontaminated food and water does not become contaminated during meal preparations.

Personal hygiene regulations are well known in the food service industry, but constant supervision is needed to ensure that those same basic food sanitation rules are followed during continuous 24 hour emergency food operations.

CHAPTER 43

# The FDA and FOOD SAFETY

• • •

**Alfred Trappey**

**DEFINITIONS:** FOOD AND DRUG ADMINISTRATION (FDA). www.fda.gov

If the bacteria is eaten and reproduces in the digestive tract, it is called a **food borne illness**. There are some bacteria that will produce toxins and when this happens, the illness is called a **food borne intoxication**.

**Contamination:** foods can be contaminated in three ways:

1) Biological: when food is contaminated with bacteria, viruses, parasites or fungi
2) Chemical: when food is contaminated by chemicals, often those commonly found in foodservice establishments, such as cleaning products, toxic metals, pesticides, sanitizers and lubricants.
3) Physical: when food is contaminated by a foreign object introduced into the food or may be naturally occurring, such as larvae.

**The keys to food safety lie in controlling time and temperature, practicing good personal hygiene and preventing cross-contamination!**

Food Services Food Safety Training: All personnel working in Hospital Food Services department must have successfully passed basic food safety training prior to being allowed to work in the department.

Food Borne Illness: It is important to understand that ensuring food safety is vital. In order to do this, there are hospital policies and procedures in place that must be followed at all times.

**There are five main reasons why food can be unsafe:**

a) It was purchased from an unsafe source
b) It was inadequately cooked
c) It was held at an improper temperature
d) It was processed in contaminated equipment
e) The food handlers had poor personal hygiene

With the exception of purchasing from an unapproved source, each factor is related to time/temperature abuse, cross-contamination or poor personal hygiene.

**Time/temperature** abuse means that it was:

a) Not properly held or stored at required temperatures or
b) Not cooked or reheated to temperatures that kill microorganisms or
c) Not cooled properly
d) And often prepared too far in advance.

**Cross-contamination** is where microorganisms are transferred from one food or surface to another. This can happen in five ways:

a) Raw contaminated ingredients are added to foods that will not be further cooked
b) Food contact surfaces are not cleaned and sanitized before touching cooked or ready to eat foods

c) Raw food is allowed to touch or drip liquids onto cooked or ready to eat foods
d) Food handler touches contaminated (usually raw) food and then touches cooked or ready to eat foods
e) Contaminated cleaning cloths are not cleaned and sanitized before being used on food-contact surfaces.

**Poor personal hygiene** by food handlers can contaminate food if:

a) food handlers fail to properly wash their hands when they are contaminated
b) they cough or sneeze on food
c) Touch or scratch sores, cuts or infections and then touch food
or report to work when they are contagious and are sick.

**NOTE:** By far the most common infectious agents causing food borne illnesses are bacteria. However, viruses, parasites, molds and fungi are also of great concern.

**The best ways to limit the growth of any of these agents are:**

a) Prevent the initial introduction of the pathogens
b) Kill pathogens by cooking if possible or
c) Reduce the growth of the pathogens by controlling <u>time and temperature</u>

It is important to understand: Bacteria will multiply when conditions are favorable. Food bacteria require protein and/or carbohydrates to grow and reproduce. Food Acidity (pH between 4.6 to 7.5 is most dangerous).

- Temperature between 41°F and 135°F is called the **temperature danger zone, the TDZ.**
- Time (limit of 4 hours in TDZ; 1 bacteria will become >1 billion in 10 hrs)
- Oxygen (most but not all need oxygen)
- Moisture (must have water activity >.85)

Of all these factors, one can best control **time and temperature**.

Keeping food out of the TDZ (between 41°F and 135°F) and limiting food in the TDZ to a **maximum of four hours!**

CHAPTER 44

# Staff Meetings

• • •

**Robert J. Muller**

KEEP THE STAFF WELL INFORMED at all times. Meet with them well in advance of any anticipated disaster and have them tuned into following a standard procedure that all emergency personnel should be aware of and adequately prepared. The best way to help a staff to prepare is to keep them educated through communications.

A **"Go Bag"** is always a <u>must</u>. This should be a medium size soft bag or suitcase, and should be part of any emergency responder's armamentarium. It should contain all personal items such as underwear (buy cheap or disposables), medications (2-4 week supply), hygiene products, extra clothes, uniforms, shoes and coat (in case of evacuation or displacement), cash ($100 minimum—in small as well as mixed bills--$1, 5, 10 and 20—as many business may not be able to make change following a disaster and credit cards may not work if there is no electricity or satellite antennas have been damaged); cell phone and charger, extra batteries as needed for any devices. See Appendix.

Arrangements should be made for staff to have access to a satellite phone. IF the situation and conditions exist when convention telephone and cellular service is non- functional; a satellite phone can be made available at certain times during the day and evening for the staff. A system should be devised in advance for use, such as, 5-6 PM staff with last names of A-G, etc. This allows for more organization and gives the staff less waiting time and thus more productiveness during working hours. A reasonable time limit for use should likewise be imposed (3-7 minutes), depending on the number of employees and the size of the facility, in order to facilitate comprehensive coverage of all personnel.

It is recommended that unless the facilities has numerous satellite phones, that the phones be kept open during normal business hours to facilitate operational continuity, and the staff only be allowed use during slack periods of time.

Pre-arranged understandings with the staff should include when the "B" team is to return for duty or how they are to be contacted for return duty.

The use of text messaging and phone trees should be encouraged; also a distant contact that could be used for a HAM operator to contact to initiate a phone tree might also be given consideration.

During a disaster it is important to keep the staff updated at least every eight hours by means of the Incident Commander, PIO, or CEO, meetings with supervisors, an intranet system, or message/bulletin boards placed around the hospital in non -public locations, such as staff lounges. It is important that the person in charge have at least one face to face meeting every 24 hours with the staff to show full engagement and commitment.

COMMUNICATION with the staff and the staff with their families is ESSENTIAL to the well- being and mental health of all personnel within the hospital environment.

The first and most essential principal is **"caring for our own".**

CHAPTER 45

# Training

• • •

Robert J. Muller

## Drills and Exercises:

Exercises provide opportunities to practice and test public information capabilities and to improve and maintain proficiency in a controlled environment. Exercises assess and validate policies, plans, and procedures, and clarify and familiarize personnel with roles and responsibilities. Exercises improve interagency coordination and communication, highlight gaps, and identify opportunities for improvement.

The topic of drills and exercises is an entire subject matter in of itself and much too detailed for the content of this book. There are several excellent works that address these subjects at great length and I refer you to the following resources for a more detailed study of this subject matter.

*Publication AHQR--#08-0019 June 2008 John Hopkins University, "Tools for Developing Core Elements of Hospital Disaster Drills".

Principles of Emergency Management, Fagel, M., CRC Press

## FEMA Courses:

FEMA offers approximately 100 self-study courses which are available from their web site and provide an immediate certificate of completion after successfully passing the final exam(1).

In addition, FEMA offers in residence courses held at the training institute located in Emmitsburg, Maryland and application can be made through your state training director by application offered on line(2).

Courses are also offered at the Center for Domestic Preparedness in Anniston, Alabama on a mostly abandoned military base, in conjunction with the Department of Homeland Security (DHS). This facility has a full scale hospital facility for medical preparedness exercises as well as providing some of the most comprehensive hazardous materials decontamination simulation, as well as direct materials exposure, offered in the United States(3).

On line training links:

1. FEMA Independent Study http://training.fema.gov/IS/
2. FEMA Emmitsburg Training Courses http://training.fema.gov/EMICourses/
3. FEMA Center for Domestic Preparedness https://cdp.dhs.gov/

Required training for the Command and General Staff: (Dependent on the facility size and community involvement and interaction with other agencies)

Introduction to the Incident Command System (ICS-100)
http://training.fema.gov/EMIWeb/IS/is100.asp
ICS for Single Resources and Initial Action Incidents (ICS-200)
http://training.fema.gov/EMIWeb/IS/is200.asp
Intermediate Incident Command System (ICS-300)

http://www.fema.gov/about/contact/statedr.shtm
National Incident Management System (NIMS), An Introduction (IS-700)
http://training.fema.gov/EMIWeb/IS/is700.asp
Recommended courses:
Basic Public Information Officers Course (G-290)
http://training.fema.gov/EMIWeb/EMICourses/E388.asp and
http://www.fema.gov/about/contact/statedr.shtm
Advanced Public Information Officer (E-388)
http://training.fema.gov/EMIWeb/EMICourses/E388.asp
Advanced Incident Command System (ICS-400)
http://www.fema.gov/about/contact/statedr.shtm
National Incident Management Systems (NIMS), Public Information Systems (IS-702)
http://training.fema.gov/EMIWeb/IS/is702.asp
National Response Plan (NRP), An Introduction (IS-800)
http://training.fema.gov/EMIWeb/IS/is800a.asp

Staff Education and Training:
"When emergencies strike, the casualties are not the only victims. Staff members in your *organization will be on the front line responding to any emergency your community faces. The* best way a health care organization can prepare staff members to meet the challenges of an emergency is to educate them in all aspects of working and protecting themselves in such a situation."

Training is essential. The absence of training is the absence of preparation. Poorly prepared and educated staff is of little value to the organization as well as a potential liability and could even pose a threat and danger to themselves as well as their coworkers.

Training may take place in many forms, including self-education through numerous web sites, in service lectures, community lectures and guest lectures. Many subject matter experts (SME) are available for training and resources may include the local as well as state agencies, communications, information technology, hazard materials and post-traumatic stress experts to name only a few.

The Federal Emergency Management Agency (FEMA) Emergency Management Institute (EMI) Independent study (IS) program (http://training.fema.gov/IS/crslist.asp) has an excellent array of online courses available. Upon successful completion a certificate may be printed. (A permanent record of training is also kept at EMI under the individual social security number for future reference) All hospital personnel should understand the basics of the Incident Command system (ICS) and thus course IS 100.HCb should be mandatory. Additional ICS courses, 200, 300 and 400 are significantly more advanced and should be required of those with Incident Command assignments on both the command staff and general staff levels. The IC should have at least the 300 level of training and someone capable of in service training should obtain the 400 level to be qualified as an instructor. Most IS courses carry the availability of college credits, and in addition, may be used by many certifying boards and organizations for continuing education credits.

In addition, the staff should be trained on IS 700 and 1900. All staff member training records must be kept either as hard copy or on computer or preferably both, for inspection by The Joint Commission should there be an inquiry.

Training cost should be a part of all hospitals budget. However, emergency management, incident command, technology, hazardous materials, chemical, radiological, explosive and bioterrorism training cost may be reimbursable through various grants, including the present Health Resources Services Administration (HRSA) grant from the Center for Disease Control (CDC) through state Departments of Health and Hospitals. This was created after the events of 911 and has been available up until the present time (2016). Its perpetuity is unknown for future planning.

Remember-there is no such thing as over training and various members of the staff should be trained for multiple positions should they be needed; a good example would be to have someone trained in helicopter landing safety and procedures besides their regular duties, and the possibility exists that this scenario may become a reality. Remember, just because a hospital does not have an official FAA heliport, does not preclude a nearby landing in a field, vacant property or the street should a dire emergency situation exist. (This is for an example only; and many other similar dual situations may likewise have more value).

CHAPTER 46

# Stress Management

• • •

**Robert J. Muller**

THE STRESS OF WORKING IN an active EOC can be equated to the stress encountered by air traffic controllers. It is ever present and constantly demanding. There is little or no options for failure and in the EOC situation there will always be some form of minor or major conflict with other coworkers.

When assigning roles for positions in the Incident Command structure the most important factor is the persons qualifications and expertise; the second most important is personality---can the person handle the job as well as the stress that goes along with its responsibility.

In order to determine these two factors it is best to create exercises that test both the competency as well as the human factor reactions to situations.

It is imperative that the personnel be given adequate breaks, keep well hydrated and eat the proper foods, and that sleep time be determined with alternating changes of shifts during the height of an event, unless a general and command staff briefing is planned to be done at one time.

If a facility has the luxury of having a staff psychiatrist or psychologist available during an event, it is worthwhile to have him/

her attend staff meetings at least once a day to pick up on any potential staff escalating stress levels.

Generally, the longer and more complex the event, the more likely there will be a command or general staff conflict. This is also more common when these staff members are not well trained and do not feel competent in their job positions, as well as those who feel they are better qualified to assume another position level, i.e. a general staff person desiring a command staff position.

It is also of great value to bring this topic up at the very first staff meeting so that the subject is breached and that all members are well aware of a potential situation and what to expect in case a situation does arise.

Upon completion of the event during the demobilization process a qualified Critical Incident Stress Management (CISM) professional should meet with the team and discuss the signs and symptoms of post-traumatic stress syndrome and provide information as to how, when and where they may obtain future help and counseling should it be needed. It is useful if the facility has a staff psychologist or psychiatrist that is available in house during or at least immediately available after the incident to help with the CISM.

CHAPTER 47

# Hospital Emergency Waste Management

• • •

**Alfred Trappey**

In the event of a natural disaster or a deliberate act of terrorism, the infrastructure that routinely deals with the storage, collection and disposal of solid and liquid waste (i.e., non-hazardous commercial and industrial waste) may be interrupted anywhere from a few days to several months. Failure of any or part of the waste collection system in a populated hospital during a catastrophic event for two to three weeks could lead to many public health-related problems. (1)

There are two basic categories of disaster impacts regarding hospital emergency waste management: First, is the disruption of the solid waste storage, collection, and disposal system that affects the ability for ongoing generation of solid waste to be managed properly. This includes hazardous solid waste generated by ongoing surgical procedures, patient care, food service activities; all during a hospital's emergency response efforts. Second, janitorial management control of large quantities of liquid waste accumulating from a blocked or damaged sewer lines or restroom facilities (i.e., toilets and laboratories).

Hospital emergency procedures may call for separating out solid materials requiring different types of containment methods, and then ensuring proper management and temporary on-site storage of each material type.

## Hospital Emergency Operations Waste Management Response

Disaster situations often result in large volumes of waste or building debris that can overburden the waste management infrastructure of a hospital and present the following potential public health concerns: insect and rodent harborage; diseases caused by environmental agents (e.g., mold); and chemical contamination. If from an earthquake, building debris in the form of dust could be contaminated with radioactive particles, lead, and mercury.

In this situation, the following procedural objectives in mitigation and response strategies need to be pre-addressed in a hospital's emergency operations response plan at various levels of activation:

1. Determine the extent of disruption to the Hospital's solid/liquid waste management system.
2. Provide information to upper level hospital administrators about potential public health concerns.
3. Ensure managerial compliance of all hospital regulatory waste disposal guidelines including use of temporary on-sight storage.
4. Temporary on-site storage of waste materials being generated by a hospital operating under emergency conditions should be pre-approved by the local and state health departments defining proper storage, collection, and management of hazardous waste.
5. Request guidance, oversight, and remember to assign a hospital staff liaison to the local office of public and environmental health.

## Waste Management Emergency Activation

Emergency waste consolidation, janitorial staff consolidation, waste accumulation segregated by hazardous class, regulatory approval to activate temporary on-site storage, hospital site security, containment and inability for off-site disposal service access must have an overall director to closely monitor waste accumulation according to "best practices".

In order to maintain a safe and effective hospital waste management service program during an on-going catastrophic patient surge, hospital leadership should also have within its Hospital Emergency Operations Plan (HEOP), a budgetary mitigation strategy to effectively manage waste generation and should consider as a viable option, the consolidation of waste collection generated daily by individual hospital departments' (in addition to ancillary support centers) into a singular emergency services solid/ liquid hazardous waste disposal program.

## Potential benefits of developing a unified emergency waste management plan:

- allow hospital administrators and department directors to make key decisions and identify roles and responsibilities prior to, during and after a catastrophic event.
- collectively, the concept of consolidation of hospital hazardous waste disposal is scalable can be pre-determined and pre-approved by local, county, state and federal regulatory agencies, all necessary hazardous waste disposal mandates!
- technical resource guidance for on-site hospital hazardous waste accumulation and pre-identified hospital physical plant storage locations to be used.
- flexibility by working from internally agreed upon consolidation of departmental directives and be willing to reallocate budgetary resources, and share on-going contracts,

collection services, vendor contracts and activation of waste management services MOUs.
- recognize and allow for potential physical, staffing and resource limitations in developing a waste management consolidation plan.

## Emergency waste management plans provide additional benefits to a hospital including:

Potential emergency waste generation estimates provided by hospital operational departments as well as pre-identifying hazardous waste classes should result in a definable (characterization) summation of the whole (i.e. solid/liquid waste) to be anticipated during emergency activation!

1. Hospital departments that have established biological, chemical and nuclear hazardous waste removal plans are better equipped to estimate waste generation levels as the intensity of the catastrophic event increases over an undetermined emergency operations time period.
2. Evaluating existing disposal resources and disposal management services helps to identify gaps prior to an incident.
3. Consolidation of planning by each contributing department towards its role in the generation of hazardous waste disposal helps hospital management understand how increases in emergency activation levels affect initial allocated hospital waste management budgets pre-established annually to accommodate normal operations.
4. The hospital's physical plant has only a finite space allocated to holding containerized hazardous waste until disposal.

## Conclusion

Emergency Waste Management Response Strategies if attached to a broader Hospital Emergency Operations Plan (HEOP) could potentially ease the burden of staff management by introducing efficiencies such as departmental consolidation of collective waste disposal services. Emergency consolidation of hazardous waste is a viable option and may be a necessary option when dealing with on-site consolidated storage of regulated solid and liquid waste. (2)

Budgetary constraints also affect the number of staff supporting waste collection as well as the inability of its hospital's administrators to project the overall cost for additional waste management resources. Specialized containment resources are needed while accumulating chemical and radiological wastes in addition to being isolated and segregated from medical waste in order to avoid dual contamination. All emergency waste stored on hospital's premises should be secure to prevent access by unauthorized persons as well as to prevent accidental spread of contamination.

Emergency waste management guidelines can be established and tested to determine if on-site hazardous waste storage is available and initiate collection services contract options for hospital hazardous waste disposal. The designated storage area for medical waste must display the appropriate warning signs using wording required by Health and Safety Codes.

In a catastrophic emergency, the potential for overloading the waste handling capacity of the hospital is greatly increased. Because of this potential, **each hospital must develop its own unique set of emergency waste management protocols** in addition to existing current waste management plans that address the challenges associated with the increased consolidated volume of medical and hazardous waste necessary for temporary emergency on-site storage. All hospital waste generated and containerized for disposal most often will be classified, handled and treated as hazardous waste. (2)

## References

1. Veterans Health Administration Center for Engineering & Occupational Safety and Health in their Emergency Management Program Guidebook, 2005. www1.va.gov/emshg/page.cfm Volume I: Hospitals, Section 5.12.1: Development of Standard Operating Procedures for Maintaining Infrastructure during a Healthcare Surge.
2. Louisianan Department of Health and Hospitals. www.new.dhh.louisiana.gov

CHAPTER 48

# Forensics and Death Investigation

• • •

## Capt. Ronald Frey (Ret.)

FROM TIME TO TIME THERE are incidents that are of a forensic nature and require proper training and handling to be compliant in the transfer of potential evidence.

The most common incidents in hospitals are victims with gunshot or knife/ice pick wounds with the cartridge or object readily visible, loose or impaled.

These objects should be treated as evidence and handled appropriately with the proper use of gloves and proper tagging, initialing and bagging to be turned over to the requesting law enforcement agency.

Sexual assault victims clothing should be collected and properly bagged according to pre designed protocols; and labeled and sealed with evidence tape in paper bags only (never use plastic bags). All evidence gathered should be **initialed** by the person who collected the evidence. **Initial** the waistband of clothing with a permanent marker, scrape your initials on the blade or handle of a knife, gun, bullet, etc. (An ice pick is excellent for this purpose).This will always answer the question asked in cases that go to court of "how do you know this is the same piece of evidence that you collected"---answer---by my initials marked on it.

The chain of evidence **MUST** be maintained and potential evidence should **NOT** be allowed to be laying on carts or tables, etc.

Once evidence is collected, each person to whom the evidence is transferred **MUST** be required to sign an evidence transfer sheet to maintain the chain. At NO time and to NO ONE should evidence be handled unless the proper transfer sheet is signed and maintained with the evidence, and a copy retained in the patient's hospital records (chart). The original evidence transfer sheet should follow the evidence and is to be signed and given to law enforcement. The last signature that should appear on the evidence transfer sheet in the patient record should be that of the law enforcement officer (LEO) accepting custody of the evidence; beyond that point it becomes the LEO responsibility to continue the chain. If for some reason the evidence is not able to be immediately transferred to a LEO, then it should be secured in a locked safe, closet, or narcotics locker with limited key access by staff members. At NO time should it be "secured" in an employee's car or trunk.

Bioterrorist and Hazardous Materials events mandate special handling of victims clothing not only from an evidence standpoint BUT also from a decontamination standpoint. Great care must be taken as well as proper training and drilling of staff to deal with such incidents prior to their occurrence. The necessary supplies and personal protective suits (PPE) must be available to deal with such incidents. A Standard Operating Procedure (SOP) must be written in conjunction with local law enforcement and fire officials as to who becomes responsible for victims clothing for evidence purposes as well as proper disposal.

## Standard Operating Procedures for Forensic Death Investigation

Forensic Fatality Incidents can occur two ways: One by man and the second by nature and both can cause massive destruction to life and property. Death caused by both will be handled in the same manner.

However, one could end up in a Criminal Court and/or Civil Court and thus precise details and protocols MUST be followed.

The hospital should have a set of Standard Operating Procedures (SOP) and a set of Administrative Operation Procedures (AOP). Each doctor and nurse that works within the emergency room setting should study and know these procedures for their protection; especially nurses if they are going to be the ones responsible for collecting items from the deceased victims.

This section will give you some ideas as what should be listed in a Standard Operation Procedure (SOP).

- Pre –assigned assignments to key personnel overall duties and per shift duties.
- One Nurse/Person should take charge and be the evidence custodial.
- Forms: ex. Chain of Evidence/Property forms, ink pens, permanent marks, permanent metal markers, should be readily available and stored in a specific area, etc.
- Supplies: Papers bags, round plastic containers, clear plastic bags, evidence tags, evidence tape, disposable scissors, disposable mask, disposable gloves and tweezers, likewise stored in one location.
- One nurse should be assigned to take charge and be the evidence custodial per shift.
- Barcode generator software and printer---if the facilities handle large volumes of forensic cases.
- Body bags.
- Refrigerated trailer should be available by a pre -established contractual arrangement with a vendor to handle potential mass fatality situations.
- Camera and most importantly, personnel trained in the technique of forensic photography.

## Photographs

Every victim that passes through the hospital in the Mass Fatalities Incident should be photographed.

First, an overall view of the deceased from the head to the foot of the body.

Second, an overall view of the deceased from the feet to the head of the body.

Third, shoot straight down looking down at the deceased's face.

Fourth, with help, roll the deceased over and get a full overall back side view.

Fifth, if there are any wounds on the body, you will need to take an overall view of the wounds and then close up views of each of the wounds.

Sixth, if anything fell from the deceased's body while in your presence, you photograph, collect, label and bag it with the proper identifying information.

Seventh, any jewelry collected from the deceased's body needs to be photographed from several different views.

Eighth, all clothing collected from the deceased's body should be photographed when collected.

All of the photographs should be entered into evidence in a clear plastic evidence bag unless the photographs are digital then a set can be printed from a computer and entered. Each printed photo should be initialed by the person who took the photograph for later verification purpose.

## Chain Of Evidence Form

This is a very important document. On the top left line of this form should be a place for an item number or incident number and on the right should be a place for the date of occurrence.

On the second line there should be a place for the name of the victim, if it is known, along with date of birth or other possible identifying data. Every item collected from the decreased body should be recorded on this form with the following information: on what date, time, place, and a description of what was collected all to be recorded on the form and repeated for each item collected.

When collecting clothes and items from the deceased's body, one should use a method that you feel safe for you. All clothing should have a marking of the person collecting the items. Using a permanent marker they should place her/his initials in a place, more commonly around the wristband, on said clothing so she/he will able to identify it should a case develop and go to trial. If you must cut the clothing off the deceased and the clothing is wet from either blood or other liquids, do not cut into the liquids if you can. Try to find a spot to cut without cutting into blood, or try removing the clothing by hand. Always remember that someone's initials need to be on the collected items.

All clothing evidence goes in paper bags. If the items are wet, double or triple bag the evidence. No exceptions. *Never put clothing in a plastic bag.*

If while collecting the clothing or other items you see pieces of hair, fiber, or items that looks out of place, **collect** them by using disposable forceps or hemostat to pick it up put and place it in a round clear plastic container; **seal** the containers with evidence tape and **label** it with the vital information; then as the final step, **log** it on the evidence sheet. Do this with each piece of evidence you remove from the deceased's body or clothing and be sure to log everything on the chain of evidence log sheet.

When collecting any gold looking jewelry you will list it as YELLOW METAL and not as gold. When collecting any silver looking jewelry, you will list it as WHITE METAL and not as silver, because you are not a certified jeweler.

The same follows for stones, diamonds, and any other valuable gems. List them by their color. Diamonds will be clear stones. You will have green stones, blue stones and red stones. Remember you are not a certified gemologist.

Upon completion, collection, initialed and recorded on the chain of evidence form, place in the evidence bags ----- complete the forms on the outside of the evidence bags that match the evidence forms.

Note: If you have several evidence bags you should set up a labeling system either by number or alphabet. This would help keep the bags in order when recording them and keeping track of them.

Now find a safe, secure, locked area that only you can access with a key and that has an alarm system. This is so only you will be able to place everything in secure storage until law enforcement personnel come collect it from you. (If you have to testify in court regarding your collection of this evidence you must be able to state ONLY you had access to this cabinet, box, locker or safe, etc.

Once you, as the evidence person, take control of the evidence either by collecting it yourself from the deceased person or receiving it from another person, **no one** is to come in contact with that evidence until you sign it over to a law enforcement officer. He/she will have to sign each of the chain of evidence sheets and you MUST retain a copy of each sheet for your records.

This sheet will release you of all responsibility should anything be reported missing before leaving your control and you have a receipt that it left your control.

## In Hospital Death Investigation

Death is a common place factor associated with hospitals, BUT death under unusual circumstances not associated with the normal causality requires special significance and handling, and requires for protocols to be in place.

A good example may be an employee that was performing a task alone and has a fatal heart attack and is either found in a remote area of the hospital (i.e. storage or maintenance area or warehouse), or falls off a balcony, etc.

There may be instances where a person dies from trauma unrelated to their original admitting diagnosis, i.e. fall out of bed or down a stairs, or situations where someone is murdered or commits suicide in the hospital or hospital grounds usually related to domestic disputes, mental patients, or prisoners in custody.

In such cases as always, the patient well-being comes first, BUT if the patient is obviously dead without hope of resuscitation, then the area should be treated as a crime scene and immediately protected by closing off the area and placing someone in charge of the area while the proper agencies and administrative personnel are notified.

The body should not be left alone once it is discovered unless there is no other means of obtaining assistance in the absence of any form of communications, and this only for the briefest period of time necessary. Once the proper investigative authorities arrive, then, with their permission, the role may be terminated.

All information and the persons' immediate findings and observations likewise must be given either in writing or verbal statement to the proper investigative authority.

Depending upon the circumstances, the employee's actions may become pertinent in either a criminal or civil court action, so my suggestions would be to have them prepare a precise signed written statement with an administrative witness. This obviously is not only for future review and recall but also for self as well as facility protection.

Always remember **DOCUMENTATION** by a witness can turn out to be your best friend in a forensic death investigation that results in criminal or civil litigation and trial proceedings.

CHAPTER 49

# Corporate Security's Response to Ebola

• • •

Michael Fagel

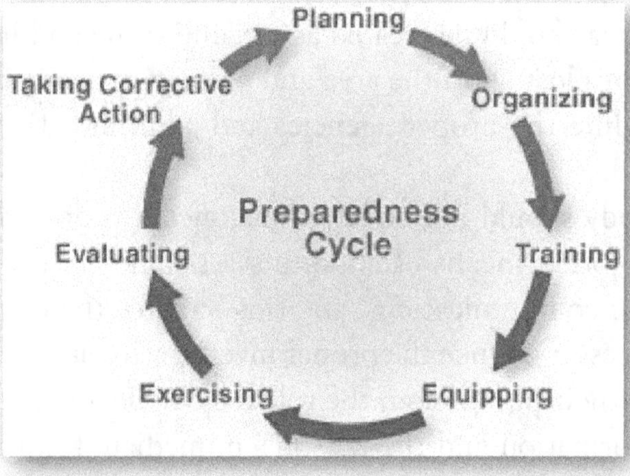


The Emergency Management Cycle is just as important to the corporate security manager as it is to any other person or agency that has a role dealing with incident response. It is only through effective and thorough planning and training, under the preparedness portion of the cycle, that security professionals will know how to adequately respond to a major incident that is clearly beyond the scope of routine emergencies, which are typically handled by local fire, police, and EMS resources.

But for incidents that are larger and global as well as local in scope, such as an Ebola outbreak, the corporate facility security manager is going to be involved in a variety of different fashions. Moreover, he or she must also be able to answer a variety of questions very quickly after an incident occurs to determine what kind of response is needed.

The following four questions are among those that corporate security managers need to consider.

## What Is the Scope of the Incident?

Ebola is an ever-present threat in Africa, but it has been moving throughout the world. Most recently, new cases were reported in Dallas, Texas, following the death of Liberian native Thomas Eric Duncan (October 2014).

It is unlikely that the local public health agency, no matter how well-equipped and organized it is, will be able to handle such cases, or a wider outbreak, on its own. In addition, a locality will rarely have sufficient supplies of the medicines needed in Ebola treatments or the protective clothing that must be used by care givers when handling the response and treatment.

The SNS was designed to be able to send needed supplies of medicines to localities within twelve hours of request. Beyond simply providing medicines, the SNS also houses supplies of antidotes, antitoxins, and medical/surgical items. It is specifically designed to bring necessary resources to localities that in most cases will not be expected to stock all such things—even though the public will need them in the case of specific types and degrees of disasters.

Initial contact with SNS officials should be made within the first six to twelve hours after an incident has occurred or discovered, to assure the most rapid delivery of supplies and medicines to those in the community that will need them immediately.

From a corporate security perspective, other concerns must be look into as the time beyond an event changes from hours to days. Has removing clothing, bedding, and medical supplies used by Ebola patients created an environmental impact and if so, what federal and state officials and agencies will need to be called in to assist in assessment, cleanup, and recovery? Is an evacuation center needed to isolate patients, and if so, how will affected people be transported to that facility?

**Exhibit 1**, Security Response Plan: Timeline, lists security concerns in the aftermath of an incident, at varying time intervals. While certain responsibilities are listed for certain time periods, keep in mind that as part of the response, those tasks that need to be taken care of early in a response will need to be continued as the response moves along, even as new responsibilities are added.

## Who Will Be Involved?

An incident commander under the nationally adopted Incident Command System (ICS) procedure is probably going to be in place by the time the corporate facility security manager gets word of a significant incident that will require his or her involvement and response. When state and federal resources are called in, a clear point of contact needs to be established to make sure everything is delivered efficiently and effectively. Certain lines of communication may have to be kept open in the wake of a medical disaster. One person needs to coordinate the information gathering and dissemination, making sure that while the public does not overly panicked, they also do not underestimate the gravity of the situation. Employees and medical personnel should be kept accurately informed of what their immediate, short-term, and long- term next steps should be.

Corporate security can assist in very specific ways to help ensure that the crisis is handled smoothly. Have training exercises and materials been developed that clearly indicate how security will be a part of the emergency management effort? Are there resources that the security team needs to access that are not immediately available in an affected area? How quickly can security provide these resources to the incident commander? Can security assist in providing transportation for a medical or research doctor from outside the area that may have particular expertise in Ebola?

The success of a security organization's response to an Ebola incident will depend greatly on the cooperation of many people. Security should look for assistance and help in coordination from a number of agencies and officials, and the lines of communication should be opened well before any incident takes place, specifically during the Preparedness phase of the Emergency Management Cycle.

The types of people that security needs to contact after an incident will always depend on the incident itself. Many crises will not require the expertise of an epidemiologist. But you can't discount the contribution that person could make in the event of the discovery of an Ebola case in your jurisdiction, Likewise personnel will vary from incident to incident.

**Exhibit 2** is a list of contacts with whom the corporate security function should have constantly open lines of communication to effectively and efficiently coordinate a fast response. The more prepared the better.

## When Can Security be the Most Helpful?

The type of response needed from a company's security team varies by the amount of time that has elapsed after an incident occurs. What is needed in the first three hours after an incident is different from what is needed after the first twelve hours, for example.

In the first hours, the corporate security team should determine if its facilities are affected and how many employees could be involved. Security will also need to know who the other responders are to the incident, as well as whom the incident commander is—if the Incident Command System has been set up at that point.

It's also important to know if an Emergency Operations Center (EOC) has been activated and if it will provide information to the security staff to help coordinate the response to the incident.

Remember, corporate security will not lead the incident response except in rare cases, so this early coordination in the first three hours after an incident is critical to assuring a cooperative, efficient, and effective response plan.

Three to six hours after the incident occurs, the security function may need to take on additional responsibilities while continuing to carry out all earlier tasks. This next period of time serves as the first window to begin seriously updating the public about what has taken place, what rescue and stability plans are in place and are being activated, if an evacuation or isolation plan is necessary, and whether avenues have been set up to receive donations of food, clothing or even blood.

Another critical function of this post-incident communication is providing direction for employees with special needs, who are disabled, or for whom English is not their first language. Communicating what has occurred and what next steps they should take is a critical part of knowing the make-up of the employee base. All employees need to know if they should stay home or take certain precautions so as to not be adversely affected by any exposure to other potentially infectious materials (OPIM), blood, or body fluids. The Occupational Safety & Health Administration (OSHA) has a set of regulations covering OPIM under 1910.1030.

Also, what may start as a local incident may become a crisis requiring a state and federal response, and these agencies may seek out their security counterparts for coordinating their actions. In light of their needs, the security staff may also discover that local supply resources and staffing needs are insufficient for this level and response, and contingency staffing plans may need to be activated.

## What Role Should Security Play?

The type of incident at hand will always determine what sort of response is needed from the corporate security team. The time to decide how to respond to an Ebola incident is not after an incident occurs. This is where the preparedness portion of the Emergency Management Cycle is critical.

As part of the training and preparedness process, the security manager must, with the cooperation of other agencies and neighboring jurisdictions, lay out specific plans for how to respond to various types of incidents. The security department must understand the fundamental ways to respond to not only the possibility of casualties, but also the potential disruption of services and supplies that the public would view as basic needs.

Another point to consider is that first responders and everyone else who will be offering some sort of assistance after an incident have probably developed their own plans for how to do so, based on what the incident is. The security aspect of the response cannot ignore the plans of everyone else. The security staff should be trained in the entire emergency operations plan for a specific facility and organization.

It is important that everyone is on the same page at all points during the response to an incident. Success in this area prevents "turf wars" between agencies and jurisdictions over who is the right person or agency to carry out a particular part of a response. Another matter to think about is that security should be involved in, or create, a continuity of operations plan that will allow the business to operate should certain personnel or departments be affected by the Ebola crisis.

For the most part, the corporate security manager is not going to be the lead in incident command. Instead, the security staff will be coordinating various aspects of the response that medical, law enforcement, and EMS crews are not going to have the time or ability to deal with, such as acquiring resources and supplies or coordinating public information.

For staff training, **Exhibit 2**, Security Response Plan: Ebola Incident, can be used to handle conditions that will vary by the severity, location, and scope of an incident. But this plan can also help security directors determine who should be involved in an incident response, what coordination needs to take place with outside agencies and jurisdictions, what safety measures need to be taken, and what other questions need to be asked immediately after an incident occurs so that the response can be efficient and effective. It is a starting point to effective planning that should also include instruction, exercises, and coordination with other likely responders.

## Training in Action, Part 1

The final section of this chapter will describe corporate security's role in an incident response- based scenario dealing with Ebola, and the confirmation of cases in the community where the company operates.

A first thought may be to skip this section; after all, as of October 2014, only two patients have been reported in the United States, and the likelihood that it would affect other communities seems very small.

But in emergency management, this is exactly where the training process begins instead of ends. The key to successful emergency management coordination is planning for everything, to the point of having a Plan X when all the other plans have failed. Two cases of Ebola, as you will see in this scenario, do not instantly set off the kind of response effort you would expect if a jetliner crashed in a densely populated residential neighborhood, such as what occurred outside New York City several years ago. However, the sequence of events and contacts that the security director must work on and with is similar and every bit as important.

One factor to consider in an Ebola incident, or similar type of disease outbreak, is that the typical first responders won't necessarily be in play. Police, fire, and EMS, who will be first on the scene in a transit accident, derailment, plane crash or explosion will not be the first ones called in should an Ebola case be discovered near a corporate facility. Instead, a public health officer is likely to be the first person made aware of the situation once the first patient who has been infected is in the hospital. From there, the scenario would look something like this.

- What medicines are available to treat the person infected in this particular case? The primary caregivers at the medical center will know what medication is immediately available to assist the patient (but not cure the disease).
- Who else in that medical center may be infected?
- Could the disease have spread to either a caregiver or another patient? How many patients have checked out of that facility in the time that this patient has been there? Thus raising the possibility (no matter how small it may be) that the disease could be carried into the general population in your area?

If there has been no apparent spread, an incident zone can be established, with many of the people who need to handle this situation already in place. Local or regional doctors and/or research experts knowledgeable about how to treat and contain Ebola should be contacted. This sort of assistance and expertise may only be available at the federal level, depending on your locality, and such contact needs to be made as quickly as possible so the proper authorities can be dispatched.

It is entirely possible, of course, that if an Ebola case has been discovered near a company's facility, others cases may be waiting in the jurisdictions around you. Word must be spread to their public health officials as quickly as possible to start any possible response and to garner help from other security professionals.

At this point, someone is going to have to speak to the public about this incident. The public, including all employees, will need to know about possible symptoms, and where to go to get assistance if they are afraid of possibly having caught the disease. The public will also want to know what precautions to take if they don't have symptoms. In this age of instant information, news will leak out, and the media will most likely converge on the corporation's site, looking for more detailed status reports and interviews.

Police as well as local and state government officials may want to discuss a possible quarantine station if other cases exist, or to remove the current case from the medical center to avoid the risk of infecting other patients or caregivers. The public will need to know where this area is so as to avoid it, and the police will be needed to not only help set it up in some cases, but also to provide protection.

Once word is released of this case, it is possible that a sort of panic will fall over the population, including employees, and anyone who feels they are suffering from symptoms similar to those described for Ebola may call in sick. The HR department should be made aware of this possibility, and a coordinated way to respond to extensive sick leave requests should be established.

Obviously, the CDC will want to know of these developments, and they will be the foremost experts in what steps the community should take next both in dealing with the patient, caregivers, and the public. They will also be able to quickly dispatch experts into the locality and may well take the lead on that side.

In addition, experts from the CDC can also advise, based on the situation, if any kind of personal protective equipment is necessary, where it can be obtained, and who should have it. Officials from the SNS can have supplies, medicines, surgical and medical equipment and other such needs delivered to your locality within twelve hours, with the help of state officials.

## Training in Action, Part 2

So, three hours have now passed. Because of the open lines of communication established during crisis management training, the security staff is getting the news from those involved in the coordinated response effort, which is operating efficiently and effectively at this point.

In the next three hours, the original patient has been successfully moved to a different facility and quarantined. The public has been informed through TV and radio about the situation and what to do if they want assistance. A call for calm has been sounded.

The SNS is sending supplies, officials from the CDC are en route, and experts in how Ebola develops and is transmitted are working with area doctors and staff to try and track down how this case ended up in your locality.

So what's next for security?

The corporate director of security will need to be constantly updated on the patient, his or her reaction, and all the steps that those involved in the response are taking. Constant communication with the designated incident commander is critical.

It is very important that corporate security interacts with employees during this time. While everyone is obviously worried about the possible spread of the disease, security can play an important role in efforts to soothe and educate employees. Remember, in this crisis the vast majority of the populace will have no idea what they should or shouldn't do in this situation to stay safe.

Panic is one of the leading risks to an effective emergency response, so information needs to be disseminated quickly, accurately, and consistently in multiple formats (and probably, multiple languages). Depending on the response of the public, or if there is a lack of resources available in your jurisdiction, be prepared for the possibility that the National Guard may be called on to assist in maintaining order.

## Training in Action, Part 3

At this point, it may be too early to tell if this crisis is just an isolated case. If the situation changes in the next six to twelve hours, however, effectively coordinating the delivery of supplies and medicines with the SNS may be needed, and security should be ready to assist.

While this crisis may initially call for an increased federal presence, the incident is still a local one. The security personnel on the scene will have first-hand information on what is happening and who can potentially be affected. Any state or federal officials that join the response during this time period will need a status report communicated to them before knowing what next steps they should take. While the security team may not be the lead the response, it will most certainly play an important role in coordinating effects within the organization, and that role doesn't diminish even when it appears that more of the response is being handled by officials and authorities from outside security's sphere of influence.

Six hours after the initial crisis, looking toward the end of the day and beyond, the security staff will now need to consider future issues. Local government officials will need to be advised on whether quarantine needs to be in effect or whether the building where this case was first discovered needs to be condemned. In all probability, such actions would only happen in extreme cases, but extreme cases are exactly what security directors have to plan for in emergency management. All other corporate facets of the response that have been discussed in the first hours after word was received of this case are progressing. To this point, the security staff has followed their training very well.

After passing the twelve-hour benchmark, it's been determined that area utilities, such as the water supply, are safe. There has been no need to call for an evacuation, and no major issues on the roads and with transit. SNS supplies and medicine reinforcements will arrive in the next couple hours, and the public has been made aware of the process for receiving the attention they need, what time that will begin, where to go, and so on.

The time leading to the twelve-hour mark and beyond is also important for another reason. Shift changes will occur, and new people will be called into the response who may not be up to speed on what has taken place to this point. You, or someone you designate, will need to update the new security staff members. And at some point, as corporate security director, you may also need to designate someone to fill in for you, someone that can handle the pressures and responsibilities that you have carried over the last days.

## The Cycle Comes Full Circle

In this Ebola scenario, one final task awaits for the security manager. He or she may be tasked with delivering the news that the person diagnosed originally has passed away. Again, a goal will be to prevent panic among employees and to stress that everyone involved in the response is doing their jobs, and that there is no further immediate threat to the public. Through communications with the Ebola expert in the community, the security director can report that this case was, in fact, an isolated incident and that there is no threat to the general population, including employees.

As the response winds down and any necessary clean up and breakdown of equipment and takes place, the Emergency Management Cycle isn't over. The Preparedness stage begins all over again. Beyond practice drills and tabletop exercises, the security director now has a live event to study, to learn what went well, what went wrong, what should be done differently, and how the emergency response should be altered should this situation occur again.

In a sense, corporate emergency management never really ends, because the security staff is always involved in a current crisis response or training for the next one. While it may seem overwhelming, this fact is the key to being a successful security leader in any organization's emergency response operation.

*This new chapter was written by Michael J. Fagel, Ph.D., CEM and will be included in future versions of his book, *Crisis Management and Emergency Planning: Preparing for Today's Challenges*, published in 2014 by CRC Press.

## Exhibit 1: Security Response Plan: Timeline

Purpose: To describe what, in general, actions should be taken in the aftermath of an incident to provide the most coordination with other local, state, and federal responders and to best serve the public's needs

0-3 Hours after Incident:

- Determine what localities are affected by the incident.
- Determine what parts of the possible security response have also been affected and/or cut off by the incident itself.
- Coordinate with other local agencies as necessary, as well as with security staffs from other jurisdictions.
- Determine who has been assigned as the incident commander.
- Determine if an Emergency Operations Center is being opened, and if so, who from corporate security will be the liaison to the EOC?

3-6 Hours after Incident:

- Assign an information officer to update employees on what has happened, the state of recovery, and any next steps they need to take (evacuation, protecting their health, etc.).
- Let employees know of any need for donated blood, food, water, and other supplies. Provide assistance to the Strategic National Stockpile agents if it's deemed necessary, based
- on the type of incident and medicinal supplies available in the locality.
- Coordinate with other jurisdictions and state and federal agencies since they will become involved, depending on the severity and type of the incident.

6-12 Hours after Incident and Beyond:

- Notify employees if shelters are up and running for the public.
- Know where facilities have been set up to handle casualties, if necessary.
- Begin consulting with environmental, transportation, utility, and facilities experts to determine what long-term plans are going to be needed for recovery, in addition to the short- term plans for continuing to deal with the aftermath of the incident for those with immediate needs.
- Determine if any other specialized assistance from state or federal agencies are necessary based on the severity/type of the incident. Know where a quarantine facility will be needed in the case of Ebola or other biological or chemical attack/incident.

## Exhibit 2: Security Response Plan: Ebola Incident

Purpose: To describe the means, organization, and process by which the Public Health agency in a jurisdiction will coordinate its role in an emergency response for this particular type of incident.

Type of Incident (Brief description of the type of incident: This job aid can be used to draw out the necessary security response for this specific incident.

Staff Needed (with contact information and particular areas of expertise): List the security staff in your company that will be critical to the emergency response. Some staff will be needed to handle daily operations, but they should still be listed here. Also list key people outside the company that will be important contacts, such as the emergency operations coordinator; police and fire chiefs; local, state, and federal government contacts; and key security contacts from nearby corporations.

Responsibilities Needed: List the responsibilities for the staff listed above.

Supplies Needed: List key supplies that either the security staff will need to provide, or that will need to be procured from volunteer organizations (blood from the Red Cross), outside jurisdictions (vehicles, blankets, food, etc.), or the federal government (the Strategic National Stockpile).

Emergency Operations Center Liaison: Name and contact information for someone in your organization who will work with the EOC to help coordinate security efforts related to the overall effort. Should Ebola case(s) be discovered in the locality, seek out an EOC liaison with research knowledge in that area, and/or knowledge of pandemics.

Lessons Learned: Has your company faced this kind of incident before? If so, what worked well, what didn't? What supplies and resources were found to be useful and whose expertise is required?

Part of being prepared is learning from the past and a brief synopsis of the response to previous incidents can be particularly useful in future training.

CHAPTER 50

# Facility Management

• • •

**Robert J. Muller**

## Hotel Management

During a crisis a hospital can soon become a hotel. Numerous people flock to the safety of a hospital for a multitude of reasons including it being a central command area. Often we see community members seeking shelter and housing during a crisis including outside law enforcement agencies, The Weather personnel, and family members of working employees to name a few.

A person within the hospital that is totally familiar with the physical layout of the facility should be designated as the "Hotel Manager". All non -utilized patient rooms as well as non- utilized areas i.e. recovery rooms, pre -operative surgical areas and common waiting areas, ultrasound and radiology rooms, etc., may be utilized for housing and bedding as long as it does not interfere with the safety and flow of hospital traffic and personnel.

The pre designated hotel manager should identify these areas for assignment and keep records as to who/whom occupy these areas. Internal retained staff working shifts may utilize the same rooms and sleep likewise in shifts --- the **doubling up effect**.

In-house law enforcement personnel should be assigned rooms that have **locks** on the doors if possible, due to the necessity for storage of their weapons.

Planning will make this situation much easier to deal with than trying to put it all together at the last moment.

Start in advance with a survey of each floor on a sheet of paper with room locations and their particular characteristics (door locks, windows, etc.) This will create a ready template when the time comes to assign rooms and fill in the name of the person(s) assigned to that particular room or area. The template could be created according to floors or to characteristics (locks, windows, showers, etc)

Another issue to be aware of for security purposes if possible is to designate certain floors or areas as **female only** --- for obvious reasons.

If the area is isolated with limited access, and adequate personnel are available, a security person may be assigned to these areas. (This is a good job to assign a family member who is willing to assume such a role).

Sample:
Room 201 (Lock) (2 persons)______________________________
__________name______________________________________
Room 202(no window)__________________________________
Ultrasound Room (no lock/no window)____________________
Mammogram Room (no window)_________________________
*See Appendix for sample registration sheet.

## Morgue Facility

Most hospitals have limited morgue facilities due to the limited time frame that body storage is normally required before being turned over to local mortuaries, funeral directors, or coroner.

In a disaster situation, this turn over may become stressed due to the inability of mortuary services to respond or their inability to process the increased number of bodies due to the disaster. Likewise the local coroner /medical examiner may be unable to handle the increased numbers in their local facility. Thus, the hospital morgue may become full with nowhere to turn for decompression.

The facility should therefore have an alternate plan for a mass causality incident until further state or federal mortuary teams can arrive on the scene and provide the necessary assistance.

Hospitals should have an adequate supply of heavy duty body bags available and should have some alternate plan for refrigerated facilities or refrigerated truck(s) for body storage.

If an excess of the normal morgue capacity become reality, then bodies should be place in body bags and stacked to the capacity of the cooler height until alternate arrangements can be made for additional facilities. The stacking of bodies is obviously not an ideal situation and should only be used as a last resort in dire situations.

All bodies as well as the bags should be properly labeled with all the necessary information for proper identification of the deceased and should be tracked as to their movement by either a manual system or a computerized tag scanning system, or both.

In a disaster, a **morgue manager** position should be identified within the Incident Command System (ICS) and all responsibilities for the operation of the morgue should be turned over to that particular individual who then becomes responsible within the ICS chain of command.

The morgue manager should maintain a community as well as regional liaison with the funeral homes and mortuaries as well as the state Mass Fatality Task Force and Federal Demort Programs.

## Hospital Inspection and Analysis

One should begin the evaluation process by a complete review of all current related emergency and disaster plans and protocols. Carefully read over and make notes of areas of possible deficiencies and other aspects of the plan that may involve further investigation. For example, the plan may state the use of an internal radio system based on a repeater within the building. Investigate how the system operates, the condition of the batteries, if the repeater is on the emergency power system should there be a power failure, and check if the system has a current valid license with the Federal Communications Commission. Evaluate the entire process and play the devils' advocate —"what IF"?

Closely evaluate the communication system, both internal and external, in every detail and evaluate for and include all possible redundancies should there be a system failure. Look at how staff will be notified in case of a disaster. Telephone lines may be destroyed and beepers may not work. Are there *alternate plans* for notification or protocols in place for the staff to automatically report for duty?

This same process should be carried out in every aspect of the plan, protocols, hospital departments, administration and external factors. At NO time should there be a "that won't happen --- attitude"--- **plan that it will --- and mitigate.**

Upon completion of the analysis--- rewrite the plans and protocols incorporating all the new found information and mitigating factors. Compose a check list for future use for all items that need periodic follow up. Reanalyze the process at least annually, preferably every six months.

Make all the necessary changes as situations change and or new situations develop, such as alterations in the physical plant layout, administrative or departmental personnel changes or contractual changes, just to name a few.

Make sure you take external and internal pictures that are time stamped of the facility, outside structures and distant ground as well as aerial shots of the facility for complete documentation.

Internal pictures should be taken of all areas that may be vulnerable to any form of damage, i.e. wind, surge, loss of structure, etc.

## Generator/Emergency Electrical Power Supply

Hospitals are required to have an emergency power supply capable of sustaining critical areas of electrical need. Most hospitals do not have generators large enough in capacity to run the entire hospital without some interruption in services; especially air conditioning and heating (HVAC).

These hospitals may have to be supplemented with rental units from national companies that have units of sufficient capacity to meet the facility demand.

Contracts with one or more of these companies should be in place before an anticipated event takes place.

Hospitals should likewise anticipate these possibilities and be properly prepared by linking their electrical system to a cross over system (switch)that can be easily "plugged" into the acquired supplemental electrical system with the proper cables. This facilitates a rapid transfer with very little interruption of services and the ability to restore the facility to total operability within a short period of time.

**Note:** the restoration of electrical service to the facility is totally dependent on the construction wiring system. Flooding in the facility above the electrical outlets will result in a shorting out of the system and pose a serious electrical as well as fire hazard, unless the system is wired as such, that segmental area cutoff switches are utilized to zone out lower areas that may be the most vulnerable.

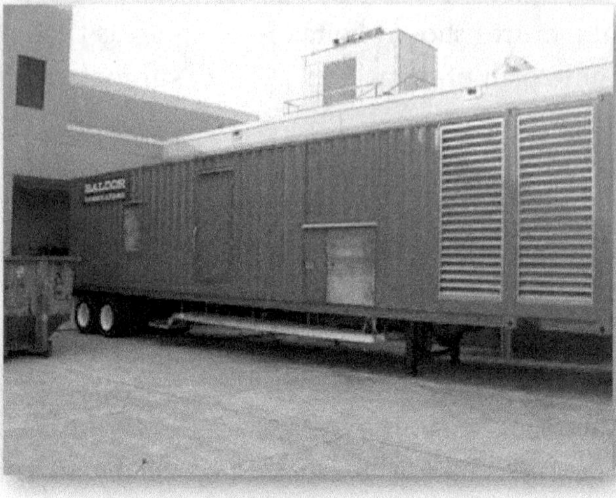

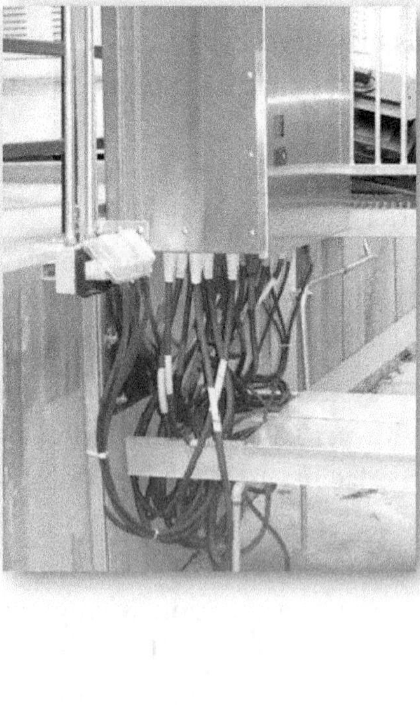

## Fuel Supply

The hospital should have an external fuel supply sufficient to operate the emergency generator capacity per hour requirements for a minimal of 72 hours. If this is not feasible, then a tank truck should be appropriated to stand by for the duration of the emergency. (If the generator burns 80 gallons per hour then a 72 hour supply would require an approximate 6000 gallon tank with some room for error. NEVER calculate down to the exact capacity as there are many variables which can alter the normal calculations.) In many cases this can be done only in anticipated emergencies such as a hurricane whereas a tornado or earthquake is like to be unanticipated.

There should be contractual **firm agreements** with fuel suppliers to be able to respond and provide for an immediate need. In case of a communications lapse, contracts should be worded as such that the company will respond despite a lack of notification---with a pre- determined fuel supply.

If an emergency can be anticipated, then all fuel tanks should be replenished to their capacity.

A supply of gasoline should also be present and kept away from the hospital, in cans, a tank or an inflatable bladder. Gasoline become necessary during prolonged emergencies to keep hospital vehicles supplied for transport, pickups and supply movements to and around the facility.

Agreements should be in place with local retail suppliers such as Texaco, Exxon, Shell, Racetrack, etc., to be able to access their station supply should their operation be abandoned in an emergency. In this situation it will be necessary to have some prearranged plan as to how the fuel can be pumped from their tanks and transported to the hospital. Company pumps may be accessed if alternate power sources are available and properly connected. In most cases it would be easier to pump from the supply tanks directly. Special pumps that are non-sparking must be utilized to pump fuel. These are readily available in various capacities and sizes. This all can be easily facilitated with preplanning as to when, where and how.

Never be afraid to think out of the box and plan according to every possible scenario.

## Helipads/Helispots

**Helipads** should be placed, constructed, lighted and licensed according to Federal Aviation Agency (FAA) standards. They should have some form of security, be away from structures that may be damaged by backwash and flying objects, and relatively close to hospital accesses either directly or indirectly. They should have established and published aviation codes and latitude and longitude designations.

According to local codes, landings may require the standby of fire equipment on a prearranged basis.

**Helispots** are temporary emergency landing sites that may include lawns, streets and parking lots. Helispots are more dangerous because they have not had the previous detailed planning and preparation as helipads and may not have adequate if any lighting. If utilized, these areas should be carefully prepared as best as possible to eliminate flying rocks and debris, lighted as best as possible with portable lighting that does not blind incoming pilots and provide a solid, flat surface for stabilization. Portable lighting likewise must also be of sufficient weight to prevent it from become a missile or sucked in the aircraft rotors and ideally should be staked or tied to a fixed object.

Areas of potential Helispots use may be identified and approximate Lat/Long coordinates obtained to be used only in cases of dire emergencies; otherwise, appropriate planning and permitting must be undertaken for the establishment of a permanent helipad.

**Landing zones** (LZ's) are areas designated for helicopter use normally in large cleared areas such as fields or on Interstate highways and are only used in critical emergency situations.

All electrical power lines around hospital potential landing sites should be marked accordingly with day markers and night lighting as required.

Hospital personnel from the emergency room, security and engineering staff should be trained in helicopter safety as well as the techniques of both day and night landing signals.

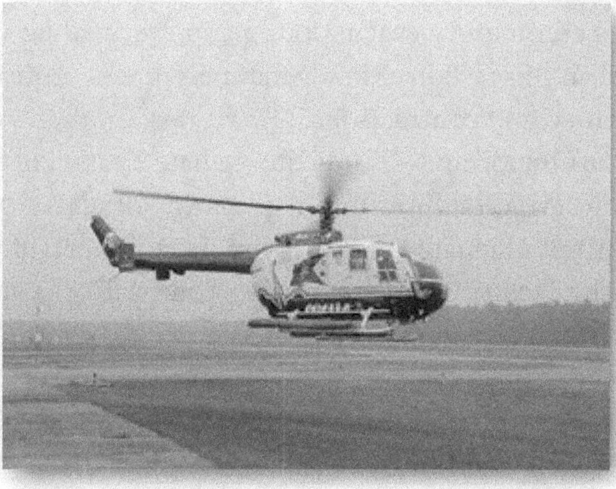

## Garbage/Waste

Following a disaster, garbage and waste may become a severe problem due to interruption of community/collection services. This should be anticipated when possible, and arrangements made by advanced ordering of addition dumpster containers to sustain for possibly as long as 7 to 30 days.

Human waste may need to be collected in garbage bags placed in toilets in cases where there is interruption of either sewer or water systems. This may be seen in cases of flooding, earthquakes, explosions, generalized or localized power failures, with disruption to sewerage collection facilities, etc.

Have a PLAN---don't think it will never happen to your facility. IT DOES. Be prepared.

## Debris Management

One of the biggest problems in the recovery phase is dealing with the clean-up process and the large amount of debris created from an event and dependent on the type of event --- from trees down to total destruction.

The large amount of debris can become problematic unless planned for in the preparatory phase. As an after event, especially following a community evacuation, manpower will be very scarce to accomplish this task in a timely manner; unless contractors have been identified and contracts let.

The most important --- is the immediate cleanup of the facility internally to avoid or limit interruption in patient services if the facility was not evacuated. The second most important is to allow access to the facility and this may be done with the use of state National Guard equipment, as well as a private contractor debris removal services.

The third most important is the cleanup of the damages to the facility itself (external), and can be done simultaneously if contracts have been vetted in advance and the contractors are able to gain reentry to begin the process, and have all the ancillary means for their personnel available to achieve the tasks, i.e. food, lodging, sanitary facilities, electrical or generator power, etc.

In my past experience, I would say to look for national recovery firms that have large crews and their own equipment and facilities self-contained and available post event on an almost immediate response basis.

There are many companies out there BUT MOST important is to have them know in advance by previous contractual arrangement, that their services are going to be required so they may mount a response team to the facility on a ASAP basis --- they are experienced and have been to the rodeo before and are totally familiar what it takes to get the job done

On January 29, 2013, the Sandy Recovery Improvement Act of 2013 (P.L. 113-2) (Sandy Act) was signed into law. This law authorizes, in part, improvements for the FEMA Public Assistance (PA) program for debris removal. Implemented as a pilot program, it provides several important provisions, including those that permit retention of income from debris recycling, reimbursement for regular time Force Account Labor, a sliding scale that increases the Federal share for accelerated debris removal and a two (2) percent incentive for Applicants who have an approved Debris Management Plan (DMP) in place before an event AND at least one pre-event prequalified debris contractor identified.

FEMA has 11 required elements in a DMP and are listed below. Four (4) of the 11 elements are NEW.

The complete elements of the plan can be found in the publication FEMA-325 Debris Management Guide (chapters noted below).

- Debris management overview (NEW)
- Events and assumptions (FEMA-325 – Chapter 6)
- Debris collection and removal plan (FEMA-325 – Chapter 7)
- Debris disposal locations and debris management sites (FEMA-325 – Chapter 8)
- Debris removal on private property (FEMA-325 – Chapter 12)
- Use and procurement of contracted services (FEMA-325 – Chapter 10)
- Use of Force Account Labor (NEW )
- Monitoring of debris operations (NEW)
- Health and safety requirements (FEMA-325 – Chapter 13)
- Environmental considerations and other regulatory requirements (NEW)
- Public information (FEMA-325 – Chapter 14)

## Water Supply

A vulnerability analysis of the facilities' water supply should be conducted and a plan formulated to maintain continuity in any way that is feasible to achieve this goal.

The hospital facility water supply should be assessed as to the possibility for loss of continuity due to any means of disruption. This may be in the form of loss of a main pump, pipeline disruption due to explosion, earthquake, or flooding of the primary service electrical supply.

Alternatives must be identified to sustain the facility ---from hours to days due to the loss; this includes having an alternate water supply, a stored water supply in tanks, bottles, bladders, tank trucks or the ability to manufacturer or purifies water from a local stream, river or lake. The use of commercial purification systems that are uniformly available may solve the emergent need of a facility and may be contracted through various vendors.

The amount of water needed will be determined by the size of the facility, census of the facility and the ability to conserve water based on need (dialysis facilities require adequate water supplies).

The loss of facility water supply, electrical and or communications can result in internal disastrous consequences other than the emergency or disaster in progress.

Alternate water sources, or the main water supply system that has possibly been damaged and comes back on line, should be tested in the laboratory, and this should be anticipated in advance as most hospital laboratories are not prepared for water testing

## Filters

Filters should be available to be utilized on incoming water supplies to the hospital. If this is not feasible, then each ice machine and water input to the food preparation area should all have individual water filters.

These can be installed with a cross over valve so that they can be utilized only during an emergency or anticipated emergency to prevent contaminated water from entering the critical areas of the hospital. This will provide some cost saving in replacing canisters.

Water supplies should be laboratory tested by the microbiologist for possible contamination, before and after the filters. The frequency should be determined depending upon the nature and severity of the events.

Only abnormally elevated contamination should be reported and documented. Specimens that have a normal range of bacteria (which most water supplies do) should be reported as "normal range" rather than documented as to actual amounts of "contamination".

Most facilities will not have the necessary testing for water, and samples may be sent out to a water reference testing laboratory and in emergency situations simple agar plating for coliforms may be done in house in all hospitals.

There may be some future legal issues associated with contaminated water, so it is important as to how this may be documented both pre and post event.

All results should be documented and kept with the incident event log for medical as well as legal purposes.

## Storage

Facility storage always seems to be at a premium and never seems to be adequately planned in facility designs.

The need for increased storage is more apparent for those hospitals that have to be self- sufficient and maintain higher par values than their larger and regionally located counterparts.

The addition of emergency management supplies as well as those in the preparation of possible chemical, biological, radiological and explosive (CBRE) events (Hazardous Materials or Bioterrorist) only causes additional shrinkage of limited facility space.

Space can be maximized by utilization of containerization of items (incident command vests, radio equipment/chargers), utilizing floor to ceiling stacking on special shelving, the use of medium to large enclosed trailers, and or the building or purchase of metal pods.

The use of outdoor storage has to be carefully planned as to the effects of temperature extremes on what may be stored within the container area. Air conditioning, heating and humidifiers may have to be additionally added in order to maintain a stable environment and preserve supplies and equipment.

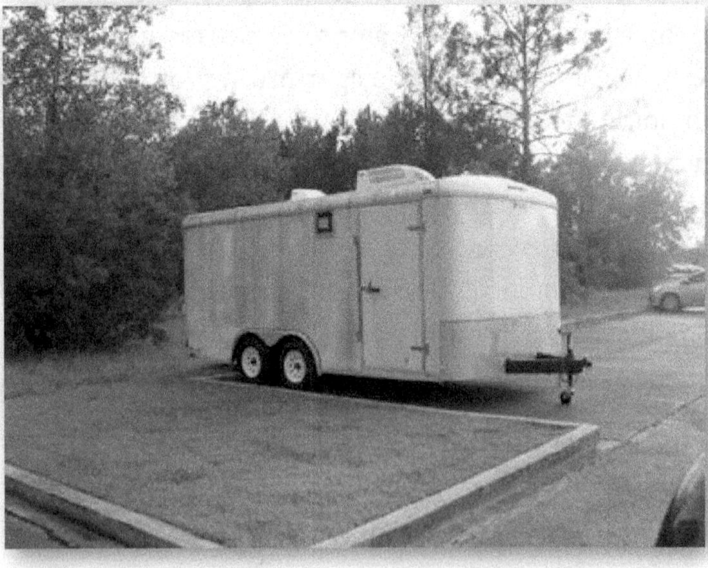

The use of trailers are particularly useful for the storage of decontamination units, tents, pools, suits and supplies; especially at facilities that do not have permanent designated decontamination areas. They can easily be stored away from the hospital and pulled into place outside of an emergency room or triage area in a relatively short time for deployment. Due to the nature of the decontamination equipment within, they must be climate controlled or else the heat will cause degeneration of the components.

**Note----Federal HRSA grant requirements mandates that all equipment purchased with those funds be physically present on the hospital premise and not stored in any off site locations.**

## Trailers

The use of portable trailers of 8-20 feet in length are excellent for storing disaster supplies in one place and is easily movable to the designated location rapidly behind a SUV or pickup truck. This is a great place for storing a Decon unit, decontamination suits and accessories, security tents, barricades, traffic cones, portable lighting and generators, portable plastic fencing and the like. They are relatively inexpensive compared to adding space or occupying internal hospital space; compact and easily inventoried and containerized as to designated supplies. The wheels can be locked for security purposes. The only drawback is the deteriorizing of items due to excess heat. They must be well vented, kept under an awning or shelter if feasible, and frequently inspected.

## Tents and Barricade Placement

Several pop tents should be available to be utilized in various established temporary locations, such as checkpoints, auxiliary registration areas, personnel screening, decontamination areas and the like. These can be easily stored in materials management or kept with the disaster response supplies.

In the situation of weather related events with possible residual wind, the tents should be secured to some form of ground attachment by posts placed in concrete and secured with large link chain with snaps secured for rapid placement and removal, but yet providing a firm reliable attachment.

Anticipate these placements according to locations, especially with barricades for traffic control around and within the campus, staking out to permanent attachments for ground placement. This may be used in locations such as streets that may need to be closed off to limit access to a particular area such as a garage or heliport area as examples.

Portable tables placed inside tents should likewise have some form of attachment available in anticipation of strong wind gusts.

The last problem that you do not want to create is that of flying projectiles that should have been secured in anticipation of possible aftermath of weather related events.

CHAPTER 51

# Communications

● ● ●

**Robert J. Muller**

THE MOST VITAL LINK IN any hospital emergency scenario is the communications network that has been previously established. It is essential to perform an analysis of not only the hospital needs, but likewise those of the community.

When performing the analysis several areas should be evaluated;

1. Internal Communications.

   The hospitals internal needs are dependent upon the hospital size as well as the physical plant layout as to hospital design.

   Multiple types of communications should be utilized to create a redundancy of systems in case of one or more system failures.

   Internal communications should likewise be **linked to the emergency power system** at all locations of base radios as well as radio chargers systems. Internal repeater systems should likewise be on the emergency power system.

   Internal communications can be linked to internal phone systems such as a Spectra link type system, internal as well as external pagers, cellular, direct connect systems such as Nextel and Verizon, and direct connect system such as portable hand held radios on VHF, UHF, CB or business band frequencies; OR preferably a multiple combination of two or three of these systems.

Before deciding which type of system is best for the hospital, make sure the system is adequately tested throughout the hospital in all possible locations, as some facilities have shielded blocking effects that do not allow certain frequencies to penetrate in various areas due to types of construction, etc.

As a general rule, the least reliable system for internal use is the CB (Citizen Band) radio and is generally only effective with limited range externally on flat topography (short line of sight).

2. External

External communications links are dependent on how sophisticated the hospital desires its system to be relevant to the community. It is imperative that an external link be established utilizing a HAM (Amateur) radio system, configured to the design of the hospital. This system requires a federally licensed operator and this person can either be trained through a training course or preferably someone within the community that does this as a full time hobby.

These people use their equipment on a regular basis, stay up on all the recent sites and developments and know and have multiple contacts within their brotherhood. Check with a local HAM club to see if anyone is interested in performing this service during an emergency for your hospital. Once this person is established, he or she should then become a part of the hospital emergency preparedness planning team and should be included in all preparedness meetings.

This person should be allowed access to the facility and to evaluate the facility for the best location to place the equipment for optimum operation. Antennae placement and distance is critical to the performance of the system. Arrangements may be made with the individual to bring his/her own equipment and utilize pre-established antennae plug type connectors, or for the hospital to purchase a system for a permanent installation. The advantage of the latter is that the system is ready to go upon arrival of an licensed operator without any set up delay, which could take up to several hours. This could be critical in case of an event such as a tornado or explosion without a preparatory notice.

Vital community links may be established with law enforcement (state, county, local), fire, EMS, county and city officials and surrounding entities as backup plans may dictate. Their frequencies and specific type of equipment may be purchased with their permission and may be able to be purchased thru the agency and their municipal discount structure with their vendors. This equipment must be kept secured at all times and not be available for any form of casual use or for monitoring purposes and this assurance must be conveyed to the agency for their assurance that this equipment will not and cannot fall into misuse.

There is NO such thing as having too much communications redundancy.

**COMMUNICATIONS** is the backbone to disaster survival and contingency planning.

## Communications 101 Basics

Hospitals should have multiple communications capabilities, both internal and external. Below are some examples of communication redundancy that need to be created to provide multiple links.

**Internal:**

1. Spectra link System
2. Nextel Direct Connect
3. UHF System
4. Internal Paging and Beeper system

**External:**

1. AT&T telephone system on TPS (Telephone Priority System—available for a monthly surcharge from your telephone carrier)
2. GETS System (Government sponsored priority system)
3. WPS (Wireless Priority System)
4. UHF---city or county system with multiple repeaters
5. VHF—HEAR system
6. 800 MHz----local, county or state law enforcement, fire or emergency management, state health agency
7. 700mmhz—local, county or state law enforcement, fire or emergency management, state health agency
8. HAM radio
9. CB and Business band radios can be used for very limited range and when clear line of site is unobstructed. They do not work well within structures.
10. Satellite telephones can be very useful but are expensive to maintain. The most cost effective way is to purchase several satellite phones with an allotment of minutes that can be used within a year period of time, and if possible can be rolled over to a subsequent year; also if you can obtain a plan with a minimum maintenance fee and a cost per minute use basis. The minutes are usually more expensive, but this way they are not lost to an expiration date.

It is also nice to have phones on more than one system (there are currently 3 systems available). Remember the limitation of satellite phones' is to have a view of "the clear sky" which is sometimes impossible during and after severe weather.

11. Marine radios and offshore high frequency radios have potential use during a disaster and may be utilized in areas where these systems are activated.

## Frequencies and What They Mean:

UHF is "Ultra High Frequency". It requires a small antenna, has limited range but penetrates building structures well. The range can be extended by the use of repeaters strategically located within a structure or surrounding area. Hospitals should have an internal repeater to extend the range for their internal UHF system to approximately 3-4 miles circumferentially.

VHF is "Very High Frequency" and is defined by higher radio power (wattage), larger antennae and operated by line of sight based on the earth azimuth. This is enhanced by placement of a larger antenna or greater antenna height placement, i.e. 150 ft. towers, etc. HEAR (Hospital Emergency Alert Radios) are on VHF frequencies.

Also on VHF are Aircraft radios which maintain a different VHF frequency grouping for aircraft, helicopter and ground crew communications---both civilian and military.

800 MHz is a system that was devised for law enforcement for continuity but became deranged when 3 separate system coding's were devised and thus intra operability was compromised. In addition cellular is also on 800.

700 MHz is the new Law Enforcement system for the State and local agencies.

HAM radio is also referred to as "amateur radio" and by FCC guideline requires licensed operators and station licensing for operation. Messages can be conveyed from the Command Center IC to the HAM via an internal UHF radio. It is much better to have HAM radios and operators in a **different location** due to the constant chatter on their frequencies which create a significant disturbance in a command center room.

## Antenna Systems:

Communications systems are totally dependent upon their antennae systems. Communication range and clarity of communications are dependent upon antennae connections, types of cable, cable lengths, connectors, and antennae height and location placement. All forms of communications are dependent upon antennas from television to HAM, with the exception of the internet which is dependent upon telephone or satellite links.

Due to the extreme significance of the antenna to communications, it is imperative that the antenna locations be carefully planned. Antenna should be placed with some form of protection, such as wind resistant webbing, etc. or even better, placed in such a way that the system can be folded or cranked down then be brought back up after the event. This of course only holds for those weather related events than can be anticipated.

In addition, in case of damage to the system in unanticipated events, backup systems should be available with quick change connectors that can facilitate rapid replacement.

REMEMBER, the most sophisticated communications is totally worthless without the proper working antenna system.

CHAPTER 52

# Contracts and Agreements

● ● ●

**Robert J. Muller**

COMMUNICATIONS----LOCAL OR REGIONAL COMPANIES FOR rental of portable radios, repeaters, cellular and satellite phones, and antennae systems.

**FUEL**--- make sure you have multiple contracts with vendors from different geographical areas to be able to access the facility in case roads are closed due to flooding or obstructions.

**Pharmaceuticals** --- local and regional suppliers; alternate contact numbers should be maintained as well as contacts via email and HAM operators.

**Sanitary** --- accessory sanitary facilities, portable toilets (consider having available outside hospital to limit traffic within the facility for use of toilets and further taxing security of the facility). This is especially important if your facility is along an evacuation route as many travelers will seek out the facility for restroom use only.

**Storage** --- metal storage (pods) for garbage, solid waste should the plumbing system fail, and pet protection (excellent when turned over on the side), refrigerated trucks for ice and body storage (not the same truck)

**Transport** --- contracts with ambulance services both locally and out of state (for transfer and evacuation), bus companies and school bus drivers, and helicopter companies if available (to possibly pick up and fly in critical supplies)

**Vendors** --- food, ice, water, milk (automatic ship agreements should be in place). Contracts should be made regionally as local companies may be inundated by the disaster and may not be able to fulfill their contracts or access may be shut off for their deliveries. Contracts should therefore be made in various geographical directions to allow for access from these different areas. Contracts with national suppliers allow some geographical variance for them to respond from their distribution warehouses in the United States. Be specific within the verbiage of the contract as to the various modes of communication that are planned to be used to contact the supplier such as telephone, email, HAM radio distant contacts, HAM radio emails, etc.

Others --- agreements as deemed individually necessary for the facility, i.e. advanced arrangement with big box stores to embed a key holder.

## Agreements

Embedding agreements with law enforcement, EMS, news and weather services, etc.

The hospital may consider agreements for embedding of key holding personnel from community stores that may be of benefit to the hospital i.e. grocery stores, Wal-Mart, Home Depot, etc.; Another excellent PR as well as community service is a verbal offer to the Weather Channel or other news media for their visiting personnel.

Local or state law enforcement may appreciate an offer to house their personnel during the height of a disaster or to give relief in shifts to personnel that have been brought in for the disaster from outside the area, as these people live a distance and usually many times lodging facilities are unavailable, i.e. state police. This should be preplanned and on as a "as space available" basis. Ancillary campus facilities such as ambulatory surgery suites and clinics may be a good place for some additional housing space.

Community agreements with local outpatient facilities (than may not be operable for services, but may be an excellent space for embedding), should be considered.

Nursing Home/Rehabilitation Facilities --- agreements with these facilities to house their patients should be discouraged due to the need for acute care space following a disaster, as well as the demand for increased staffing due to the acuity of this category of patients. If agreements are made with these facilities then agreements should be made with them to also send their own staffing to accompany their patients.

Parking --- agreements with local governmental agencies to house their vehicles.

*Transfer agreement --- agreements should be made with local, regional and distant hospital facilities to send or accept patients in transfer in the event of an impending disaster or an internal event such as a fire, explosion, contamination, etc. Agreements should be made appropriately regarding sending or NOT to send staffing with the patients, or likewise to provide staffing services to distant shelters or off site facilities or campuses (clinics), as it will become necessary to keep sufficient staffing within the facility to deal with the possible influx of acute care patients post disaster in the affected area.

*See appendix for sample agreement

CHAPTER 53

# Security

●●●

**Robert J. Muller**

Hospital security is of vital importance on a daily basis as well as in the chaos of a disaster when many of the safeguards of daily routine become extremely relaxed either due to the increase demands or lack of manpower or BOTH.

Security plans should be completed in advance and done with the help of or with consultant professionals, especially for larger facilities with multi-complex situations that could affect the well-being of the entire facility.

A plan should be established starting with the basics; an evaluation of the facility location, street access, parking access, locations of the various departments of the hospital requiring public access, i.e. radiology and laboratory, etc.) and the numbers of ingress points within the hospital.

It is important when determining a facility disaster security plan to always keep employee and patient safety at the forefront as well as all local and state fire regulation codes.

A plan for increased security staffing should be put together knowing in actuality that an alternate plan may need to be formulated due to the planned personnel not being able to show up to the facility due limited access created by the very disaster planned for at the time.

Thus an alternate "bare bones" plan should likewise be created utilizing minimum numbers and possibly planning for other staff members to assist with the security task despite other jobs they may be performing. Also allow and plan for volunteers to assist with the task and have a plan for them to assume the secondary or tertiary roles rather than primary roles.

Husbands, relatives, and other family members 21 years old or greater, are perfect for many roles, i.e. providing security for a secondary entry point, or handling traffic entering a parking facility, etc.

Volunteers should not be allow to be armed---unless they are likewise valid and licensed security personnel, prior law enforcement or military and have a current firearms license and certifications and are needed to provide this function, i.e. providing security for the hospital safe that has an increased amount of cash on hand to provide for in house pay day loan payments to employees; or guarding as for cache of the National Stockpile delivered to the hospital, etc.

Someone with NO previous security experience should not be chosen to work any MAJOR security function ALONE. If utilized, place these people in positions to provide security to egress point for staff but do not place them on any major ingress flow points.

Ingress points should be limited to as few as possible, and predesignated as employee check-in and public check-in points as well as limiting or locking egress points as allowed by fire codes.

If egress points are unable to be locked, then they should be manned by security personnel to prevent a breach from someone gaining access to the facility when someone is exiting.

ALL hospital personnel should have some form of VISIBLE identification on their person, such as an ID badge or some other form such as special shirts or uniforms. Scrub suits are NOT to be considered a valid uniform as they can be purchased by anyone at multiple facilities within a community. (See section on Uniforms)

Validation stickers may be applied during an emergency to personnel ID cards showing a bright orange or lime green sicker visible from a distance of 6 feet or more. This validates an employee's presence specific to the event and helps with the possibility of lost or old hospital ID badges being utilized from past employees, etc.

Visitor wrist banding works very well is efficient, easily recognizable and cost efficient.

One color may be utilized or multiple colors to signify different areas for security purposes. For example a patient may be banded at the security with a blue wrist band to indicate they are going for a radiology procedure. If they are seen wondering around the third floor patient area by a staff member or security person, then they immediately know this person should not be in that area.

Multiple color bands should be kept in general stores inventory or in the pre designated area for disaster equipment and supplies. (See references for a source)

Hospital access is of the utmost importance and depending on the locale and physical setup, pre-determined access routes could be determined and marked by property signage for the general public, employees and emergencies presenting to the hospital.

There are multiple security issues that hospitals face on a daily basis and this should be evaluated well in advance of any and all possible disaster situations---again advanced **planning** is the key to success

## Hospital Identification Systems

All staff hospital personnel should have some form of picture identification card, including administrative staff, physicians and board members; frequent hospital contractors may likewise be given a different color ID with or without a picture but redeemable upon demand as well as a predetermined expiration date. After the expiration date on ID cards, a different color card should be used. The "RepTrack" type system may also be effectively utilized if in place within the hospital.

If it is not hospital policy for ID cards to be returned upon completion or termination of employment, then a 6 month revalidation process must take place. This can easily be done by placing a validation sticker on the front of the ID card with a different color (that can be easily recognized from a distance of 6-10 feet) with an expiration date printed on it. This keeps all ID cards current without the expense of remaking new ID cards for all employees.

Generic ID cards (without a picture) can be printed in advance and kept for use by volunteers, family members and law enforcement or security personnel. They should be of a particular color or design with large distinct lettering on them, such as "LEO" (law enforcement officer); "V" (volunteer), "G" (guest) or "FM" (family member) for some examples.

Colored wrist bands may be used as an alternate, particularly for guests and visitors, with specific color designated for different floors or areas of the hospital, i.e. blue-first floor, orange-emergency room, etc.

**Everyone who is in the hospital during a disaster and particular any type of national security event should have some form of ID visible to internal hospital security.** Anyone who does not have some form of authorized ID should be reported to, and stopped and questioned by security. All plain clothed law enforcement officers (local, state or federal) should have their badge displayed on their shirt, hanging on a lanyard around their neck, or displayed on their belt facing forward so they are readily visible. All experienced law enforcement will have some form of badge or ID in their possession at all times. If someone should present stating they are law enforcement and do not possess any form of valid ID and or badge, they should be thoroughly questioned before assuming their validity.

Identification as to group: FM=Family Member; V=Volunteer; LEO=Law Enforcement Office (especially internal security); C=Contractor, etc.

Note: Expiration Date sticker to be upgraded every 6 months if necessary

## Parking

Garages --- those facilities that have parking in garage facilities should have some form of security in terms of either manned security or automated gated security to both enter and exit the facility. In a disaster, parking garages may become inundated with locals who desire to secure their vehicles from flying debris and or rising water, etc., especially if it is a free parking garage. Also garage space may be reserved for police and fire agencies as well as public works, to safeguard their vehicles for immediate utilization post disaster. Pre -arranged agreements with the various agencies are highly recommended.

Also garage entry points into the hospital or clinic facilities should have some form of planned security or closed to prevent unauthorized or undetected entry.

Parking Lots --- should likewise be reserved and secured for facility personnel by utilizing locking barricades or some other form of permanent delineation as to the designated site. Metal pipes should be secured in concrete well in advance of any type of event and utilized to chain the barricades to prevent them from become projectiles. These areas should be inspected for any loose objects or objects that may become projectiles. In situations of wind related disasters it may be suggested in advance for employees to purchase some form of locking car covers to help preserve their vehicles from flying debris. (A small pebble at 100 miles per hour can do severe damage to windows and painted surfaces.)

## Uniforms:

The use of some form of uniforms is extremely important to the security of a hospital, no matter what size the hospital, they allow easy identification of personnel from a patient perspective, as well as other **employees in larger facilities.**

Today scrub suits are readily purchased in every type of store from uniform stores to grocery stores, and this allows unlimited access to the general public.

The elderly patients in a hospital have a tendency, because of previously established norms, to identify scrubs suits on personnel as being "doctors". Today many hospitals allow the wearing of scrub suits from their nursing staff to their janitorial staff. Unless some form of parameter is set up within the hospital, this can be a serious breach of security and safety for the hospital as well as the patient.

At one hospital, a female patient had a "consultant" come into her room one night and performed a breast examination on her; only to find out the next morning that no such consultation was requested by her admitting physician. The only description that she could remember was that other than being a male, he was a "doctor in a scrub suit".

Security may be best established with types of uniforms required of certain department personnel, like engineering, housekeeping, janitorial, etc.; while professional staffing may wear the traditional white nursing apparel or if scrub suits are permitted for these people, then a color should be established.

This may be based on departments, i.e. nurses-white, physical therapist-blue, and respiratory therapist-green, laboratory-black, etc. Likewise, colors may be differentiated by floors or units, such as nurses in different color pants and shirts, i.e. ICU white pants, blue tops; OB pink, etc.

During times of high level security this uniformity can be a great help in identifying potential breaches within the hospital system, and is an easy as well as a very cost effective system to implement.

## Signage

The liberal use of signage in and around a facility is imperative on a daily basis but even more so important in an emergent situation when people awareness levels have been dulled from whatever means.

The signage should be easily visible, easy to read, contrasting colors and very specific with directional arrows and directed instructions. The reader should not have to ask anyone what the sign means or is referring to----it should be distinctively obvious.

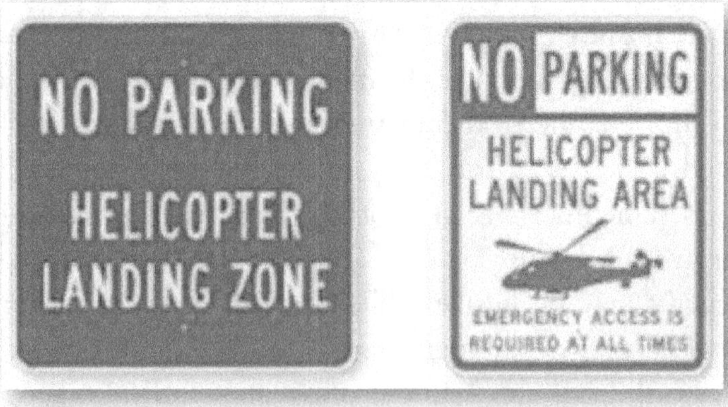
NO PARKING
HELICOPTER
LANDING ZONE
NO PARKING
HELICOPTER
LANDING AREA
EMERGENCY ACCESS IS
REQUIRED AT ALL TIMES

# Appendix

# APPENDIX 1

## Communications
## Telephone Priority Restoration (TPS)

TPS IS A POST DISASTER restoration program that requires authorization through a federal congressman or senator (paperwork) verifying the nature of the facility and authorizing the telephone carrier to prioritize post disaster repairs to the facility equipment and service lines.

This service is NOT a free service and is charged to the facility on a monthly basis and a per line basis that is eligible for restoration.

Thus a facility may have 30 lines coming in @ $3- $5 per month fee; or in the case of post disaster use and to keep facility cost within budgets, the facility could opt to pay for 3 or 5 lines to be restored in a priority mode post disaster.

The options for the facility are purely up to the facility management and the service is optional and does not have to be utilized, but is sure nice to have in place when and IF needed.

Discuss with your local carrier as to fee structures as these vary from time to time and place to place.

The necessary paper work can be obtained on line and then approval must be signed off by a state official as designated by the carrier.

http://www.fcc.gov/encyclopedia/telecommunications-service-priority

APPENDIX 2

• • •

## GETS Program Information

### The GETS Concept

THE GOVERNMENT EMERGENCY TELECOMMUNICATIONS SERVICE (GETS) is a White House-directed emergency phone service provided by the National Communications System (NCS) in the Office of Cybersecurity and Communications Division, National Protection and Programs Directorate, Department of Homeland Security. GETS supports Federal, State, local, and tribal government, industry, and non-governmental organization (NGO) personnel in performing their National Security and Emergency Preparedness (NS/EP) missions. GETS provides emergency access and priority processing in the local and long distance segments of the Public Switched Telephone Network (PSTN). It is intended to be used in an emergency or crisis situation when the PSTN is congested and the probability of completing a call over normal or other alternate telecommunication means has significantly decreased.

GETS is necessary because of the increasing reliance on telecommunications. The economic viability and technical feasibility of such advances as nationwide fiber optic networks, high-speed digital switching, and intelligent features have revolutionized the way we communicate. This growth has been accompanied by an increased vulnerability to network congestion and system failures.

Although backup systems are in place, disruptions in service can still occur. Recent events have shown that natural disasters, power outages, fiber cable cuts, and software problems can cripple the telephone services of entire regions. Additionally, congestion in the PSTN, such as the well-documented "Mother's Day phenomenon," can prevent access to circuits. However, during times of emergency, crisis, or war, personnel with NS/EP missions need to know that their calls will go through. GETS addresses this need. Using enhancements based on existing commercial technology, GETS allows the NS/EP community to communicate over existing PSTN paths with a high likelihood of call completion during the most severe conditions of high-traffic congestion and disruption. The result is a cost-effective, easy-to-use emergency telephone service that is accessed through a simple dialing plan and Personal Identification Number (PIN) card verification methodology. It is maintained in a constant state of readiness as a means to overcome network outages through such methods as enhanced routing and priority treatment.

GETS uses these major types of networks:

- The local networks provided by Local Exchange Carriers (LECs) and wireless providers, such as cellular carriers and personal communications services (PCS)
- The major long-distance networks provided by Interexchange Carriers (IXCs) - AT&T, Verizon Business, and Sprint - including their international services
- Government-leased networks, such as the Federal Technology Service (FTS), the Diplomatic Telecommunication Service (DTS), and the Defense Switched Network (DSN)

GETS is accessed through a universal access number using common telephone equipment such as a standard desk set, STU-III, facsimile, modem, or wireless phone. A prompt will direct the entry of your PIN and the destination telephone number. Once you are authenticated as a valid user, your call is identified as an NS/EP call and receives special treatment.

The **Nationwide Wireless Priority Service** (WPS) is a system in the United States that allows high-priority emergency telephone calls to avoid congestion on wireless telephone networks. This complements the Government Emergency Telecommunications Service (GETS), which allows such calls to avoid congestion on landline networks. The service is overseen by the Federal Communications Commission and administered by the National Communications System in the Department of Homeland Security.

During a local or national emergency, wireless telephone networks are likely to become congested with calls. Even absent emergencies, some towers and networks receive more calls than they can handle. WPS allows high-priority calls to bypass that congestion and receive priority by dialing *+272+*DST_NUMBER*+send (the 'star' key followed by 272 followed by the destination number followed by the dial key). The system is authorized only for use by National Security and Emergency Preparedness personnel, classified into five categories:

- Executive leadership and policy makers (e.g. the President of the United States and members of Congress)
- Disaster response/military command and control
- Public Health, safety, and law enforcement command
- Public services/utilities and public welfare
- Disaster recovery

Unlike the GETS system, which provides landline priority telephone calls, participation in the *WPS* system is optional for telephone companies. As such, support is only available on selected networks and usually requires additional fees for activation, availability, and use.

Before using the system, each user must receive authorization from the National Communications System and subscribe to the service with a participating provider. Once authorized, a user simply needs to prepend calls the vertical service code of "*272" to receive priority consideration on the wireless network.

Although the system is said to ensure a high probability of call completion, it is not without serious limitations. The WPS will not preempt calls in progress, so the user will have to wait for bandwidth to open. It is also not yet supported by all carriers. In order for a call to work, telephone infrastructure must be powered and functioning. Finally, a call that receives priority using WPS does not automatically get priority on landline networks. Therefore, congestion on the Public Switched Telephone Network may prevent the call from completion unless the user makes additional steps to access the GETS service for landline calls as well. Because of these and other limitations, the WPS explicitly does not guarantee call completion.

## APPENDIX 3

• • •

Communications Worksheet

Name of Hospital/Facility __________ Parish/County __________

Facility Tier Level I II (circle one)

Form Completed By __________ Licensed Bed Capacity __________

Please Complete the Communications Available at your Hospital/ Facility: (Circle Choices)

HEAR Radio: Base Handheld Power (watts output) __________

Roof Antennae: Y N (circle)

VHF Frequency: Transmit ______ Receive ______ PL Code ______

UHF Frequency: Transmit ______ Receive ______ PL Code ______

Repeater: Internal External Radio Range __________ mile(s)

800mhz Analog Digital TYPE: Motorola Erickson Johnson Icom Other __________

HAM Frequency: Transmit ______ Receive ______ Antennae Type: External (roof) Portable

Nextel/Verizon Direct Connect Code # ________________

# APPENDIX 4

• • •

EMERGENCY TELEPHONE NUMBERS: (INCLUDE PROPER area codes)
Command Center Telephone Numbers

Administration ____________________________________________
Emergency Room __________________________________________

Hospital Emergency Lines _______________________________

Emergency Cellular Lines _______________________________

Satellite Phone Number _________________________________
FAX Telephone Numbers

Command Center ______________________________
Administration _______________________________
Emergency Room ______________________________
Does your Facility have Telephone Priority System (TPS)? Y N
Does your Facility participate in the Satellite Emergency Communications System? Y N

# APPENDIX 5

## Phonetic Alphabet

Word list adopted by the
International Telecommunications Union

A – ALFA
B – BRAVO
C – CHARLIE
D – DELTA
E – ECHO
F – FOXTROT
G – GOLF
H – HOTEL
I – INDIA
J – JULIET
K – KILO
L – LIMA
M – MIKE
N – NOVEMBER
O – OSCAR
P – PAPA
Q – QUEBEC
R – ROMEO
S – SIERRA
T – TANGO
U – UNIFORM
V – VICTOR
W – WHISKEY
X – X-RAY
Y – YANKEE
Z - ZULU

# APPENDIX 6

• • •

## Examples of Radio Identification Coding

The numbers in ( ) match the numbers on the physical radios.

Green VHF---GE MPA (8)

Gold UHF---Motorola Radius CP200 (4)

White Kentwood (1)

Red VHF---Motorola—JT 1000 (12)
Icom—Marine/Weather

Yellow 700/800 Motorola XTS 5000R (2)

Blue Aircraft --- Bendix King Air KX 99 (9)

Black 800 mhz MaCom (3)

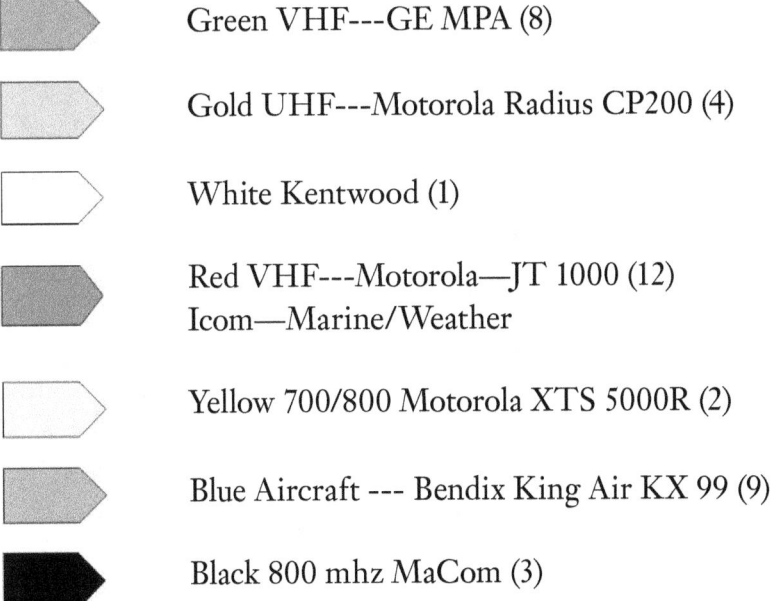

Color coding by placing a piece of colored tape on the antennae to match the corresponding chart is an excellent system to identify types of radios, radio frequencies and what they are used in conjunction with; the-y also may be numbered (#) with stick on numbers that can be obtained from any office supply store. This allows for the person who is not totally familiar with the communications operations system to immediately identify and "fill in", until a more qualified person becomes available to assume command or at least the communication role.

APPENDIX 7

• • •

**Checklists**

# PIO Major Responsibilities Checklist

DETERMINE FROM THE IC IF there are any limits on information release.

Develop material for use in media briefings. Establish an area to hold media briefings that is easily accessible to the media, yet distant from the operation center location.

Obtain IC approval of media releases.

Inform the media and conduct media briefings.

Arrange for tours and other interviews or briefings, as necessary. A tour of the operation center (EOC) is advisable but the EOC should not be used as a location for briefings.

Evaluate the need for and, as appropriate, establish and operate a JIC (Joint Information Center).

Establish a JIC, as necessary, to coordinate and disseminate accurate and timely incident-related information.

Maintain current information summaries and/or displays on the incident.

Provide information on the status of the incident to assigned personnel.

Maintain an Activity Log (ICS form 214).

Manage media and public inquiries.

APPENDIX 8

# Hospital Emergency Manager Checklist

**Hurricane Preparedness Checklist**
***(Circle when addressed)***

| | | | | | | |
|---|---|---|---|---|---|---|
| ***Generator*** | Crossover Plan | | | | | |
| ***Fuel*** | Diesel | Gas | Contracts | Alternate | | |
| ***Water*** | Bladder | Bottled | Testing | Ice | Filters | |
| ***Food*** | Schedule | EOC | | | | |
| ***Sleeping*** | Cots | | | | | |
| ***Pets*** | Registration | Location | Cages | Food | | |
| ***Communications*** | Antenna | HAM | Satellite | Batteries | Adapters | Signout |
| | Aircraft | Liaison | Radio checks | Phone tree | | |
| ***Command Center*** | Vests | Phones | Computer wifi | Control access | Meeting times/locations | |
| | Intranet | | | | | |
| ***Washer Dryer*** | Soap | Assign times | | | | |
| ***Finance*** | Cash | Safe/valuables | | | | |
| ***ER*** | Supplies | Vests | Staff | | | |
| ***Pharmacy*** | Tetanus | Snakebite antibiotic par | | | | |
| ***Surgery*** | Supplies | | | | | |
| ***Staffing*** | Hospitalist Oral | Psych | Vet | Dialysis | Census | |
| | Sat comm | Reentry | | | | |
| ***Morgue*** | # | Empty | CO Liaison | Funeral homes | | |
| ***Gen Stores*** | Refer truck | Ice | Garbage | Fans | Extension | Par values |
| ***Hotel Mgmt*** | Room assignments | | | | | |
| ***Logistics*** | Trailers | Generator | Surg suite | Sleeping | | |
| ***Visitors*** | Bands | Assignments | Heliport mgr | Personnel pool | Childcare | |
| ***Admissions*** | Paper entry | | | | | |
| ***PR*** | Digital picture documentation | | Location | Interviews | | |
| ***Personal*** | Supplies | Clothing | Family | Communications | Pets | |

# APPENDIX 9

## Decontamination Guidelines

1. All hospitals shall be prepared to decontaminate ambulatory and non-ambulatory patients presenting and seeking emergency care.
2. Clothing control should be a focus of decontamination efforts. Contingency plans should include a way for large numbers of patients to remove clothing ('dry decon') while maintaining privacy (e.g.: large trash bag).
3. Each hospital should be prepared to contain 55 gallons of wash water from decontamination operations based on standard HAZMAT events.
4. Hospitals are encouraged to have contingency plans and facilities for large numbers of victims presenting after a community disaster rather than depending on public safety resources.
5. Hospitals should not plan to control wash water during mass casualty decontamination operations (i.e.: in excess of capacity outlined above) per the EPA Good Samaritan Clause.
6. Hospitals should immediately notify the State Duty Officer of any contaminated wash water that goes down a sewer drain.
7. Hospitals should preferentially direct wash water to sanitary containers rather than storm sewer when containment

capacity is exceeded if possible and feasible---see number 3 and 5 above.

8. Hospitals should place absorbent barriers around drains when organic and non-water soluble agents are known or suspected to be involved.

## Background:

With increasing attention being paid to the possibility of mass decontamination following exposure to a potentially hazardous substance the control of the wash water generated becomes a significant issue. Guidelines are needed to ensure that public safety and hospitals providing decontamination services to the public are not held to unrealistic expectations regarding their ability to contain wash water generated in the process of emergency patient care. The containment of wash water accounts for substantial (and in some cases, a majority of) project costs for facilities that seek to increase decontamination capacity for mass exposure incidents.

According to ATSDR HSEES data from 2001, of 710 hazardous materials incidents that resulted in injury, 558 were fixed facility, which are more likely to be employees and better controlled at the scene. These events involved 1 victim in 62% of cases, 2 in 16.5% of cases, 3 in 7.6% of cases, 4 in 3.2% of cases, and >4 in 10.7% of cases (all of which involved gas exposures, for example, chlorine). This is consistent with prior year's data which shows that the vast majority of HAZMAT incidents resulting in injury involve a few persons, and those that involve many persons are nearly always gas exposures, which do not require technical decontamination.

The U.S. Environmental Protection Agency's Good Samaritan Language (CERCLA Sec. 107(d)(1) holds harmless from Federal action any facility or agency that makes a good faith attempt to contain wash water during patient decontamination operations but is unable to due to the volume of patients encountered. EPA 550-F-00-009 July 2000 states 'the EPA will not pursue enforcement actions against state and local responders for the environmental consequences of necessary and appropriate emergency response actions'. The question remains open as to what is a reasonable target for wash water containment for public safety services and hospitals providing decontamination as a part of patient care activities (life safety activities). This is not to be confused with mitigation activities or control activities undertaken by public safety agencies.

Due to clothing removal approximately 90% of contaminant will be eliminated prior to wet decontamination. The larger the number of persons seeking decontamination, the less contaminant that is actually present per person in the wash water stream due to the self-referral of non-poisoned casualties and less deposition of vapor or gas on the persons affected.

Example

Assuming an incident in which the nerve agent VX (more persistent than Sarin) was used in an attack which resulted in 1000 persons seeking decontamination of which 100 were actually contaminated with 25% of the LD50 for VX (2.5mg). 90% of the contaminant was confined to clothing.

1000 persons x 10 gal/person = 10000 gal = 37854 liters wash water

100 contaminated persons x 2.5 mg/person = 250 mg on persons and clothing

250 mg x 0.10 (disrobing reduction) = 25 mg residual on persons

25 mg agent / 37854 L = 0.00066 mg/L (L/1000 g) (g/0.001 mg) = 0.00066 ppm

= 0.66 ppb concentration in wash water

0.66ppb concentration in wash water at its most concentrated point in the disposal process.

# APPENDIX 10

## Decontamination Units

DECONTAMINATION PRESENTS CHALLENGES FROM VARIOUS aspects and each hospital should have its own plan as well as a community plan for decontamination of affected persons.

The size and location of the facility, along with the hazard and vulnerability analysis of the community should dictate as to the needs of the hospital with planning, staffing and securing the proper equipment for the decontamination process.

It should never be ASSUMED that a patient arriving at the hospital ER has already been completely decontaminated.

Many hospitals will have a permanent Decon area or section built in to the flow of the system; MOST will not - it is these that will require the use of portable decontamination showers and have the need to store, rapidly locate and deploy, assemble and mobilize this equipment - before the hospital facility becomes contaminated by victims entering before being properly decontaminated.

Time and availability of trained personnel can become the enemy in critical situations.

One suggestion that may be useful is for the assembly of portable units to become more users friendly. This can be achieved in several ways including frequent training which can become labor intensive projects, and the use of assembly systems to attempt to make the assembly as fool proof as possible.

One such systems to think about, it to assemble the portable unit as a training exercise with various people in attendance that may be required to perform such a task in emergency and disaster situations and when the "regular staff" (maintenance/engineering) is unavailable, etc.

Upon assemble of the equipment and units is a non-stress situation, mark all the conjoined joints and segments with different color paints, then label them appropriately with strong stick on commercial labels. Use subsets if they are three way joints. An example of this would be to use bright-- highly visible colors, such as white, red, orange, lime, etc. Then label the area with numbers and or letters, such as 1-1, 2-2, A-A; three or four way joints could be labels 1-1A-1B-1-C, etc. Use a rotational system, such a clockwise would be 1-1A, 1-1B in a clockwise assembly manner. The bottom line is whatever system works and is understood by the personnel is the system that is best utilized.

This will save invaluable time, reduce stress and make assembly much easier for those unfamiliar with the setup in situations where the normally trained personnel are unavailable and time when the trained personnel are available.

The location of the equipment and all the ancillary equipment such as soap, buckets, brushes, containment device, garbage bags, etc. should be known to the Decon team as well as those that may not be team members but someday may be called into emergency service.

## Irrigation

There are many well-read protocols regarding decontamination utilizing "copious amounts" of irrigation. However, there are no strict definitions as to what this terminology means of refers to in terms of water flow, time or pressure.

Based on military protocol, acceptable decontamination is irrigation for 10 minutes with normal shower heads which produce 3.5 gallons per minute of flow. Shower heads of 20 gallons per minute are available but require adequate water supply.

There are no tested protocols available for comparison of increased flow per minute for a shorter period of time versus reduced flow for longer period of time. It is however theorized that increase flow is likely to cause increase scatter of the contaminate thus partially defeating the principles of decontamination and or to drive the contaminate thru clothing and the skin.

## Heads:

3-3.5 gallons per minute (GPM) positioned 82" from ground level Spray pattern minimum distance of 20" at 60" above ground level. Flow rate of 3+ gallons per minute require approximate 60 pounds per square inch (psi) pressure---in some instances this may be too much pressure and cause additional non contained dispersion of contaminate.

## Water Temperature

*ANSIZ358.1 standards states the use of "tepid" water. However, there is no temperature range defined for this term----thus use caution with the temperature range utilized, especially with eye irrigation so not to result in the activation of any additional chemical reaction that maybe heat responsive as well as to cause increase skin burning along with the irritation effect of the chemical compound.

*(American National Standards Institute, New York. (212 642-4900) 1998

## Water Pressure Calculation

For the evaluation and placement of the proper decontamination equipment, the adequate supply of water pressure and volume must be appropriate to the supply source.

Gallons per minute through a pipe may be calculated by:

$$GPM = 29.83 \times C \times d^2 \times P$$

Where 29.83 is a constant
C is the nozzle coefficient of 1 for practical purposed
D is orifice diameter in inches
P is the pressure
Therefore GPM is 29.7 x $d^2$ x P
1 gallon of water equals 231 cubic inches and is equal to 8.333 pounds
1 pound of water is 27.7 cubic inches
1 cubic foot of water equals 7.7 gallons and weighs 62.5 pounds
The pounds per square inch at the bottom of a column of water equals the height of the column in feet x 0.434.

APPENDIX 11

• • •

# Vulnerability Analysis

## (Enter Year Here) "XYZ" Hospital HAZARD AND VULNERABILITY ASSESSMENT TOOL

### Instructions:

Evaluate potential for event and response among the following categories using the hazard specific scale.

Issues to consider for **probability** include, but are not limited to:

1 Known risk
2 Historical data
3 Manufacturer/Vendor statistics

Issues to consider for **response** include, but are not limited to:

1 Time to marshal an on-scene response
2 Scope of response capability
3 Historical evaluation of response success

Issues to consider for **human impact** include, but are not limited to:

1. Potential for staff death or injury
2. Potential for patient death or injury

Issues to consider for **property impact** include, but are not limited to:

1. Cost to replace
2. Cost to set up temporary replacement
3. Cost to repair

Issues to consider for **business impact** include, but are not limited to:

1. Business interruption
2. Employees unable to report to work
3. Customers unable to reach facility
4. Company in violation of contractual agreements
5. Imposition of fines and penalties or legal costs
6. Interruption of critical supplies
7. Interruption of product distribution

Issues to consider for **preparedness** include, but are not limited to:

1. Status of current plans
2. Training status
3. Insurance
4. Availability of back-up systems
5. Community resources

Issues to consider for **internal resources** include, but are not limited to:

1 Types of supplies on hand
2 Volume of supplies on hand
3 Staff availability
4 Coordination with MOB's

Issues to consider for **external resources** include, but are not limited to:

1 Types of agreements with community agencies
2 Coordination with local and state agencies
3 Coordination with proximal health care facilities
4 Coordination with treatment specific facilities

Complete all worksheets including Natural, Technological, Human and Hazmat. The summary section will automatically provide your specific and overall relative threat.

APPENDIX 12

# "XYZ" Hospital
# Vulnerability Analysis Checklist

## Buildings and Structures

- ☐ Dams
- ☐ Monuments/Museums/Parks
- ☐ Convention Centers
- ☐ Sports and Entertainment Complexes/Casinos

## Facilities

- ☐ Chemical Plants
- ☐ Munitions Plants
- ☐ Hotels
- ☐ Hospitals
- ☐ Law Enforcement Complexes
- ☐ Experimental Laboratories
- ☐ Communication Facilities
- ☐ Office Building Complexes, esp. High Rise and High Profile

**Government**

- ☐ **Military Bases/Complexes**
- ☐ **Government Buildings and Facilities – i.e. State Department, NASA, Embassy, FBI/DEA Field Offices, State Capitol**

**Industry**

- ☐ **Trucking and Shipping Facilities/Depots**
- ☐ **Refineries**
- ☐ **Manufacturing Facilities**
- ☐ **Distribution Sites**
- ☐ **Factories (esp. high profile manufacturing)**

**Transportation**

- ☐ **Airports**
- ☐ **Bus Depots**
- ☐ **Train Stations, Railways and Switching Yards**
- ☐ **Truck Stops**
- ☐ **Interstate Highways**
- ☐ **Ports and Waterways; Cruise Ship Terminals**
- ☐ **Bridges**
- ☐ **Lakes and Marinas**

APPENDIX 13

# Hazard Checklist

## Hazard:______________________________
## Brief description of scenario:

**Location:**
**Characterization**
❐ natural ❐ technological ❐ human ❐ secondary ❐ complex

**Probability of occurrence**
❐ calculated ❐ hypothesized ❐ unknown ❐ independent of past events ❐ dependent of past events

**Frequency**
❐ regular (e.g. seasonal) ❐ some regularity ❐ random

**Pattern of impact**
❐ sudden catastrophe ❐ rapid build-up (<24h) ❐ slow build-up

**Duration**
❐ seconds ❐ minutes ❐ hours ❐ days ❐ weeks ❐ months ❐ years

**Area of Impact**
❐ widespread ❐ local ❐site specific

**Short-term predictability (forecast capability)**
**Location** ❐ predictable ❐ variable but generally known ❐ unpredictable
**Timing** ❐ highly predictable ❐ very predictable ❐ somewhat predictable ❐ highly unpredictable

**Warning capability**
❐ very high ❐ high ❐ moderate ❐ low ❐ very low

**Controllability (can physical process be stopped?)**
❐ definitely ❐ probably ❐ possibly ❐ no

**General assessments**
**Vulnerability** ❐ very high ❐ high ❐ moderate ❐ low ❐ very low
**Risk levels** ❐ very high ❐ high ❐ moderate ❐ low ❐ very low

**Preparedness levels**
❐ very effective ❐ effective ❐ unknown ❐ ineffective ❐ lacking

**Structural and semi-structural preparedness**
❐ very effective ❐ effective ❐ unknown ❐ ineffective ❐ lacking
**Infrastructure preparedness**
❐ very effective ❐ effective ❐ unknown ❐ ineffective ❐ lacking

**Probable future impact levels**
❐ very effective ❐ effective ❐ unknown ❐ ineffective ❐ lacking

**Staff awareness of hazard**
❐ very effective ❐ effective ❐ unknown ❐ ineffective ❐ lacking

**Support for mitigation and preparedness measures**
❐ very effective ❐ effective ❐ unknown ❐ ineffective ❐ lacking

**General assessment of mitigation situation for this hazard**
❐ very effective ❐ effective ❐ unknown ❐ ineffective ❐ lacking

# Summary Of "XYZ" Hospital Hazards Analysis

| | Natural | Technologica l | Human | Hazmat | Total for Facility |
|---|---|---|---|---|---|
| **Probability** | 0.00 | 0.00 | 0.00 | 0.00 | 0.00 |
| **Severity** | 0.00 | 0.00 | 0.00 | 0.00 | 0.00 |
| **Hazard Specific Relative Risk:** | 0.00 | 0.00 | 0.00 | 0.00 | 0.00 |

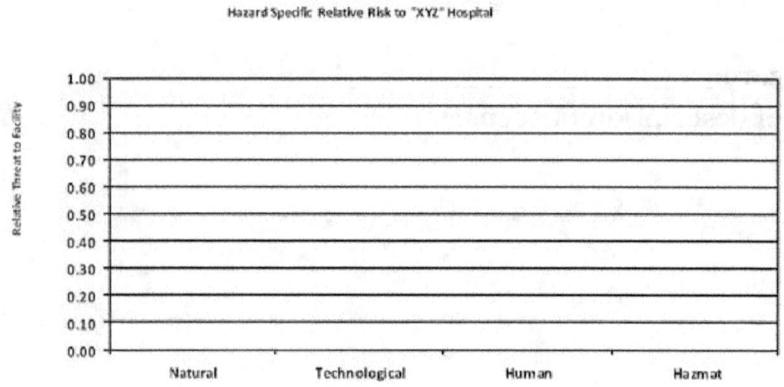


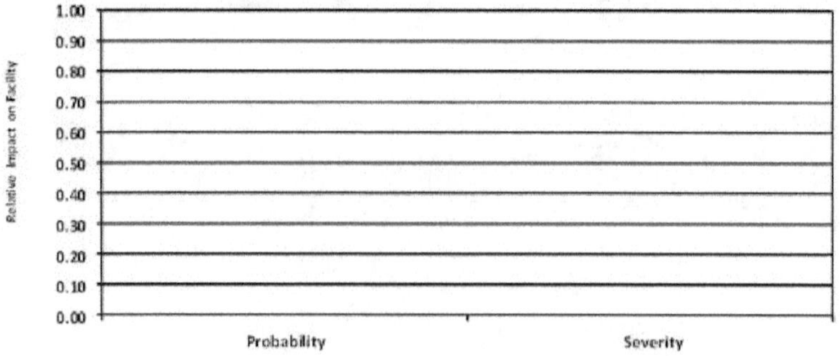

## HAZARD PROFILE WORKSHEET

***HAZARD:***

***POTENTIAL MAGNITUDE*** **(Percentage of the facility that may be affected):**

- ○ **Catastrophic:** More than 50 %
- ○ **Critical:** 25 to 50%
- ○ **Limited:** 10 to 25%
- ○ **Negligible:** Less than 10%

***FREQUENCY OF OCCURRENCE:***

- ○ **Highly likely:** Near 100% probability in next year.
- ○ **Likely:** Between 10 and 100% probability in next year, or at least one chance in next 10 years.
- ○ **Possible:** Between 1 and 10% probability in next year, or at least one chance in next 100 years.
- ○ **Unlikely:** Less than 1% probability in next 100 years.

***PATTERN:***

***AREAS LIKELY TO BE AFFECTED:***

***PROBABLE DURATION:***

***POTENTIAL SPEED OF ONSET (Probable amount of warning time):***

- ○ Minimal (or no) warning
- ○ 6 to 12 hours warning
- ○ 12 to 24 hours warning
- ○ More than 24 hours warning

***EXISTING WARNING MECHANISMS:***

***COMPLETE VULNERABILITY ANALYSIS:***

- ○ Yes
- ○ No

# APPENDIX 14

• • •

## EOC Evaluation Tool

Observer: Date:_/_____/_____

Where is the EOC Location?

Primary: Building____Room______

Alternate: Building____Room______

Was an Incident Commander designated? ☐Yes ☐No

If yes, who?__

Were other members of the incident command center easily identifiable? ☐Yes ☐No

| Role | Check if position filled | Comments |
|---|---|---|
| Incident Commander | ☐ | ______ |
| Public Information Officer | ☐ | ______ |
| Liaison | ☐ | ______ |
| Safety | ☐ | ______ |
| Police | ☐ | ______ |
| Operations Chief | ☐ | ______ |
| Logistics Chief | ☐ | ______ |
| Planning Chief | ☐ | ______ |
| Facilities Management | ☐ | ______ |
| Communications | ☐ | ______ |
| Patient Transportation | ☐ | ______ |

| **Role** | **Check if position filled** | **Comments** |
|---|---|---|
| Supply | ☐ | ____________________ |
| Nutrition & Food Service | ☐ | ____________________ |
| Labor Pool | ☐ | ____________________ |
| Medical Staff | ☐ | ____________________ |
| Nursing | ☐ | ____________________ |
| Ancillary Services Director (Laboratory, radiology, pharmacy, etc.) | ☐ | ____________________ |
| Human Services Director (staff and psychological support) | ☐ | ____________________ |
| Recorder | ☐ | ____________________ |
| Other (Specify):__________________ | ☐ | ____________________ |
| Other (Specify):__________________ | ☐ | ____________________ |
| Other (Specify):__________________ | ☐ | ____________________ |
| Other (Specify):__________________ | ☐ | ____________________ |

**EOC Operations**

Time EOC Activated:__________AM/PM

Was the hospital disaster plan available? ☐Yes ☐No

If the hospital disaster plan was available, what was its format? (Hardcopy, electronic, etc.)

____________________

Was the space allocated for the EOC adequate? ☐Yes ☐No

If not enough space for the EOC, where did EOC activities overflow to?___________

Average number of people in the incident command center.

☐< 5 ☐6 – 10 ☐11 - 20 ☐>20

Did the noise level in the incident command center interfere with effective communication?

☐Yes ☐No

If the noise level interfered with communications, were steps taken to correct the problem?

☐Yes ☐No

If yes what steps were taken?________________________________

## Communications

| Device | Used | Comments |
| --- | --- | --- |
| ☐2-way radio | ☐ | ______________ |
| ☐Ham Radio | ☐ | ______________ |
| ☐AM/FM radio(s) | ☐ | ______________ |
| ☐E-mail and Internet access | ☐ | ______________ |
| ☐Direct line(s) | ☐ | ______________ |
| ☐FAX machine(s) | ☐ | ______________ |
| ☐Intercom | ☐ | ______________ |
| ☐Landline phone(s) | ☐ | ______________ |
| ☐Megaphone(s) | ☐ | ______________ |
| ☐Numeric paging | ☐ | ______________ |
| ☐Overhead paging | ☐ | ______________ |
| ☐Runner(s) | ☐ | ______________ |
| ☐Television(s) | ☐ | ______________ |
| ☐Text paging | ☐ | ______________ |
| ☐Wireless/cell phone(s) | ☐ | ______________ |
| ☐Other (Specify): | ☐ | ______________ |

How was incoming information to the EOC recorded?

☐Computer (other electronic device)

☐Notepaper

☐Posted paper

☐White board/chalk board

☐Not recorded

☐Other (Specify):

## Information Flow

Were problems created by delays in receiving information?

☐ Yes ☐ No

How often was the following information received by the incident command center?

| **Information Received** | **Source** | | **Frequency** | |
|---|---|---|---|---|
| | **Internal** | **External** | **Once** | **Other (list frequency)** |
| Available operating rooms | ☐ | ☐ | ☐ | ☐______ |
| Available staffed floor beds | ☐ | ☐ | ☐ | ☐______ |
| Available staffed intensive care beds | ☐ | ☐ | ☐ | ☐______ |
| Available staffed isolation beds | ☐ | ☐ | ☐ | ☐______ |
| Number of arriving victims | ☐ | ☐ | ☐ | ☐______ |
| Estimated time of victims' arrival | ☐ | ☐ | ☐ | ☐______ |
| Expected triage level of victims | ☐ | ☐ | ☐ | ☐______ |
| Number of victims Emergency | ☐ | ☐ | ☐ | ☐______ |
| Department can accept | ☐ | ☐ | ☐ | ☐______ |
| Clinical staff available (e.g., physicians, nurses) | ☐ | ☐ | ☐ | ☐______ |
| Total number of expected victims | ☐ | ☐ | ☐ | ☐______ |
| Potential discharges of 'actual' patients | ☐ | ☐ | ☐ | ☐______ |

| **Information Received** | **Source** | | **Frequency** | |
|---|---|---|---|---|
| | **Internal** | **External** | **Once** | **Other (list frequency)** |
| Support staff available (e.g., registrar, security) | ☐ | ☐ | ☐ | ☐______ |
| Other (Specify): | ☐ | ☐ | ☐ | ☐______ |
| Other (Specify): | ☐ | ☐ | ☐ | ☐______ |
| Other (Specify): | ☐ | ☐ | ☐ | ☐______ |

Was the EOC in communication with outside agencies?
☐Yes ☐No

| Outside Agencies | Contacted | Communication Issues |
|---|---|---|
| Ambulance systems | ☐ | ______________ |
| Disaster response agency (state or federal) (e.g., FEMA) | ☐ | ______________ |
| Fire | ☐ | ______________ |
| Health department (local, state, or federal) | ☐ | ______________ |
| Media | ☐ | ______________ |
| Military | ☐ | ______________ |
| Other hospitals | ☐ | ______________ |
| Police | ☐ | ______________ |
| Other (specify):______________ | ☐ | ______________ |
| Other (specify):______________ | ☐ | ______________ |

## Security

Were security personnel present in the EOC? ☐ Yes ☐ No

If security personnel were present, what type of security?

☐ VA Police

☐ Other________________________________________

Did all security staff present have a portable means of communication? ☐ Yes ☐ No

Were entrances and exits strictly controlled in this area?

☐ Yes ☐ No

Did any security issues arise in this EOC? ☐ Yes ☐ No

If yes, did security respond? ☐ Yes ☐ No

If yes, was the situation effectively mitigated ☐ Yes ☐ No

Description of issue and measures taken:____________________

## Rotation of Staff

Was there a staff rotation/shift change? ☐ Yes ☐ No

If there was a staff rotation, did the officially designated person in charge of the EOC change? ☐ Yes ☐ No

If there was a staff rotation, did problems arise? ☐ Yes ☐ No

Describe______________________________

How were incoming staff updated?

- ☐ Group briefing
- ☐ Individual briefing
- ☐ Written notes
- ☐ Not updated
- ☐ Other (Specify):

## EOC Disruption

Was there a plan in place to relocate the primary EOC if necessary? ☐ Yes ☐ No

Did the primary EOC close at any time during the drill? ☐ Yes ☐ No

If the primary EOC closed during the drill, what was the reason for closing?

Describe______________________________

If the primary EOC closed during the drill, were other EOCs notified? ☐ Yes ☐ No

Was an alternate EOC site determined and opened? ☐ Yes ☐ No

If yes, state location:______________________________

Were operations interrupted until the alternate EOC opened? ☐ Yes ☐ No

Were other EOCs notified when the alternate EOC opened? ☐ Yes ☐ No

Were any critical issues observed with opening this EOC? ☐ Yes ☐ No

If yes, describe____________________________________

APPENDIX 15

## Incident Command
## Who Is In Charge?

ONE OF THE BIGGEST ADMINISTRATIVE problems unless adequately planned, trained and executed is --- "Who Is in Charge"? In emergency situations there is always the questions asked why Joe is the IC or Sam the Ops director, or why am "I" not in charge of some form of command position. This is best determined well before hand and exercised so that the entire staff can become familiar with who will occupy a certain position in an emergency situation and what their capabilities are as well as their short comings.

In national /federal emergencies the personnel staff is very well trained in all positions and occupies a particular position for the particular incident. Many times the positions can be switched in prolonged incidents but most of the time the chosen person occupies a leadership position and has a deputy or assistant, etc. as their backup.

In the national incident, all are used to working with each other in the various roles, trained together, and are familiar with each other and hence no or limited animosities exist.

There is always the difficulty of persons being placed in a zone to which they are uncomfortable and not familiar and thus their stress levels are accelerated.

While this is difficult to totally eliminate, adequate choices of personnel for position placement along with training and exercising will eliminate a great majority of the problems in anticipation of their occurrence with an event. The Hospital Emergency Incident Command System Job Action Sheets

(The following text is excerpted and edited from the HEICS Plan Version 3, Part I Manual available at www.heics.com)

The Job Action Sheets, or job descriptions, are the essence of the HEICS program. This is the component that tells your responding personnel "what they are going to do; when they are going to do it; and, who they will report it to after they have done it."

Each position does not necessarily represent a person and each position must be filled as soon as possible. Each crisis is unique. Those positions, which will be immediately needed to manage the emergency will be the first assignments made. One person may hold more than one position. There are some positions or roles, which are not needed for hours or days after the onset of the emergency. Some may not be needed at all.

Each hospital is encouraged to create a" Crosswalk". The crosswalk is a listing of day-today positions as they may relate to the ICS positions as found in the Job Action Sheets. For example, the CFO may crosswalk to the Finance Section Chief. While it is not recommended that these be the only people trained for each position, it is reasonable to visualize how these individuals may be a logical first choice for filling a particular role. It must be remembered that the Incident Commander will assign Officers and Chiefs and they in turn will assign the positions under them.

## Job Action Sheets

The Job Action Sheets were the basis for the first HEICS manual, written in the spring of 1991. These sheets should be altered to meet the needs of the facility. There are two components of the Job Action Sheets, which should not be changed: job titles and the mission statement.

The universal titles and mission statements, found in HIECS, allow emergency responders from a variety of organizations to communicate quickly and clearly with other users of ICS. Changing job titles and mission statements will go against the very purpose of having common terminology and structure.

The National Incident Management System (NIMS) now formalizes ICS as the structure to be used by all agencies, involved in a response.

## Incident Commander

Mission: Organize and direct Emergency Operations Center (EOC). Give overall direction for hospital operations and if needed, authorize evacuation.

Immediate Responsibilities: Initiate the Hospital Emergency Incident Command System by assuming role of Emergency Incident Commander. Read this entire Job Action Sheet. Put on position identification vest. Appoint all Section Chiefs and the Medical Staff Director positions; distribute the four section packets which contain: Job Action Sheets for each position, Identification vest for each position, Forms pertinent to Section & positions Appoint Public Information Officer, Liaison Officer, and Safety and Security Officer; distribute Job Action Sheets. (May be pre-established.) Announce a status/action plan meeting of all Section Chiefs and Medical Staff Director to be held within 5 to 10 minutes. Assign someone as Documentation Recorder/Aide. Receive status report and discuss an initial action plan with Section Chiefs and Medical Staff Director. Determine appropriate level of service during immediate aftermath. Receive initial facility damage survey report from Logistics Chief, and, if applicable, evaluate the need for evacuation. Obtain patient census and status from Planning Section Chief. Emphasize proactive actions within the Planning Section. Call for a hospital-wide projection report for 4, 8, 24 & 48 hours from time of incident onset. Adjust projections as necessary. Authorize a patient prioritization assessment for the purposes of designating appropriate early discharge, if additional beds needed. Assure that contact and resource information has been established with outside agencies through the Liaison Officer.

Intermediate Responsibilities: Authorize resources as needed or requested by Section Chiefs. Designate routine briefings with Section Chiefs to receive status reports and update the action plan regarding the continuance and termination of the action plan. Communicate status to chairperson of the Hospital Board of Directors or the designee. Consult with Section Chiefs on needs for staff, physician, and volunteer responder food and shelter. Consider needs for dependents. Authorize plan of action.

Extended Responsibilities: Approve media releases submitted by P.I.O. Observe all staff, volunteers and patients for signs of stress and inappropriate behavior. Report concerns to Psychological Support Unit Leader. Provide for staff rest periods and relief.

## Public Information Officer (PIO)

You Report To: Incident Commander

Mission: Provide information to the news media.

Immediate Responsibilities: Receive appointment from Incident Commander. Read this entire Job Action sheet and review organizational chart on back. Put on position identification vest. Identify restrictions in contents of news release information from Incident Commander. Establish a Public Information area away from E.O.C. and patient care activity.

Intermediate Responsibilities: Ensure that all news releases have the approval of the Incident Commander. Issue an initial incident information report to the news media with the cooperation of the Situation-Status Unit Leader. Relay any pertinent data back to Situation-Status Unit Leader. Inform on-site media of the physical areas which they have access to and those which are restricted. Coordinate with Safety and Security Officer. Contact other at-scene agencies to coordinate released information, with respective P.I.O.s. Inform Liaison Officer of action.

Extended Responsibilities: Obtain progress reports from Section Chiefs as appropriate. Notify media about casualty status. Direct calls from those who wish to volunteer for Labor Pool. Contact Labor Pool to determine requests to be made to the public via the media. Observe all staff, volunteers and patients for signs of stress and inappropriate behavior. Report concerns to Psychological Support Unit Leader. Provide for staff rest periods and relief.

## Liaison Officer

You Report To: Incident Commander

Mission: Function as incident contact person for representatives from other agencies.

Immediate Responsibilities: Receive appointment from Incident Commander. Read this entire Job Action Sheet and review organizational chart on back. Put on position identification vest. Obtain briefing from Incident Commander. Establish contact with Communications Unit Leader in E.O.C. Obtain one or more aides as necessary from Labor Pool. Review county and municipal emergency organizational charts to determine appropriate contacts and message routing. Coordinate with Public Information Officer. Obtain information to provide the interhospital emergency communication network, municipal E.O.C. and/or county E.O.C as appropriate, upon request. The following information should be gathered for relay: The number of "RED" and "YELLOW" patients that can be received and treated immediately. Any current or anticipated shortage of personnel, supplies, etc. Current condition of hospital structure and utilities (hospital's overall status). Number of patients to be transferred by wheelchair or stretcher to another hospital. Any resources which are requested by other facilities (i.e., staff, equipment, supplies). Establish communication with the assistance of the Communication Unit Leader with the interhospital emergency communication network, municipal E.O.C. or with county E.O.C./County Health Officer. Relay current hospital status. Establish contact with liaison counterparts of each assisting and cooperating agency (i.e., municipal E.O.C.). Keeping governmental Liaison Officers updated on changes and development of hospital's response to incident.

Intermediate Responsibilities: Request assistance and information as needed through the interhospital emergency communication network or municipal/county E.O.C. Respond to requests and complaints from incident personnel regarding interorganization problems. Prepare to assist Labor Pool Unit Leader with problems encountered in the volunteer credentialing process. Relay any special information obtained to appropriate personnel in the receiving facility (i.e., information regarding toxic decontamination or any special emergency conditions).

Extended Responsibilities: Assist the Medical Staff Director and Labor Pool Unit Leader in soliciting physicians and other hospital personnel willing to volunteer as Disaster Service Workers outside of the hospital, when appropriate. Inventory any material resources, which may be sent upon official request and method of transportation, if appropriate. Supply casualty data to the appropriate authorities; prepare the following minimum data: Number of casualties received and types of injuries treated, Number hospitalized and number discharged to home or other facilities, Number dead, Individual casualty data: name or physical description, sex, age, address, seriousness of injury or condition, Observe all staff, volunteers and patients for signs of stress and inappropriate behavior. Report concerns to Psychological Support Unit Leader. Provide for staff rest periods and relief.

## Safety And Security Officer

You Report To: Incident Commander

Mission: Monitor and have authority over the safety of rescue operations and hazardous conditions. Organize and enforce scene/ facility protection and traffic security.

Immediate Responsibilities: Receive appointment from Incident Commander. Read this entire Job Action sheet and review organizational chart on back. Put on position identification vest. Obtain a briefing from Incident Commander. Implement the facility's disaster plan emergency lockdown policy and personnel identification policy. Establish Security Command Post. Remove unauthorized persons from restricted areas. Establish ambulance entry and exit routes in cooperation with Transportation Unit Leader. Secure the E.O.C., triage, patient care, morgue and other sensitive or strategic areas from unauthorized access.

Intermediate Responsibilities: Communicate with Damage Assessment and Control Officer to secure and post no entry signs around unsafe areas. Keep Safety and Security staff alert to identify and report all hazards and unsafe conditions to the Damage Assessment and Control Officer. Secure areas evacuated to and from, to limit unauthorized personnel access. Initiate contact with fire, police agencies through the Liaison Officer, when necessary. Advise the Incident Commander and Section Chiefs immediately of any unsafe, hazardous or security related conditions. Assist Labor Pool and Medical Staff Unit Leaders with credentialing/screening process of volunteers. Prepare to manage large numbers of potential volunteers. Confer with Public Information Officer to establish areas for media personnel. Establish routine briefings with Incident Commander. Provide vehicular and pedestrian traffic control. Secure food, water, medical, and blood resources. Inform Safety & Security staff to document all actions and observations. Establish routine briefings with Safety & Security staff. Observe all staff, volunteers and patients for signs of stress and inappropriate behavior. Report concerns to Psychological Support Unit Leader. Provide for staff rest periods and relief.

## Logistics Section Chief

You Report To: Incident Commander

Mission: Organize and direct those operations associated with maintenance of the physical environment, and adequate levels of food, shelter and supplies to support the medical objectives.

Immediate Responsibilities: Receive appointment from the Incident Commander. Obtain packet containing Section's Job Action Sheets, identification vests and forms. Read this entire Job Action Sheet and review organizational chart on back. Put on position identification vest. Obtain briefing from Incident Commander. Appoint Logistics Section Unit Leaders: Facilities Unit Leader, Communications Unit Leader, Transportation Unit Leader, Material's Supply Unit Leader, Nutritional Supply Unit Leader; distribute Job Action Sheets and vests. (May be pre-established.) Brief unit leaders on current situation; outline action plan and designate time for next briefing. Establish Logistics Section

Center in proximity to E.O.C. Attend damage assessment meeting with Incident Commander, Facility Unit Leader and Damage Assessment and Control Officer.

Intermediate Responsibilities: Obtain information and updates regularly from unit leaders and officers; maintain current status of all areas; pass status info to Situation-Status Unit Leader. Communicate frequently with Incident Commander. Obtain needed supplies with assistance of the Finance Section Chief, Communications Unit Leader and Liaison Unit Leader.

Extended Responsibilities: Assure that all communications are copied to the Communications Unit Leader. Document actions and decisions on a continual basis. Observe all staff, volunteers and patients for signs of stress and inappropriate behavior. Report concerns to Psychological Support Unit Leader. Provide for staff rest periods and relief.

## Planning Section Chief

You Report To: Incident Commander

Mission: Organize and direct all aspects of Planning Section operations. Ensure the distribution of critical information/data. Compile scenario/resource projections from all section chiefs and effect long range planning. Document and distribute facility Action Plan.

Immediate Responsibilities: Receive appointment from Incident Commander. Obtain packet containing Section's Job Action Sheets. Read this entire Job Action Sheet and review organizational chart on back. Put on position identification vest. Obtain briefing from Incident Commander. Recruit a documentation aide from the Labor Pool Appoint Planning unit leaders: Situation - Status Unit Leader, Labor Pool Unit Leader, Medical Staff Unit Leader, Nursing Unit Leader; distribute the corresponding Job

Action Sheets and vests. (May be pre-established.) Brief unit leaders after meeting with Incident Commander. Provide for a Planning/ Information Center. Ensure the formulation and documentation of an incident-specific, facility Action Plan. Distribute copies to Incident Commander and all section chiefs. Call for projection reports (Action Plan) from all Planning Section unit leaders and section chiefs for scenarios 4, 8, 24 & 48 hours from time of incident onset. Adjust time for receiving projection reports as necessary. Instruct Situation - Status Unit Leader and staff to document/update status reports from all disaster section chiefs and unit leaders for use in decision making and for reference in post-disaster evaluation and recovery assistance applications.

Intermediate Responsibilities: Obtain briefings and updates as appropriate. Continue to update and distribute the facility Action Plan. Schedule planning meetings to include Planning Section unit leaders, section chiefs and the Incident Commander for continued update of the facility Action Plan.

Extended Responsibilities: Continue to receive projected activity reports from section chiefs and Planning Section unit leaders at appropriate intervals. Assure that all requests are routed/documented through the Communications Unit Leader. Observe all staff, volunteers and patients for signs of stress and inappropriate behavior. Report concerns to Psychological Support Unit Leader. Provide for staff rest periods and relief.

## Finance Section Chief

You Report To: Incident Commander

Mission: Monitor the utilization of financial assets. Oversee the acquisition of supplies and services necessary to carry out the hospital's medical mission. Supervise the documentation of expenditures relevant to the emergency incident.

Immediate Responsibilities: Receive appointment from Incident Commander. Obtain packet containing Section's Job Action Sheets. Read this entire Job Action Sheet and review organizational chart on back. Put on position identification vest. Obtain briefing from Incident Commander. Appoint Time Unit Leader, Procurement Unit Leader, Claims Unit Leader and Cost Unit Leader; distribute the corresponding Job Action Sheets and vests. (May be pre-established.) Confer with Unit Leaders after meeting with Emergency Incident Commander; develop a section action plan. Establish a Financial Section Operations Center. Ensure adequate documentation/recording personnel.

Intermediate Responsibilities: Approve a "cost-to-date" incident financial status report submitted by the Cost Unit Leader every eight hours summarizing financial data relative to personnel, supplies and miscellaneous expenses. Obtain briefings and updates from Emergency Incident Commander as appropriate. Relate pertinent financial status reports to appropriate chiefs and unit leaders. Schedule planning meetings to include Finance Section unit leaders to discuss updating the section's incident action plan and termination procedures.

Extended Responsibilities: Assure that all requests for personnel or supplies are copied to the Communications Unit Leader in a timely manner. Observe all staff, volunteers and patients for signs of stress and inappropriate behavior. Report concerns to Psychological Support Unit Leader. Provide for staff rest periods and relief.

## Operations Section Chief

You Report To: Incident Commander

Mission: Organize and direct aspects relating to the Operations Section. Carry out directives of the Incident Commander.

Coordinate and supervise the Medical Services Subsection, Ancillary Services Subsection and Human Services Subsection of the Operations Section.

Immediate Responsibilities: Receive appointment from Incident Commander. Obtain packet containing Section's Job Action Sheets. Read this entire Job Action Sheet and review organizational chart on back. Put on position identification vest. Obtain briefing from Incident Commander. Appoint Medical Staff Director, Medical Care Director, Ancillary Services Director and Human Services Director and transfer the corresponding Job Action Sheets. (May be pre-established.) Brief all Operations Section directors on current situation and develop the section's initial action plan. Designate time for next briefing. Establish Operations Section Center in proximity to E.O.C. Meet with the Medical Staff Director, Medical Care Director and Nursing Unit Leader to plan and project patient care needs.

Intermediate Responsibilities: Designate times for briefings and updates with all Operations Section directors to develop/update section's action plan. Ensure that the Medical Services Subsection, Ancillary Services Subsection and Human Services Subsection are adequately staffed and supplied. Brief the Emergency Incident Commander routinely on the status of the Operations Section.

Extended Responsibilities: Assure that all communications are copied to the Communications Unit Leader; document all actions and decisions. Observe all staff, volunteers and patients for signs of stress and inappropriate behavior. Report concerns to Psychological Support Unit Leader. Provide for staff rest periods and relief.

APPENDIX 16

• • •

## Incident Types

INCIDENTS MAY BE TYPED IN order to make decisions about resource requirements. Incident types are based on the following five levels of complexity. (Source: U.S. Fire Administration)

### TYPE 5

The incident can be handled with one or two single resources with up to six personnel. Command and General Staff positions (other than the Incident Commander) are not activated. No written Incident Action Plan (IAP) is required. The incident is contained within the first operational period and often within an hour to a few hours after resources arrive on scene. Examples include a vehicle fire, an injured person, or a police traffic stop.

### TYPE 4

Command staff and general staff functions are activated only if needed. Several resources are required to mitigate the incident. The incident is usually limited to one operational period in the control phase. The agency administrator may have briefings, and ensure the complexity analysis and delegation of authority are updated. No written Incident Action Plan (IAP) is required but a documented operational briefing will be completed for all incoming resources. The role of the agency administrator includes operational plans including objectives and priorities.

## Type 3

When capabilities exceed initial attack, the appropriate ICS positions should be added to match the complexity of the incident. Some or all of the Command and General Staff positions may be activated, as well as Division/Group Supervisor and/or Unit Leader level positions. A Type 3 Incident Management Team (IMT) or incident command organization manages initial action incidents with a significant number of resources, an extended attack incident until containment/control is achieved, or an expanding incident until transition to a Type 1 or 2 team. The incident may extend into multiple operational periods. A written IAP may be required for each operational period.

## Type 2

This type of incident extends beyond the capabilities for local control and is expected to go into multiple operational periods. A Type 2 incident may require the response of resources out of area, including regional and/or national resources, to effectively manage the operations, command, and general staffing. Most or all of the Command and General Staff positions are filled. A written IAP is required for each operational period. Many of the functional units are needed and staffed. Operations personnel normally do not exceed 200 per operational period and total incident personnel do not exceed 500 (guidelines only). The agency administrator is responsible for the incident complexity analysis, agency administrator briefings, and the written delegation of authority.

### Type 1

This type of incident is the most complex, requiring national resources to safely and effectively manage and operate. All Command and General Staff positions are activated. Operations personnel often exceed 500 per operational period and total personnel will usually exceed 1,000. Branches need to be established. The agency administrator will have briefings, and ensure that the complexity analysis and delegation of authority are updated. Use of resource advisors at the incident base is recommended. There is a high impact on the local jurisdiction, requiring additional staff for office administrative and support functions.

APPENDIX 17

• • •

## Strategic National Stockpile Material Listing

| Description | Unit Pack |
| --- | --- |
| APS (Automated Packaging System) prescription packaging machine | 1/EA |
| APS Compressor | 1/EA |
| APS Spare Parts Kit | 1/EA |
| Abdominal pad, sterile, 8"x 10", 320's | 320/CS |
| Aero Chamber Plus | 10 |
| Aero Chamber, lg | 10 |
| Aero Chamber, md | 10 |
| Albuterol metered dose inhaler, 17gm, 72's | 72/CS |
| Amoxicillin 200mg chewable tablet, #75 tab unit of use bottle (40/cs) | 40 |
| Amoxicillin 500mg oral capsule unit of use #30 cap bottle (40/cs) | 40 |
| Amoxicillin 500mg oral capsule unit of use #30 cap bottle (480/cs) | 480 |
| Amoxicillin 500mg oral capsule unit of use #30 cap bottle (80/cs) | 80 |
| Atropine 0.4mg/ml x 20ml soln. for inj., multi-dose vial, 100's | 100/CS |
| Bottle, Qorpack 48's | 48/CS |

| | |
|---|---|
| CO2 detector, Easy cap II ( use with MPR), 24's | 24/CS |
| Carpuject Device, 50's | 50/CS |
| Ciprofloxacin 250mg/5ml oral suspension, powder, 100ml bottle, 24's | 24/CS |
| Ciprofloxacin 500mg oral tablet #20 tab unit of use bottle (100/cs) | 100 |
| Ciprofloxacin 500mg oral tablet #20 tab unit of use bottle (400/cs) | 400 |
| Ciprofloxacin 500mg oral tablet, 100# tablet bottle 144's | 144 |
| Ciprofloxacin soln. for inj., 400mg in D5W 200ml flexi-bag, 24's | 24/CS |
| Container "A" Tall | 1/EA |
| Container "A" Tall, 5-DOOR, APS | 1/EA |
| Container "B" Short | 1/EA |
| Diazepam soln. for inj., 5mg/ml x 2ml auto-injector, (Ea) | 1 |
| Diazepam soln. for inj., 5mg/ml, x 10ml multi-dose vial, 25's | 25/BX |
| Dopamine soln. for inj., 400mg (40mg/ml x 10ml) vial, 50's | 50/CS |
| Doxycycline 100mg oral tablet #20 tab unit of use (100/cs) | 100 |
| Doxycycline 100mg oral tablet #20 tab unit of use (400/cs) | 400 |
| Doxycycline 100mg oral tablet, #500 tab bottle 24's | 24 |
| Doxycycline 100mg powder vial for injection, 100's | 100/CS |
| Doxycycline 25mg/5ml oral suspension, powder, 60ml bottle, 48's | 48/CS |
| Duct tape, roll | 1/EA |
| Endotracheal tube guide (Stylet), 10FR, (adult), 200's | 200/CS |
| Endotracheal tube guide (Stylet), 6Fr, (infant, pediatric), 200's | 200/CS |
| Endotracheal tube guide (Stylet), 8Fr (pediatric), 200's | 200/CS |

| | |
|---|---|
| Endotracheal tube, 3mm ID, uncuffed, (infant), 10's | 10/BX |
| Endotracheal tube, 4mm ID, uncuffed, (infant), 10's | 10/BX |
| Endotracheal tube, 5mm ID, uncuffed, (pediatric), 10's | 10/BX |
| Endotracheal tube, 6mm ID, cuffed (pediatric, small adult), 10's | 10/BX |
| Endotracheal tube, 7mm ID, cuffed (adult), 10's | 10/BX |
| Endotracheal tube, 8mm ID, cuffed (adult), 10's | 10/BX |
| Epinephrine HCl 1:10000 (10ml) syringe/needle for injection, 50's | 50/CS |
| Epinephrine soln., 0.15mg auto-injector (1:2000), 12's | 12/BX |
| Epinephrine soln., 0.3mg auto-injector (1:1000), 12's | 12/BX |
| Extension cord, heavy-duty, 25 ft. 1/EA | |
| Fan, Port-A-Cool 48" 3-Speed, (Air cooling unit) 1/EA | |
| Gauze bandage, conforming 4" x 180", 96's | 96/CS |
| Gauze dressing, sterile, (sponge) 4"x 4", 1200's | 1,200/CS |
| Gentamicin soln. for inj., 40mg/ml x 20ml multi-dose vial, 100's | 100/CS |
| Gloves, large, non-sterile, powder-free, non-latex, 1000's | 1,000/CS |
| Gloves, medium, non-sterile, powder free, non-latex, 1000's | 1,000/CS |
| IV Intermittent injection site, long, with Luer-Lok, 200's | 200/CS |
| IV administration set, 10 drop/ml, unvented, 48's | 48/CS |
| IV administration set, 10 drop/ml, vented, 48's | 48/CS |
| IV administration set, 60 drop/ml, unvented, 48's | 48/CS |
| IV administration set, 60 drop/ml, vented, 48's | 48/CS |
| IV administration set, butterfly, 21G x 3/4", 120's | 120/CS |
| IV catheter/needle, 18G x 1 1/4", 200's | 200/CS |
| IV catheter/needle, 18G x 2", 200's | 200/CS |
| IV catheter/needle, 20G x 1 1/4", 200's | 200/CS |
| IV catheter/needle, 24G x 5/8", 200's | 200/CS |

| | |
|---|---|
| IV site transparent dressing 2 3/8"x2 3/4", 600's | 600/CS |
| Ink pad, black | 1/EA |
| Isopropyl alcohol pads, 70%, 1 1/4" x 2 1/2", 3000's | 3,000/CS |
| Label-Avery Name Badge, 2000's | 2000/CS |
| Laryngoscope handle/blade, disposable, large (Mac 3), 10's | 10/BX |
| Laryngoscope handle/blade, disposable, small (Mac 2), 10's | 10/BX |
| Laryngoscope illuminator (fits in handle) | 1/EA |
| Manual pulmonary resuscitator (MPR), adult, w/ bag, mask, valve, 12's | 12/CS |
| Manual pulmonary resuscitator (MPR), pediatric, w/ bag, mask, valve, 12's | 12/CS |
| Mark 1 (600mg pralidoxime/2mg atropine) auto-injector, (Each) | 1 |
| Methylprednisolone - (2ml) powder/diluent vial for inj 25's | 25/BX |
| Nasal cannula, with tubing, adult, 50's | 50/CS |
| Nasogastric tube, adult, 14Fr., 50's | 50/CS |
| Nasogastric tube, adult, 16Fr., 50's | 50/CS |
| Nasogastric tube, pediatric, 10Fr., 50's | 50/CS |
| Oropharyngeal airway, Berman, 40mm (infant), 12's | 12/CS |
| Oropharyngeal airway, Berman, 60mm, (pediatric), 12's | 12/CS |
| Oropharyngeal airway, Berman, 90mm, (adult), 12's | 12/CS |
| Oxygen mask, non-rebreather, adult, 50's | 50/CS |
| Oxygen mask, non-rebreather, pediatric, 50's | 50/CS |
| Oxygen tubing, 7 ft., 50's | 50/CS |
| Polymixin/bacitracin antibiotic ointment, 0.9gm packet, 1728's | 1728/CS |
| Povidone Iodine swabsticks, 10%, triple paks, 750's | 750/CS |
| Power strip, electric | 1/EA |
| Pralidoxime 1gm powder vial for injection, 276's | 276/CS |

| | |
|---|---|
| Prescription dispensing bag, plastic, 3" x 5", zipper seal, 10,000's | 10,000/CS |
| Prescription dispensing bag, plastic, 3" x 5", zipper seal, 2ML, 20,000's | 20,000/CS |
| Safety cap removal device | 1/EA |
| Sodium Chloride 0.9% 3ml Carpuject (IV Flush, Preservative Free), 300's | 300/CS |
| Sodium Chloride for inj., 0.9%, 1000ml flexi-bag, 12's | 12/CS |
| Sodium Chloride for inj., 0.9%, 100ml flexi-bag, 96's | 96/CS |
| Stamper, Bates Model 7AMULT | 1/EA |
| Sterile water for injection, preservative free, 10ml vial, 400's | 400/CS |
| Suction catheter 14Fr, sterile, flexible, with control valve, 50's | 50/CS |
| Suction catheter 18Fr, sterile, flexible, with control valve, 50's | 50/CS |
| Suction, Yankauer, with control vent, 50's | 50/CS |
| Syringe 10ml, 20G x 1 1/2" needle, 600's | 600/CS |
| Syringe, oral dosing, calibrated 10ml, 500's | 500/CS |
| Tablet counting machine, Kirby Lester | 1/EA |
| Tape, cloth, 1" x 10 yd, roll (Durapore or equivalent), 120's | 120/CS |
| Tourniquet, latex-free, 3/4" x 18", 1000's | 1,000/CS |
| Tweezers (removal cotton from tablet bottles) | 1/EA |
| Volumetric Devices | 1/EA |
| Water tank, Port-A-Fill 50 gallon (for use with port-a-cooler) | 1/EA |

## APPENDIX 18

• • •

# The "GO-BAG"

EVERYONE WORKING IN ANY FIELD dealing with emergencies requiring their immediate deployment should be ready to "GO" in just a matter of minutes. This concept was adopted from the National Transportation Safety Board Go Team that is required to deploy to a site within 60 minutes of being notified.

This likewise works well for all persons that live and or work in an area that may have a high vulnerability index for disasters and emergencies, such as tornados, hurricanes, earthquakes, landslides, and chemical and explosive proximities.

Below is a suggested list, but each person MUST personalize their own Go-Bag to meet their needs.

Each 6 to 12 months the bag should be inventoried, items replaced or refreshed as necessary to keep the contents up to date and ready for immediate use should that become necessary.

Each hospital employee should have such a kit readily available, and many hospitals have given their employees such a bag as Christmas presents so there would be uniformity within their system.

Each employee should keep the kit readily available in the automobiles or lockers, etc., especially during peak seasons or in critical events that may result in major hospital surge, i.e., pandemics, major sporting events or seasonal activities.

## Personal Supplies:

Prescription Rx medications in a small amount in separate containers; extra contact lens or glasses.

Cash $50-100 in small bills $1, 5 and 10; as credit cards may not work at point of sales in disaster areas due to the devastation or loss of electrical power.

Sleeping Bag

Change of clothes, include cheap or disposable sets of underwear; jacket or raincoat as maybe needed.

Moist towelettes and few garbage bags for personal sanitation

Personal hygiene items

Cell phone battery or charger

Small roll of duct tape

Manual can opener, flashlight, N-95 mask

Personalized Items individualized to needs, wishes and desires

Place items in individual zip lock bags with all the air squeezed out to reduce size as well as keep moisture out.

## APPENDIX 19

• • •

### Weather Facts and Information
### Saffir Simpson Wind Scale

THE SAFFIR-SIMPSON HURRICANE WIND SCALE was first developed in the early 1970s by Herbert Saffir, a consulting engineer who lived in Florida, and Dr. Robert Simpson, who was then director of the National Hurricane Center.

The current version is strictly a wind scale. Previous versions listed central pressures typically associated with each category due to a relationship that exists between pressure and wind, but the details can vary quite a bit depending on the nature of each particular hurricane. Also, storm surge was quantified by category.

However, hurricanes with wind fields which are very large in size can produce storm surge heights that are much higher than is average for a give category, such as was the case with Category 2 Hurricane Ike in 2008.

Conversely, very compact hurricanes, even if extremely strong wind-wise and with very low central pressures as was the case with Hurricane Charley in 2004, can produce surges substantially lower than what was included in the original scale.

Today, the Saffir-Simpson Hurricane Wind Scale is a 1 to 5 categorization based on the hurricane's intensity at the indicated time. The scale provides examples of the type of damage and impacts in the United States associated with winds of the indicated intensity. In general, damage rises by about a factor of four for every category increase.

The scale was modified slightly in 2012. Category 3 hurricanes now have a wind speed range of 111-129 mph (previously 111-130 mph). Category 4 hurricanes now have a wind speed range of 130-156 mph (previously 131-155 mph). Category 5 hurricanes now have winds of 157+ mph (previously 156+ mph).

This modification was done in order to help resolve rounding issues from knots to mph in the advisories The National Hurricane Center issues. An example of this is when a hurricane has an intensity of 115 knots. Although 115 knots is within the Category 4 range, it converts to 132.3 mph, which rounds down to 130 mph. This would classify a hurricane as a Category 3 in the old scale when using mph. The National Hurricane Center would then have to incorrectly covert 115 knots to 135 mph in their advisory products to work around this issue.

## Category 1: Very dangerous winds will produce some damage

People, livestock, and pets struck by flying or falling debris could be injured or killed.

Older (mainly pre-1994 construction) mobile homes could be destroyed, especially if they are not anchored properly as they tend to shift or roll off their foundations.

Newer mobile homes that are anchored properly can sustain damage involving the removal of shingle or metal roof coverings, and loss of vinyl siding, as well as damage to carports, sunrooms, or lanais.

Some poorly constructed frame homes can experience major damage, involving loss of the roof covering and damage to gable ends as well as the removal of porch coverings and awnings. Unprotected windows may break if struck by flying debris.

Masonry chimneys can be toppled. Well-constructed frame homes could have damage to roof shingles, vinyl siding, soffit panels, and gutters.

Failure of aluminum, screened-in, swimming pool enclosures can occur. Some apartment building and shopping center roof coverings could be partially removed. Industrial buildings can lose roofing and siding especially from windward corners, rakes, and eaves.

Failures to overhead doors and unprotected windows will be common. Windows in high-rise buildings can be broken by flying debris. Falling and broken glass will pose a significant danger even after the storm. There will be occasional damage to commercial signage, fences, and canopies. Large branches of trees will snap and shallow rooted trees can be toppled. Extensive damage to power lines and poles will likely result in power outages that could last a few to several days.

Hurricane Dolly (2008) is an example of a hurricane that brought Category 1 winds and impacts to South Padre Island, Texas.

## Category 2: Extremely dangerous winds will cause extensive damage

There is a substantial risk of injury or death to people, livestock, and pets due to flying and falling debris. Older (mainly pre-1994 construction) mobile homes have a very high chance of being destroyed and the flying debris generated can shred nearby mobile homes.

Newer mobile homes can also be destroyed. Poorly constructed frame homes have a high chance of having their roof structures removed especially if they are not anchored properly. Unprotected windows will have a high probability of being broken by flying debris.

Well-constructed frame homes could sustain major roof and siding damage. Failure of aluminum, screened-in, swimming pool enclosures will be common. There will be a substantial percentage of roof and siding damage to apartment buildings and industrial buildings. Unreinforced masonry walls can collapse.

Windows in high-rise buildings can be broken by flying debris. Falling and broken glass will pose a significant danger even after the storm. Commercial signage, fences, and canopies will be damaged and often destroyed.

Many shallowly rooted trees will be snapped or uprooted and block numerous roads. Near-total power loss is expected with outages that could last from several days to weeks. Potable water could become scarce as filtration systems begin to fail.

Hurricane Frances (2004) is an example of a hurricane that brought Category 2 winds and impacts to coastal portions of Port St. Lucie, Florida with Category 1 conditions experienced elsewhere in the city.

## Category 3: Devastating damage will occur

There is a high risk of injury or death to people, livestock, and pets due to flying and falling debris. Nearly all older (pre-1994) mobile homes will be destroyed. Most newer mobile homes will sustain severe damage with potential for complete roof failure and wall collapse.

Poorly constructed frame homes can be destroyed by the removal of the roof and exterior walls. Unprotected windows will be broken by flying debris. Well-built frame homes can experience major damage involving the removal of roof decking and gable ends.

There will be a high percentage of roof covering and siding damage to apartment buildings and industrial buildings. Isolated structural damage to wood or steel framing can occur. Complete failure of older metal buildings is possible, and older unreinforced masonry buildings can collapse.

Numerous windows will be blown out of high-rise buildings resulting in falling glass, which will pose a threat for days to weeks after the storm. Most commercial signage, fences, and canopies will be destroyed. Many trees will be snapped or uprooted, blocking numerous roads. Electricity and water will be unavailable for several days to a few weeks after the storm passes.

Hurricane Ivan (2004) is an example of a hurricane that brought Category 3 winds and impacts to coastal portions of Gulf Shores, Alabama with Category 2 conditions experienced elsewhere in this city.

## Category 4: Catastrophic damage will occur

There is a very high risk of injury or death to people, livestock, and pets due to flying and falling debris. Nearly all older (pre-1994) mobile homes will be destroyed. A high percentage of newer mobile homes also will be destroyed.

Poorly constructed homes can sustain complete collapse of all walls as well as the loss of the roof structure. Well-built homes also can sustain severe damage with loss of most of the roof structure and/or some exterior walls.

Extensive damage to roof coverings, windows, and doors will occur. Large amounts of windborne debris will be lofted into the air. Windborne debris damage will break most unprotected windows and penetrate some protected windows.

There will be a high percentage of structural damage to the top floors of apartment buildings. Steel frames in older industrial buildings can collapse. There will be a high percentage of collapse to older unreinforced masonry buildings. Most windows will be blown out of high-rise buildings resulting in falling glass, which will pose a threat for days to weeks after the storm.

Nearly all commercial signage, fences, and canopies will be destroyed. Most trees will be snapped or uprooted and power poles downed. Fallen trees and power poles will isolate residential areas. Power outages will last for weeks to possibly months. Long-term water shortages will increase human suffering. Most of the area will be uninhabitable for weeks or months.

Hurricane Charley (2004) is an example of a hurricane that brought Category 4 winds and impacts to coastal portions of Punta Gorda, Florida with Category 3 conditions experienced elsewhere in the city.

## Category 5: Catastrophic damage will occur

People, livestock, and pets are at very high risk of injury or death from flying or falling debris, even if indoors in mobile homes or framed homes. Almost complete destruction of all mobile homes will occur, regardless of age or construction.

A high percentage of frame homes will be destroyed, with total roof failure and wall collapse. Extensive damage to roof covers, windows, and doors will occur. Large amounts of windborne debris will be lofted into the air.

Windborne debris damage will occur to nearly all unprotected windows and many protected windows. Significant damage to wood roof commercial buildings will occur due to loss of roof sheathing. Complete collapse of many older metal buildings can occur. Most unreinforced masonry walls will fail which can lead to the collapse of the buildings.

A high percentage of industrial buildings and low-rise apartment buildings will be destroyed. Nearly all windows will be blown out of high-rise buildings resulting in falling glass, which will pose a threat for days to weeks after the storm.

Nearly all commercial signage, fences, and canopies will be destroyed. Nearly all trees will be snapped or uprooted and power poles downed. Fallen trees and power poles will isolate residential areas. Power outages will last for weeks to possibly months. Long-term water shortages will increase human suffering. Most of the area will be uninhabitable for weeks or months.

Hurricane Andrew (1992) is an example of a hurricane that brought Category 5 winds and impacts to coastal portions of Cutler Ridge, Florida with Category 4 conditions experienced elsewhere in south Miami-Dade County.

Source: National Hurricane Center

APPENDIX 20

• • •

## How to Read the Public Advisory Text
## Reading a Tropical Cyclone Public Advisory

THE TCP BEGINS WITH A headline, followed by these sections: summary, watches and warnings, discussion and outlook, hazards, and next advisory. Each section of the TCP begins with a specific header text string. Each header is preceded by two blank lines, and is followed by a line of dashes (to give the appearance of an underline).

1. **Summary**. This section summarizes the essential facts of the tropical cyclone (location, intensity, etc.) in a fixed format.
   - Header (example): SUMMARY OF 500 AM EDT...0900 UTC...INFORMATION
   - In the summary section header, UTC time will always be given with four characters (e.g., 0300 UTC). No other numerical values in this section will appear with leading zeros.
   - The summary section follows a fixed format, containing lines for the location, geographical reference(s), maximum winds, direction of movement, and minimum pressure. The section will always contain at

least one geographical reference, but not more than two. Geographical reference lines begin with the keyword ABOUT. In the summary section, all directions are abbreviated (e.g., N, NNE, NE, ENE, E, etc.) If the forward speed is zero, the motion will be given as STATIONARY.

2. **Watches and Warnings**. This is a free text section that makes use of keywords to identify specific content regarding watches and warnings. Watch/warning definitions and call to action statements may also appear in this section.
   - Header: WATCHES AND WARNINGS
   - Whenever watches or warnings are issued, continue in effect, or are discontinued, the watch/warning section will contain the following two keyword strings:
   - CHANGES WITH THIS ADVISORY...
   - SUMMARY OF WATCHES AND WARNINGS IN EFFECT...
   - Changes to watches and warnings since the last TCP or TCU (Tropical Cyclone Update) will be listed in paragraph form, one change per paragraph.
   - The summary of active watches and warnings will appear as a bulleted list, grouped by warning type. Each grouping will begin with a statement such as A HURRICANE WARNING IS IN EFFECT FOR.... Each watch or warning segment that follows will appear on a separate line beginning with an asterisk. However, watches or warnings that encompass entire islands or jurisdictions may be grouped together as a single segment, e.g.:
   - A TROPICAL STORM WARNING IS IN EFFECT FOR...
   - * ANTIGUA...BARBUDA...ANGUILLA...AND ST. MARTIN

- o A TROPICAL STORM WARNING IS IN EFFECT FOR...
- o * THE CUBAN PROVINCES OF GUANTANAMO AND HOLGUIN
- o When a watch or warning is introduced for a new major geographical area, the watch/warning section should contain a definition of the watch or warning. These definitions may also be included at other times. The definitions will appear after the list of active watches and warnings in effect. Other statements (e.g., "INTERESTS IN THE LEEWARD ISLANDS SHOULD MONITOR THE PROGRESS OF BILL...") may also appear in this location.

3. **Discussion and outlook**. This is a free text section with no keywords. It will describe the current location and motion, maximum winds, extent of hurricane and tropical storm winds, and minimum pressure. It will provide a general outlook for the track and intensity of the cyclone over the next 24-48 hours.
   - o Header: DISCUSSION AND 48-HOUR OUTLOOK
4. **Hazards**. A free text section that uses keywords to identify the typical threats of a tropical cyclone.
   - o Header: HAZARDS AFFECTING LAND
   - o Most paragraphs in this section will begin with one of the following keywords: STORM SURGE, WIND, RAINFALL, TORNADOES, SURF, or OTHER.
5. **Next advisory**: This free text section will indicate the time of the next complete advisory, and intermediate advisory(ies), if any. If this is the last advisory, and the system will be discussed subsequently in another NWS product, that product will be identified.
   - o Header: NEXT ADVISORY

## TCP Example 1

000
WTNT34 KNHC 120241
TCPAT4

BULLETIN
HURRICANE IKE ADVISORY NUMBER 44
NWS NATIONAL HURRICANE CENTER MIAMI FL AL092008
1000 PM CDT THU SEP 11 2008

...IKE CONTINUES TO GROW IN SIZE BUT HAS NOT STRENGTHENED YET...
...HURRICANE WARNING ISSUED FOR NORTHWESTERN GULF COAST...

SUMMARY OF 1000 PM CDT...0300 UTC...INFORMATION

---

LOCATION...25.5N 88.4W
ABOUT 580 MI...930 KM ESE OF CORPUS CHRISTI TEXAS
ABOUT 470 MI...760 KM ESE OF GALVESTON TEXAS
MAXIMUM SUSTAINED WINDS...100 MPH...160 KM/H
PRESENT MOVEMENT...WNW OR 290 DEGREES AT 10 MPH...17 KM/H
MINIMUM CENTRAL PRESSURE...945 MB...27.91 INCHES

WATCHES AND WARNINGS

---

CHANGES WITH THIS ADVISORY...

A HURRICANE WARNING HAS BEEN ISSUED FROM MORGAN CITY LOUISIANA TO BAFFIN BAY TEXAS.

A TROPICAL STORM WARNING HAS BEEN ISSUED FROM SOUTH OF BAFFIN BAY TO PORT MANSFIELD TEXAS.

SUMMARY OF WATCHES AND WARNINGS IN EFFECT...

A HURRICANE WARNING IS IN EFFECT FOR...
* MORGAN CITY LOUISIANA TO BAFFIN BAY TEXAS

A TROPICAL STORM WARNING IS IN EFFECT FOR...
* EAST OF MORGAN CITY TO THE MISSISSIPPI-ALABAMA BORDER...INCLUDING THE CITY OF NEW ORLEANS AND LAKE PONTCHARTRAIN

* SOUTH OF BAFFIN BAY TO PORT MANSFIELD
A HURRICANE WARNING MEANS THAT HURRICANE CONDITIONS ARE EXPECTED SOMEWHERE WITHIN THE WARNING AREA. A WARNING IS TYPICALLY ISSUED 36 HOURS BEFORE THE ANTICIPATED FIRST OCCURRENCE OF TROPICAL-STORM-FORCE WINDS... CONDITIONS THAT MAKE OUTSIDE PREPARATIONS DIFFICULT OR DANGEROUS. PREPARATIONS TO PROTECT LIFE AND PROPERTY SHOULD BE RUSHED TO COMPLETION.

A TROPICAL STORM WARNING MEANS THAT TROPICAL STORM CONDITIONS ARE EXPECTED SOMEWHERE WITHIN THE WARNING AREA WITHIN THE NEXT 36 HOURS.

FOR STORM INFORMATION SPECIFIC TO YOUR AREA... INCLUDING POSSIBLE INLAND WATCHES AND WARNINGS...PLEASE MONITOR PRODUCTS ISSUED BY YOUR LOCAL WEATHER OFFICE.

DISCUSSION AND 48-HOUR OUTLOOK

---

AT 1000 PM CDT...0300 UTC...THE CENTER OF HURRICANE IKE WAS LOCATED NEAR LATITUDE 25.5 NORTH...LONGITUDE 88.4 WEST. IKE IS MOVING TOWARD THE WEST-NORTHWEST NEAR 10 MPH...17 KM/H. A GENERAL WEST- NORTHWESTWARD MOTION IS EXPECTED OVER THE NEXT DAY OR SO... AND THE CENTER OF IKE SHOULD BE VERY NEAR THE COAST BY LATE FRIDAY.

MAXIMUM SUSTAINED WINDS ARE NEAR 100 MPH...160 KM/H...WITH HIGHER GUSTS. IKE IS A CATEGORY TWO HURRICANE ON THE SAFFIR-SIMPSON SCALE.
IKE IS FORECAST TO BECOME A MAJOR HURRICANE PRIOR TO REACHING THE COASTLINE.

IKE REMAINS A VERY LARGE TROPICAL CYCLONE. HURRICANE FORCE WINDS EXTEND OUTWARD UP TO 115 MILES...185 KM...FROM THE CENTER...AND TROPICAL STORM FORCE WINDS EXTEND OUTWARD UP TO 275 MILES...445 KM.

THE LATEST MINIMUM CENTRAL PRESSURE REPORTED BY A NOAA HURRICANE HUNTER AIRCRAFT WAS 945 MB...27.91 INCHES.

HAZARDS AFFECTING LAND

STORM SURGE...STORM SURGE WILL RAISE WATER LEVELS AS MUCH AS 10 TO 15 FT ABOVE GROUND LEVEL ALONG THE COAST WITHIN THE HURRICANE WARNING AREA...WITH LARGE AND DANGEROUS BATTERING WAVES...NEAR AND TO THE EAST OF WHERE THE CENTER OF IKE MAKES LANDFALL. STORM SURGE WILL RAISE WATER LEVELS AS MUCH AS 5 TO 7 FEET ABOVE GROUND LEVEL ALONG THE COAST WITHIN THE TROPICAL STORM WARNING AREA ALONG THE NORTHERN GULF COAST. THE SURGE COULD PENETRATE AS FAR INLAND AS ABOUT 10 MILES FROM THE SHORE WITH DEPTH GRADUALLY DECREASING AS THE WATER MOVES INLAND.

WIND...BECAUSE IKE IS A VERY LARGE TROPICAL CYCLONE...WEATHER WILL DETERIORATE ALONG THE COASTLINE LONG BEFORE THE CENTER REACHES THE COAST. HURRICANE CONDITIONS ARE EXPECTED TO REACH NORTHWESTERN GULF COAST WITHIN THE WARNING AREA FRIDAY AFTERNOON. WINDS ARE EXPECTED TO FIRST REACH TROPICAL STORM STRENGTH FRIDAY MORNING...MAKING OUTSIDE PREPARATIONS DIFFICULT OR DANGEROUS. PREPARATIONS TO PROTECT LIFE AND PROPERTY SHOULD BE RUSHED TO COMPLETION.

RAINFALL...IKE IS EXPECTED TO PRODUCE RAINFALL AMOUNTS OF 5 TO 10 INCHES ALONG THE CENTRAL AND UPPER TEXAS COAST AND OVER PORTIONS

OF SOUTHWESTERN LOUISIANA...WITH ISOLATED MAXIMUM AMOUNTS OF 15 INCHES POSSIBLE. RAINFALL AMOUNTS OF 1 TO 2 INCHES ARE POSSIBLE OVER PORTIONS OF THE YUCATAN PENINSULA.

NEXT ADVISORY

---

NEXT INTERMEDIATE ADVISORY...100 AM CDT.
NEXT COMPLETE ADVISORY...400 AM CDT.

$$
FORECASTER FRANKLIN

# APPENDIX 21

CONVERTING ZULU TIME TO LOCAL TIME

NOAA satellites use Zulu Time or Coordinated Universal Time (UTC) as their time reference. The satellite images that appear on NOAA's Web sites are stamped in Zulu time. To make the conversion to your local time, see the chart below. Find your local time in the first column. If you are on Eastern Daylight Saving Time (EDT), you would use the second column to find your Zulu Time/UTC. For instance, if it's 11 a.m. Eastern Daylight Saving Time in Washington, D.C., it's 1500 hours in Zulu time/UTC. See legend below. (Back to Hurricanes Page.)

| LOCAL | EDT | EST | CDT | CST | MDT | MST | PDT | PST |
|---|---|---|---|---|---|---|---|---|
| Midnight | 0400 | 0500 | 0500 | 0600 | 0600 | 0700 | 0700 | 0800 |
| 1 a.m. 0500 | 0600 | 0600 | 0700 | 0700 | 0800 | 0800 | 0900 | |
| 2 a.m. 0600 | 0700 | 0700 | 0800 | 0800 | 0900 | 0900 | 1000 | |
| 3 a.m. 0700 | 0800 | 0800 | 0900 | 0900 | 1000 | 1000 | 1100 | |
| 4 a.m. 0800 | 0900 | 0900 | 1000 | 1000 | 1100 | 1100 | 1200 | |
| 5 a.m. 0900 | 1000 | 1000 | 1100 | 1100 | 1200 | 1200 | 1300 | |
| 6 a.m. 1000 | 1100 | 1100 | 1200 | 1200 | 1300 | 1300 | 1400 | |
| 7 a.m. 1100 | 1200 | 1200 | 1300 | 1300 | 1400 | 1400 | 1500 | |
| 8 a.m. 1200 | 1300 | 1300 | 1400 | 1400 | 1500 | 1500 | 1600 | |
| 9 a.m. 1300 | 1400 | 1400 | 1500 | 1500 | 1600 | 1600 | 1700 | |
| 10 a.m.1400 | 1500 | 1500 | 1600 | 1600 | 1700 | 1700 | 1800 | |
| 11 a.m.1500 | 1600 | 1600 | 1700 | 1700 | 1800 | 1800 | 1900 | |
| NOON 1600 | 1700 | 1700 | 1800 | 1800 | 1900 | 1900 | 2000 | |
| 1 p.m. 1700 | 1800 | 1800 | 1900 | 1900 | 2000 | 2000 | 2100 | |
| 2 p.m. 1800 | 1900 | 1900 | 2000 | 2000 | 2100 | 2100 | 2200 | |
| 3 p.m. 1900 | 2000 | 2000 | 2100 | 2100 | 2200 | 2200 | 2300 | |
| 4 p.m. 2000 | 2100 | 2100 | 2200 | 2200 | 2300 | 2300 | 2400 | |
| 5 p.m. 2100 | 2200 | 2200 | 2300 | 2300 | 2400 | 2400 | 0100 | |
| 6 p.m. 2200 | 2300 | 2300 | 2400 | 2400 | 0100 | 0100 | 0200 | |
| 7 p.m. 2300 | 2400 | 2400 | 0100 | 0100 | 0200 | 0200 | 0300 | |
| 8 p.m. 2400 | 0100 | 0100 | 0200 | 0200 | 0300 | 0300 | 0400 | |
| 9 p.m. 0100 | 0200 | 0200 | 0300 | 0300 | 0400 | 0400 | 0500 | |
| 10 p.m. | 0200 | 0300 | 0300 | 0400 | 0400 | 0500 | 0500 | 0600 |
| 11 p.m. | 0300 | 0400 | 0400 | 0500 | 0500 | 0600 | 0600 | 0700 |
| LOCAL | EDT | EST | CDT | CST | MDT | MST | PDT | PST |

LEGEND:

EDT = Eastern Daylight Saving Time
EST = Eastern Standard Time
CDT = Central Daylight Saving Time
CST = Central Standard Time
MDT = Mountain Daylight Saving Time
MST = Mountain Standard Time
PDT = Pacific Daylight Saving Time
PST = Pacific Standard Time

# APPENDIX 22

• • •

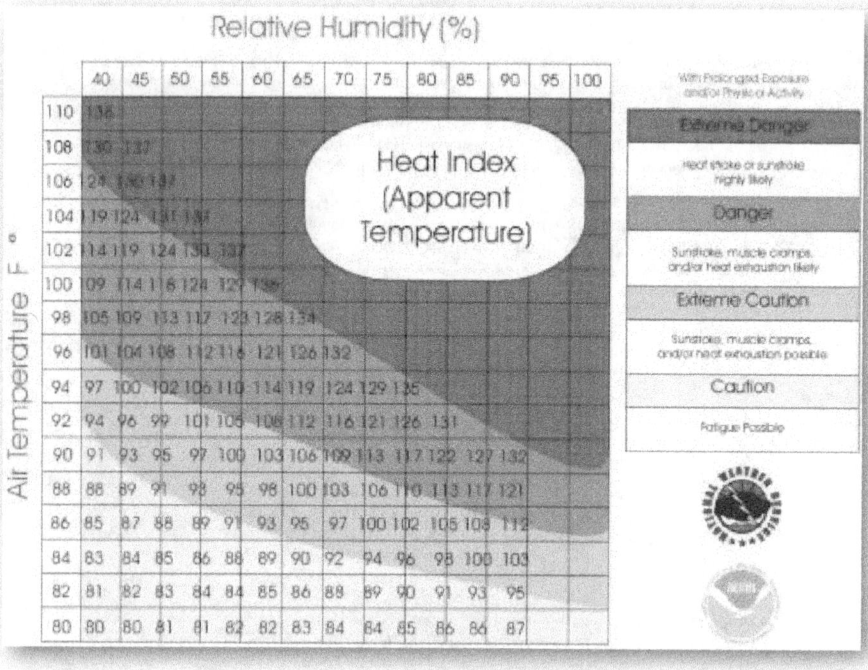

Relative Humidity (%)

| Air Temperature F° | 40 | 45 | 50 | 55 | 60 | 65 | 70 | 75 | 80 | 85 | 90 | 95 | 100 |
|---|---|---|---|---|---|---|---|---|---|---|---|---|---|
| 110 | 136 | | | | | | | | | | | | |
| 108 | 130 | 137 | | | | | | | | | | | |
| 106 | 124 | 130 | 137 | | | | | | | | | | |
| 104 | 119 | 124 | 131 | 137 | | | | | | | | | |
| 102 | 114 | 119 | 124 | 130 | 137 | | | | | | | | |
| 100 | 109 | 114 | 118 | 124 | 129 | 136 | | | | | | | |
| 98 | 105 | 109 | 113 | 117 | 123 | 128 | 134 | | | | | | |
| 96 | 101 | 104 | 108 | 112 | 116 | 121 | 126 | 132 | | | | | |
| 94 | 97 | 100 | 102 | 106 | 110 | 114 | 119 | 124 | 129 | 135 | | | |
| 92 | 94 | 96 | 99 | 101 | 105 | 108 | 112 | 116 | 121 | 126 | 131 | | |
| 90 | 91 | 93 | 95 | 97 | 100 | 103 | 106 | 109 | 113 | 117 | 122 | 127 | 132 |
| 88 | 88 | 89 | 91 | 93 | 95 | 98 | 100 | 103 | 106 | 110 | 113 | 117 | 121 |
| 86 | 85 | 87 | 88 | 89 | 91 | 93 | 95 | 97 | 100 | 102 | 105 | 108 | 112 |
| 84 | 83 | 84 | 85 | 86 | 88 | 89 | 90 | 92 | 94 | 96 | 98 | 100 | 103 |
| 82 | 81 | 82 | 83 | 84 | 84 | 85 | 86 | 88 | 89 | 90 | 91 | 93 | 95 |
| 80 | 80 | 80 | 81 | 81 | 82 | 82 | 83 | 84 | 84 | 85 | 86 | 86 | 87 |

Heat Index (Apparent Temperature)
With Prolonged Exposure and/or Physical Activity
Extreme Danger
Heat stroke or sunstroke highly likely
Danger
Sunstroke, muscle cramps, and/or heat exhaustion likely
Extreme Caution
Sunstroke, muscle cramps, and/or heat exhaustion possible
Caution
Fatigue Possible

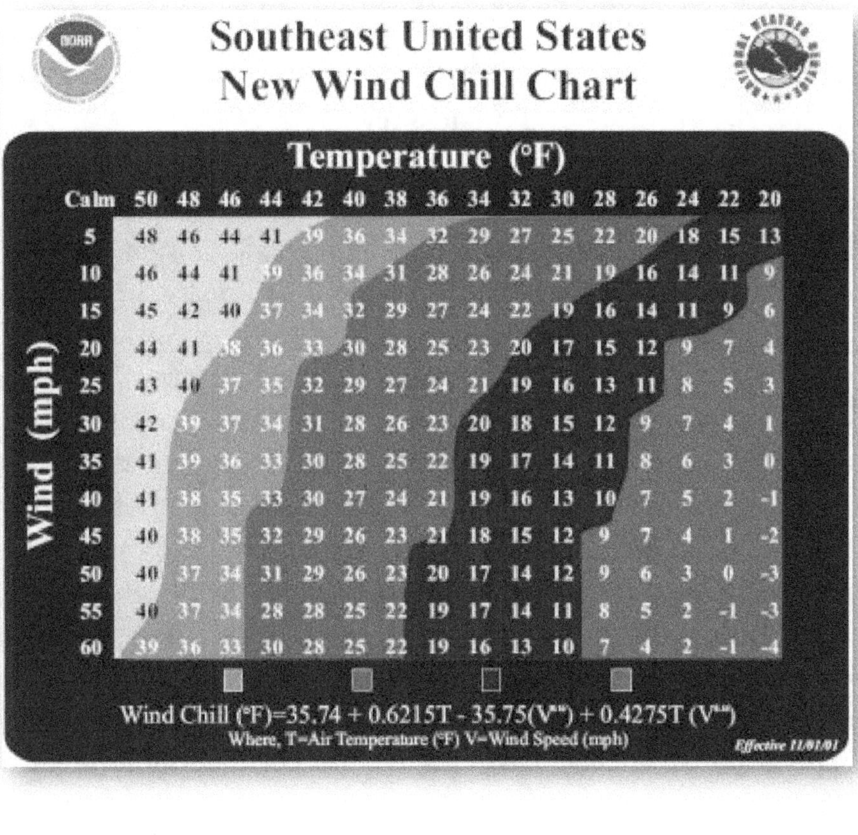

## Southeast United States New Wind Chill Chart

Temperature (°F)

| Wind (mph) | Calm 50 | 48 | 46 | 44 | 42 | 40 | 38 | 36 | 34 | 32 | 30 | 28 | 26 | 24 | 22 | 20 |
|---|---|---|---|---|---|---|---|---|---|---|---|---|---|---|---|---|
| 5 | 48 | 46 | 44 | 41 | 39 | 36 | 34 | 32 | 29 | 27 | 25 | 22 | 20 | 18 | 15 | 13 |
| 10 | 46 | 44 | 41 | 39 | 36 | 34 | 31 | 28 | 26 | 24 | 21 | 19 | 16 | 14 | 11 | 9 |
| 15 | 45 | 42 | 40 | 37 | 34 | 32 | 29 | 27 | 24 | 22 | 19 | 16 | 14 | 11 | 9 | 6 |
| 20 | 44 | 41 | 38 | 36 | 33 | 30 | 28 | 25 | 23 | 20 | 17 | 15 | 12 | 9 | 7 | 4 |
| 25 | 43 | 40 | 37 | 35 | 32 | 29 | 27 | 24 | 21 | 19 | 16 | 13 | 11 | 8 | 5 | 3 |
| 30 | 42 | 39 | 37 | 34 | 31 | 28 | 26 | 23 | 20 | 18 | 15 | 12 | 9 | 7 | 4 | 1 |
| 35 | 41 | 39 | 36 | 33 | 30 | 28 | 25 | 22 | 19 | 17 | 14 | 11 | 8 | 6 | 3 | 0 |
| 40 | 41 | 38 | 35 | 33 | 30 | 27 | 24 | 21 | 19 | 16 | 13 | 10 | 7 | 5 | 2 | -1 |
| 45 | 40 | 38 | 35 | 32 | 29 | 26 | 23 | 21 | 18 | 15 | 12 | 9 | 7 | 4 | 1 | -2 |
| 50 | 40 | 37 | 34 | 31 | 29 | 26 | 23 | 20 | 17 | 14 | 12 | 9 | 6 | 3 | 0 | -3 |
| 55 | 40 | 37 | 34 | 28 | 28 | 25 | 22 | 19 | 17 | 14 | 11 | 8 | 5 | 2 | -1 | -3 |
| 60 | 39 | 36 | 33 | 30 | 28 | 25 | 22 | 19 | 16 | 13 | 10 | 7 | 4 | 2 | -1 | -4 |

Wind Chill (°F) $= 35.74 + 0.6215T - 35.75(V^{0.16}) + 0.4275T(V^{0.16})$

Where, T=Air Temperature (°F) V=Wind Speed (mph)

*Effective 11/01/01*

APPENDIX 23

• • •

# Glossary

*Act of God*: An unintentional hazard event (usually a natural hazard) whereby society feels that no individual or organization is responsible for the hazard occurrence or its impact, i.e., an "accident." This is an increasingly narrow category of hazards in the U.S., as society has begun to view almost all hazards or their impact as predictable, and that mitigation actions could be undertaken. In particular, risk management has presented the view that technological hazards are expected outcomes of planned risk behavior, and even that technological failure from a natural hazard is usually predictable and could have been avoided. For example, almost all motor vehicle crashes are now viewed as expected outcomes of speed, substance use, distracted drivers or other behavior, failure of mechanical equipment or road design, and are now referred to as "crashes"" rather than motor vehicle accidents

***Activate*** (emergency management definition): To begin the process of mobilizing a response team, or to set in motion an emergency response or recovery plan, process, or procedure for an exercise or for an actual hazard incident ***Advisory***: A notification category that provides urgent information about an unusual occurrence or threat of an occurrence, but no activation of the notified entity is ordered or expected at that time. An advisory can be used for notification that something has occurred or is anticipated, and provide actionable information for notified personnel even though the response entity is not being activated. For example, a weather advisory that includes recommended actions for individuals. (See "update" - "alert" – "activation" for contrast between the other notification categories.)

***After Action Report (AAR)***: The document that describes the incident response and findings related to system response performance (see AAR process).

***Agency***: A division of government with a specific function offering a particular kind of assistance. In ICS, agencies are defined either as jurisdictional (having statutory responsibility for incident management) or as assisting or cooperating (providing resources or other assistance).

***Agency, Assisting***:

- An agency directly contributing tactical or service resources to another agency.
  *(FIRESCOPE/NIIMS 1999)*
- An agency or organization providing personnel, services, or other resources to the agency with direct responsibility for incident management. (*NIMS*) See also Supporting Agency.

***Agency, Cooperating***:

- An agency supplying assistance other than direct operational or support functions or resources to the incident management effort. (*NIMS*)
- An Agency supplying assistance including but not limited to direct tactical or support functions or resources to the

incident control effort (e.g. Red Cross, law enforcement agency, telephone company, etc.). *(FIRESCOPE/NIIMS 1999)*

***Agency, Supporting***: An agency providing suppression or other support and resource assistance to a protecting [fire] agency. *(FIRESCOPE/NIIMS 1999*

***Agency Representative***: A person assigned by a primary, assisting, or cooperating Federal, State, local, or tribal government agency or private entity that has been delegated authority to make decisions affecting that agency's or organization's participation in incident management activities following appropriate consultation with the leadership of that agency. *(NIMS)*

***All-hazards***: A descriptor that denotes a specific strategy for managing activities in an emergency management program. Throughout the four phases of EM, management structure, processes and procedures are developed so they are applicable to every significant identified hazard. The remaining hazard specific interventions are layered on top of the basic components as indicated and presented through "incident" annexes in the emergency operations plan (EOP). For example, the procedures for notifying appropriate personnel during EOP activation would use the same process across all hazard types, even though the types of personnel notified and mobilized may vary by hazard.

***Area Command*** (***Unified Area Command***): An organization established (1) to oversee the management of multiple incidents that are each being handled by an ICS organization or (2) to oversee the management of large or multiple incidents to which several Incident Management Teams have been assigned. Area Command has the responsibility to set overall strategy and priorities, allocate critical resources according to priorities, ensure that incidents are properly managed, and ensure that objectives are met and strategies followed. Area Command becomes Unified Area Command when incidents are multijurisdictional. Area Command may be established at an emergency operations center facility or at some location other than an incident command post. (*NIMS*)

***Badging***: The act of providing an identification badge to physically identify personnel who have been privileged to access a specific incident or to access a specific incident location

***Branch***: The organizational level having functional or geographical responsibility for major aspects of incident operations. A branch is organizationally situated between the section and the division or group in the Operations Section, and between the section and units in the Logistics Section. Branches are identified by the use of Roman numerals or by functional area. *(NIMS)*

***Capability, Surge***: The ability to manage patients requiring unusual or very specialized medical evaluation and care. Surge requirements span the range of specialized medical and health services (expertise, information, procedures, equipment, or personnel) that are not normally available at the location where they are needed (e.g., pediatric care provided at non-pediatric facilities or burn care services at a non-burn center). Surge capability also includes patient problems that require special intervention to protect medical providers, other patients, and the integrity of the medical care facility.

***Capacity, Surge***: The ability to evaluate and care for a markedly increased volume of patients—one that challenges or exceeds normal operating capacity. The surge requirements may extend beyond direct patient care to include such tasks as extensive laboratory studies or epidemiological investigations.

***Command Staff***: In an incident management organization, the Command Staff consists of the Incident Command and the special staff positions of Public Information Officer, Safety Officer, Liaison Officer, and other positions as required, who report directly to the Incident Commander. They may have an assistant or assistants, as needed. *(NIMS)*

***Credentialing***: According to the NIMS: "Credentialing involves providing documentation that can authenticate and verify the certification and identity of designated incident command staff and emergency responders. This system helps ensure that personnel representing various jurisdictional levels and functional disciplines possess a minimum common level of training, currency, experience, physical and medical fitness, and capability for the incident management or emergency responder position they are tasked to fill.

***Decontamination***: The reduction or removal of a chemical, biological, or radiological material from the surface of a structure, area, object, or person. *(FEMA State and Local Guide 101)*

***Deputy***: A fully qualified individual who, in the absence of a superior, can be delegated the authority to manage a functional operation or perform a specific task. In some cases, a deputy can act as relief for a superior and, therefore, must be fully qualified in the position. Deputies can be assigned to the Incident Commander, General Staff, and Branch Directors. *(NIMS)*

***Drill***: A training application that develops a combination or series of skills (for example – a drill of mobilizing the decontamination area). It can also be referred to as an "instructional drill" for clarity. A drill conducted primarily for evaluation rather than training should be referred to as an "evaluative drill."

***Emergency Management***: The science of managing complex systems and multidisciplinary personnel to address emergencies and disasters, across all hazards, and through the phases of mitigation, preparedness, response, and recovery.

***Emergency Management Assistance Compact (EMAC)***: A congressionally ratified organization that provides form and structure to interstate mutual aid. Through EMAC, a disaster impacted state can request and receive assistance from other member states quickly and efficiently, resolving two key issues upfront: liability and reimbursement. *(EMAC web site).*

***Emergency Management Operations***: A term that can be used to denote the activities that occur during the response phase of an emergency event, based at the Emergency Operations Center and managed and directed by an Emergency Management Team. Emergency Management Operations include management of the EOC and activities administered by the Emergency Support Functions. Emergency Management Operations are intended to support the incident management team and the incident response, address countywide incident-related issues that are outside the scope of the incident management team, support the coordination with other jurisdictions and levels of government, and assist with keeping political authorities adequately informed.

***Emergency Management Program***: A program that implements the organization's mission, vision, management framework, and strategic goals and objectives related to emergencies and disasters. It uses a comprehensive approach to emergency management as a conceptual framework, combining mitigation, preparedness, response, and recovery into a fully integrated set of activities. The "program" applies to all departments and organizational units within the organization that have roles in responding to a potential emergency. *(NFPA 1600, 2004 and the VHA Guidebook, 2004)*

***Emergency Manager***: The person who has the day-to-day responsibility for emergency management programs and activities. The role is one of coordinating all aspects of a jurisdiction's mitigation, preparedness, response, and recovery capabilities. The local emergency management position is referred to with different titles across the country, such as civil defense coordinator or director, civil preparedness coordinator or director, disaster services director, and emergency services director. It now commonly is referred to as homeland security director. Within organizations, this person may be the safety director, emergency program coordinator (VA Medical Centers) or another title.

***Emergency Operations Center (EOC)***:

- The physical location at which the coordination of information and resources to support domestic incident management activities normally takes place. An EOC may be a temporary facility or may be located in a more central or permanently established facility, perhaps at a higher level of organization within a jurisdiction. EOCs may be organized by major functional disciplines (e.g., fire, law enforcement, and medical services), by jurisdiction (e.g., Federal, State, regional, county, city, tribal), or some combination thereof. (*NIMS*)
- An emergency operations center (EOC) is a location from which centralized emergency management can be performed during response and recovery. The use of EOCs is a standard practice in emergency management, and is one type of multiagency coordinating entity. Local governments should have designated EOCs. The physical size, staffing, and equipping of a local government EOC will depend on the size and complexity of the local government and the emergency operations it can expect to manage. The level of EOC staffing will also vary with the specific emergency situation.

  A local government's EOC facility should be capable of serving as the central point for:
- Coordination of all the jurisdiction's emergency operations.
- Information gathering and dissemination.
- Coordination with other local governments and the operational area. *(SEMS)*

***Emergency Operations Plan (EOP)***:

- The "response" plan that an entity (organization, jurisdiction, State, etc.) maintains for responding to any hazard event. It provides action guidance for management and emergency response personnel during the response phase of Comprehensive Emergency Management.
- An all-hazards document that specifies actions to be taken in the event of an emergency or disaster event; identifies authorities, relationships, and the actions to be taken by whom, what, when, and where, based on predetermined assumptions, objectives, and existing capabilities. (*FEMA Higher Education Project*)
- The "steady-state" plan maintained by various jurisdictional levels for responding to a wide variety of potential hazards. (*NIMS*)

***Emergency Preparedness***: Activities and measures designed or undertaken to prepare for or minimize the effects of a hazard upon the civilian population, to deal with the immediate emergency conditions which would be created by the hazard, and to effectuate emergency repairs to, or the emergency restoration of, vital utilities and facilities destroyed or damaged by the hazard. (*Stafford Act*)

***Emergency Support Function (ESF)***: A grouping of government and certain private-sector capabilities into an organizational structure to provide support, resources, and services. *(NRP)*

***Exercise, Functional***: The scenario-based execution of specific tasks and/or more complex activity within a functional area of the EOP. This is typically conducted under increased levels of stress and genuine constraints that provide increased realism, and so is less reliant upon orally presented simulation. Collaboration and cooperation and interactive decision-making are more focused within the exercised function and accomplished in real-time. Interaction with other functions and "outside" personnel are simulated, commonly through the play of exercise controllers.

***Exercise, Full-Scale***: A scenario-based extension of a functional exercise to include all or most of the functions and complex activities of the EOP. It is typically conducted under high levels of stress and very real-time constraints of an actual incident. Interaction across all functions by the players decreases the artificial (oral) injects by controllers, and make the overall scenario much more realistic. Because of this, the full-scale exercise is a more comprehensive evaluation/validation of the EOP, its policies and procedures, in the context of emergency conditions.

***Expert***: An individual who meets some defined level of knowledge, skills and abilities (i.e., competencies) that usually have been demonstrated by the expert's past experiences.

***Facility Emergency Plan (FEP)***: A support annex to the EOP that describes the initial evacuation, shelter in place, and other reactive measures during the life-safety stages of an emergency that directly affects the facility. Also referred to by VHA as Emergency Safety Procedures for Building Occupant, and by GSA as the Occupant Emergency Plan.

***Federal Disaster Area***: An area of a state (often times defined by counties) that is declared eligible for federal disaster relief under the Stafford Act. These declarations are made by the President usually as a result of a request made by the governor of the affected state. *(VHA Emergency Management Guidebook 2005)*

***Federal Response Plan (FRP)***: A national level plan developed by the Federal Emergency Management Agency (FEMA) in coordination with 26 federal departments and agencies plus the American Red Cross. This plan was developed in 1992 and updated in 1999 to implement the Stafford Act in the provision of federal disaster to states and local communities in a Presidential declared disaster. It was superseded by the National Response Plan in March 2004. *(VHA Emergency Management Guidebook 2005)*

***Field Operations***: Field Operations are all activities within the defined scope of the "incident" (the incident scope is delineated by the incident commander through incident control and operational objectives). The Incident Management Team manages field operations, which are the for direct incident-scene actions for management of the emergency situation. The Incident Commander is the leader of Field Operations.

***Finance/Administration***: The ICS functional area that addresses the financial, administrative, and legal/regulatory issues for the incident management system. It monitors costs related to the incident, and provides accounting, procurement, time recording, cost analyses, and overall fiscal guidance

***Four Phases***: The time and function-based divisions within Comprehensive Emergency Management: Mitigation, Preparedness, Response and Recovery.

***Function***:

- Function refers to the five major activities in ICS: Command, Operations, Planning, Logistics, and Finance/Administration. The term function is also used when describing the activity involved, e.g., the planning function. A sixth function, Intelligence, may be established, if required, to meet incident management needs. (*NIMS*)
- In the Incident Command System, refers to the five major activities (i.e., Command, Operations, Plans/Information, Logistics, and Finance/Administration). The term function is also used when describing the activity involved (e.g., the planning function). Intelligence is not considered a separate function under ICS.

***Gale***: Wind with a speed between 34 and 40 knots

***Global Patient Movements Requirements Center (GPMRC)***: A component of the United States Transportation Command (USTRANSCOM) that has the responsibility for the management of DoD, VA and NDMS beds, regulating of military and NDMS domestic casualties to those beds, and arranging for the transportation of the casualties to the facilities in which the beds are located. (*VHA Emergency Management Guidebook 2005*)

***Group***: Established to divide the incident management structure into functional areas of operation. Groups are composed of resources assembled to perform a special function not necessarily within a single geographic division. Groups, when activated, are located between branches and resources in the Operations Section.

***Hazard Vulnerability Analysis (HVA)***: A systematic approach to identifying all hazards that may affect an organization and/or its community, assessing the risk (probability of hazard occurrence and the consequence for the organization) associated with each hazard and analyzing the findings to create a prioritized comparison of hazard vulnerabilities. The consequence, or "vulnerability," is related to both the impact on organizational function and the likely service demands created by the hazard impact.

***Healthcare facility***: Any asset where point-of-service medical care is regularly provided or provided during an incident. It includes hospitals, integrated healthcare systems, private physician offices, outpatient clinics, long-term care facilities and other medical care configurations. During an incident response, alternative medical care facilities and sites where definitive medical care is provided by EMS and other field personnel would be included in this definition.

***Health Insurance Portability and Accountability Act (HIPAA)***: Public Law 104-191 (August 21, 1996) addresses many aspects of healthcare practice and medical records. This federal act most notably addresses the privacy of personal health information, and directs the development of specific parameters as to how personal health information may be shared.

***Healthcare system***: A system that may include one or several healthcare facilities that provides patient evaluation and medical interventions (for illness and injury) and/or preventive medicine/health services.

***Horizontal Evacuation***: Partial evacuation of personnel and/or patients from one area of the health care facility to another – typically on the same floor, using fire doors as barriers from the hazard impact.

***Hotwash***: A systems performance review that is generally less formal and detailed than the After-Action Report (AAR) meeting, and occurs in close proximity to the end of the incident or exercise.

Preparation for a hot wash is commonly less extensive than for an AAR meeting. The results of the hot wash may serve as a starting point for a later, more formal AAR meeting. It should never be considered the endpoint to an after-action report process for an incident or exercise, or replace formal AAR meetings.

***Incident Action Plan (IAP)***:

- An oral or written plan containing general objectives reflecting the overall strategy for managing an incident. It may include the identification of operational resources and assignments. It may also include attachments that provide direction and important information for management of the incident during one or more operational periods. (*NIMS*) See also "Action Plan."
- The document in ICS/IMS that guides the response for that operational period. It contains the overall incident objectives and strategy, general tactical actions and supporting information to enable successful completion of objectives.

The IAP may be oral or written. When written, the IAP may have a number of supportive plans and information as attachments (e.g., traffic plan, safety plan, communications plan, and maps). There is only one "incident action plan" at an incident, all other "action plans" are subsets of the IAP and their titles should be qualified accordingly.

***Incident Commander*** **(*IC*)**: The individual responsible for all incident activities, including the development of strategies and tactics and the ordering and the release of resources. The IC has overall authority and responsibility for conducting incident operations and is responsible for the management of all incident operations at the incident site. (*NIMS*)

***Incident Objectives***: "statements of guidance and direction necessary for selecting appropriate strategy(s) and the tactical direction of resources. Incident objectives are based on realistic expectations of what can be accomplished have been effectively deployed (sic). Incident objectives must be achievable and measurable, yet flexible enough to allow strategic and tactical alternatives." (*NIMS*)

***Lat/Long:*** an abbreviation used to signify the latitude and longitude of a location.

***Liaison*** *(Noun)*: In ICS, it is a position(s) assigned to establish and maintain direct coordination and information exchange with agencies and organizations outside of the specific incident's ICS/IMS structure. (*NIMS*)

***Liaison Officer***: A member of the Command Staff responsible for coordinating with representatives from cooperating and assisting agencies. (*NIMS*)

***Logistics***: Providing resources and other services to support incident management. Logistics Section: The [ICS] section responsible for providing facilities, services, and material support for the incident. (*NIMS*)

***Management*** *(general)*: Management consists of decision-making activities undertaken by one or more individuals to direct and coordinate the activities of other people in order to achieve results that could not be accomplished by any one person acting alone. Effective management focuses on group effort, various forms of coordination, and the manner of making decisions. Management is required whenever two or more persons combine their efforts and resources to accomplish a goal that cannot be accomplished by acting alone. Coordination is necessary when the actions of group participants constitute parts of a total task. If one person acts alone to accomplish a task, no coordination may be required; but when that person delegates a part of the task to others, the individual efforts must be coordinated. (*Unknown source*)

***Management*** *(ICS/IMS –noun)*: The IMS/ICS function related to directing and coordinating resources while establishing overall response objectives. Typically objectives are defined in a manner so that they are measurable and achievable within a defined period of time.

***Mass casualty incident (MCI)***: A casualty-creating hazard incident in which the available organizational and medical resources (both "first" and "second response"), or their management systems, are severely challenged or become insufficient to adequately meet the medical needs of the affected population. Insufficient management, response, or support capability or capacity can result in increased morbidity and mortality among the impacted population. "Mass casualty" equates to a "disaster," whereas "multiple casualty incident" equates to an "emergency."

***Mitigation***:

- The phase of Comprehensive Emergency Management that encompasses all activities that reduce or eliminate the probability of a hazard occurrence, or eliminate or reduce the impact from the hazard if it should occur. In comprehensive emergency management, mitigation activities are undertaken during the time period prior to an imminent or actual hazard impact. Once an imminent or actual hazard impact is recognized, subsequent actions are considered response actions and are not called "mitigation" – this avoids the confusion that occurs with the HAZMAT discipline's use of mitigation, which applies to response actions that reduce the impact of a hazardous materials spill.

- Activities taken to eliminate or reduce the probability of the event, or reduce its severity or consequences, either prior to or following a disaster/emergency. *(NFPA 1600, 2004)*
- The activities designed to reduce or eliminate risks to persons or property or to lessen the actual or potential effects or consequences of an incident. Mitigation measures may be implemented prior to, during, or after an incident. Mitigation measures are often informed by lessons learned from prior incidents. Mitigation involves ongoing actions to reduce exposure to, probability of, or potential loss from hazards. Measures may include zoning and building codes, floodplain buyouts, and analysis of hazard- related data to determine where it is safe to build or locate temporary facilities. Mitigation can include efforts to educate governments, businesses, and the public on measures they can take to reduce loss and injury. (*NIMS*)

***National Disaster Medical System (NDMS)***:

- A cooperative, asset-sharing partnership between the Department of Health and Human Services, the Department of Veterans Affairs, the Department of Homeland Security, and the Department of Defense. NDMS provides resources for meeting the continuity of care and mental health services requirements of the Emergency Support Function 8 in the Federal Response Plan. (*NIMS*)

- A federally coordinated initiative to augment the nation's emergency medical response capability by providing medical assets to be used during major disasters or emergencies. NDMS has three major components: Disaster Medical Assistance Teams and Clearing-Staging Units to provide triage, patient stabilization, and austere medical services at a disaster site; an evacuation capability for movement of patients from a disaster area to locations where definitive medical care can be provided; and a voluntary hospital network to provide definitive medical care. NDMS is administered by the Department of Health and Human Services/U.S. Public Health Service, in cooperation with the Department of Defense, the Department of Veterans Affairs, FEMA, State and local governments, and the private sector.

***National Incident Management System (NIMS)***: A system mandated by HSPD-5 that provides a consistent nationwide approach for Federal, State, local, and tribal governments; the private sector, and nongovernmental organizations to work effectively and efficiently together to prepare for, respond to, and recover from domestic incidents, regardless of cause, size, or complexity. To provide for interoperability and compatibility among Federal, State, local, and tribal capabilities, the NIMS includes a core set of concepts, principles, and terminology. HSPD-5 identifies these as the ICS; multiagency coordination systems; training; identification and management of resources (including systems for classifying types of resources); qualification and certification; and the collection, tracking, and reporting of incident information and incident resources. National Response (*NIMS*)

***National Response Plan (NRP)***: The National Response Plan establishes a comprehensive all hazards approach to enhance the ability of the United States to manage domestic incidents. The plan incorporates best practices and procedures from incident management disciplines— homeland security, emergency management, law enforcement, firefighting, public works, public health, responder and recovery worker health and safety, emergency medical services, and the private sector—and integrates them into a unified structure. It forms the basis of how the federal government coordinates with state, local, and tribal governments and the private sector during incidents.

***Planning Section***: Responsible for the collection, evaluation, and dissemination of operational information related to the incident, and for the preparation and documentation of the IAP. This section also maintains information on the current and forecasted situation and on the status of resources assigned to the incident. (*NIMS*)

***Position Description***: Position description is a written summary of the critical features of an emergency response or recovery job, including the nature of the work performed and the specific duties and responsibilities. It is intended to help assigned personnel understand their specific role and to clarify relationships between positions. The position description is augmented by position qualifications or competencies.

***Privileging***: The process where appropriately credentialed personnel (see credentialing) are accepted into an incident to participate as an assigned resource in the response. This process may include both confirmation of a responder's credentials and a determination that an incident need exists that the responder is qualified to address. Privileging is associated with a separate process, badging (see badging), which indicates that a person has been privileged to access a specific incident or to access a specific location.

***Public Information Officer***: A member of the Command Staff responsible for interfacing with the public and media or with other agencies with incident-related information requirements. (*NIMS*)

***Qualification***:

- A term indicating that an individual has met all the requirements of training plus the requirements for physical and medical fitness, psychological fitness, strength/agility, **experience** or other necessary requirements/standards for a position. "Qualification" therefore indicates that the individual possesses all the competencies required for the response position. In some job categories, qualification is demonstrated by obtaining a professional license.

***Recovery***:

- The phase of Comprehensive Emergency Management that encompasses activities and programs implemented during and after response that are designed to return the entity to its usual state or to a "new normal." For response organizations, this includes return-to readiness activities.
- Activities and programs designed to return conditions to a level that is acceptable to the entity. *(NFPA 1600, 2004)*
- The development, coordination, and execution of service- and site-restoration plans; the reconstitution of government operations and services; individual, private- sector, nongovernmental, and public-assistance programs to provide housing and to promote restoration; long-term care and treatment of affected persons; additional measures for social, political, environmental, and economic restoration; evaluation of the incident to identify lessons learned;

post-incident reporting; and development of initiatives to mitigate the effects of future incidents. (*NIMS*)

***Risk Analysis***: A detailed examination performed to understand the nature of unwanted, negative consequences to human life, health, property, or the environment; an analytical process to provide information regarding undesirable events; the process of quantification of the probabilities and expected consequences for identified risks. *(Gratt 1987)*

***Safety Officer (SO)***: A member of the Command Staff responsible for monitoring and assessing safety hazards or unsafe situations and for developing measures for ensuring personnel safety.

***Situation Analysis***: The process of evaluating the severity and consequences of an incident and communicating the results. *(NFPA 1600, 2004)*

***Situation assessment***: An assessment produced during emergency response and recovery that combines incident geography/topography, weather, hazard, hazard impact, and resource data to provide a balanced knowledge base for decision-making. Adequate situation assessment and dissemination of a comprehensive situation assessment (through situation reports and other means) creates the "common operating picture."

***Span of Control***: The number of individuals a supervisor is responsible for, usually expressed as the ratio of supervisors to individuals. (Under the NIMS, an appropriate span of control is between 1:3 and 1:7.) (*NIMS*)

***Stafford Act***: 1) The Robert T. Stafford Disaster Relief and Emergency Assistance Act, Public Law 93-288, as amended. 2) The Stafford Act provides an orderly and continuing means of assistance by the Federal Government to State and local governments in carrying out their responsibilities to alleviate the suffering and damage which result from disaster. The President, in response to a State Governor's request, may declare an "emergency" or "major disaster" in order to provide Federal assistance under the Act. The President, in Executive Order 12148, delegated all functions, except those in Sections 301, 401, and 409, to the Director, of FEMA. The Act provides for the appointment of a Federal Coordinating Officer who will operate in the designated area with a State Coordinating Officer for the purpose of coordinating state and local disaster assistance efforts with those of the Federal Government. (*44 CFR 206.2*)

***Staging Area***: Location established where resources can be placed while awaiting a tactical assignment. The Operations Section manages Staging Areas [where assets assigned to operations are staged]. (*NIMS*)

***Standardized Emergency Management Systems (SEMS)***: As defined in Section 2401 of Title 19 of the California Code of Regulations – A system for managing response to multi-agency and multi-jurisdiction emergencies in California. SEMS consists of five organizational levels that are activated as necessary: Field Response, Local Government, Operational Area, Region, and State:

- Field Response Level: The level where emergency response personnel and resources carry out tactical decisions and activities in direct response to an incident or threat.
- Local Government Level: Cities, counties and special districts; local governments manage and coordinate the overall emergency response and recovery in their jurisdictions.
- Operational Area Level: A county and all political subdivisions within the county area.
- Regional Level: An area defined by state OES for the purpose of efficiently administering disaster services, includes multiple operational areas.

- State Level: The state level manages state resources in response to needs of other levels; coordinates the mutual aid program; and serves as coordination and communication link with the federal disaster response system.

***Strike Team***: A set number of resources of the same kind and type that have an established minimum number of personnel. *(NIMS)*

***Tactics***: Tactics in incident management are specific actions, sequence of actions, procedures, tasks, assignments and schedules used to fulfill strategy and achieve objectives.

***Tactical element***: Tactical elements of ICS are specific organizational elements that execute the tactics (see tactics) set by a management element.

***Task***: A clearly defined and measurable activity accomplished by organizations or some subset thereof (sections, functions, teams, individuals and others). It is the lowest behavioral level in a job or unit that is performed for its own sake.

***Task Force***: Any combination of resources assembled to support a specific mission or operational need. All resource elements within a Task Force must have common communications and a designated leader. (*NIMS*)

***Team*** *(emergency management)*: A nonspecific term for a group of personnel who work as a unit management. The term may also be used as a shortened meaning for "strike team" (see "strike team")

***Terrorism***:

- Under the Homeland Security Act of 2002, terrorism is defined as activity that involves an act dangerous to human life or potentially destructive of critical infrastructure or key resources and is a violation of the criminal laws of the United States or of any State or other subdivision of the United States in which it occurs and is intended to intimidate or coerce the civilian population or influence a government or affect the conduct of a government by mass destruction, assassination, or kidnapping. (*NIMS*)

- "The unlawful use of force or violence against persons or property to intimidate or coerce a government, the civilian population, or any segment thereof, in furtherance of political or social objectives (FBI). **Domestic** terrorism involves groups or individuals who are based and operate entirely within the United States and U.S. territories without foreign direction and whose acts are directed at elements of the U.S. government or population." *(FEMA 2001)*

***TRAC2ES* (United States Transportation Command [USTRANSCOM] Command and Control Evacuation System)**: Automated system used by DoD to regulate patients to health care facilities that have the capacity to treat the patient. The system also integrates the regulating of those patients with available transport assets and provides the ability to track the patient from point of origin to final destination. This system is used by VA Primary Receiving Centers to report available beds under the VA/DoD Contingency Plan and by VA Federal Coordinating Centers for reporting of private hospital sector NDMS beds.

***Type***: A classification of resources in the ICS that refers to capability. Type 1 is generally considered to be more capable than Types 2, 3, or 4, respectively, because of size; power; capacity; or, in the case of incident management teams, experience and qualifications.

***Unified Area Command***: A Unified Area Command is established when incidents under an Area Command are multijurisdictional. (*NIMS*)

***Unified Command***:

- An application of ICS used when there is more than one agency with incident jurisdiction or when incidents cross political jurisdictions. Agencies work together through the designated members of the UC, often the senior person from agencies and/or disciplines participating in the UC, to establish a common set of objectives and strategies and a single IAP. (*NIMS*)
- This management structure brings together the Incident Managers of all major organizations involved in the incident, to coordinate an effective response while allowing each manager to carry out his/her own jurisdictional or discipline responsibilities. UC links the organizations responding to the incident at the leadership level, and it provides a forum for these entities to make consensus decisions. Under UC, the various jurisdictions and/or agencies and nongovernment responders may blend together throughout the organization to create an integrated response team. UC may be used whenever multiple jurisdictions or response agencies are involved in a response effort. UC may be established to overcome divisions from:
  - Geographic boundaries;
  - Government levels;
  - Functional and/or statutory responsibilities; or
  - Some combination of the above. (*U.S. Coast Guard*)

***Unity of Command***: The concept by which each person within an organization reports to one and only one designated person. The purpose of unity of command is to ensure unity of effort under one responsible commander for every objective. (*NIMS*)

***Vertical Evacuation***: The evacuation of persons from an entire area, floor, or wing of a hospital to another floor (either higher or lower based upon the threat/event). (*VHA Emergency Management Guidebook 2005*).

***Vulnerability***: The likelihood of an organization being affected by a hazard, and its susceptibility to the impact and consequences (injury, death, and damage) of the hazard. *(Adapted from the VHA Emergency Management Guidebook 2005*)

***Vulnerability Analysis***: The process of estimating the vulnerability to potential disaster hazards of specified elements at risk. For engineering purposes, vulnerability analysis involves the analysis of theoretical and empirical data concerning the effects of particular phenomena on particular types of structures. For more general socio-economic purposes, it involves consideration of all significant elements in society, including physical, social and economic considerations (both short and long term), and the extent to which essential services (and traditional and local coping mechanisms) are able to continue functioning. (*Simeon Institute 1998*)

***Vulnerability Assessment***: A vulnerability assessment presents "the extent of injury and damage that may result from a hazard event of a given intensity in a given area. The vulnerability assessment should address impacts of hazard events on the existing and future built environment." (*FEMA 2001 (August)*, 7)

***Warning***: Dissemination of notification message signaling imminent hazard which may include advice on protective measures. See also "alert." *(Adapted from U.N. 1992*). For example, a warning is issued by the National Weather Service to let people know that a severe weather event is already occurring or is imminent, and usually provides direction on protective actions. A "warning" notification for individuals is equivalent to an "activation" notification for response systems.

***Watch***: A watch is a notification issued by the National Weather Service to let people know that conditions are right for a potential disaster to occur. It does not mean that an event will necessarily occur. People should listen to their radio or TV to keep informed about changing weather conditions. A watch is issued for specific geographic areas, such as counties, for phenomena such as hurricanes, tornadoes, floods, flash floods, severe thunderstorms, and winter storms. ( *Simeon Institute 1992*). As such, a "watch" notification for individuals is equivalent to an "alert" notification for response systems.

***Weapons of Mass Destruction (WMD)***: Generally refers to chemical, nuclear, biological agents or explosive devices that could be deployed against civilian populations (differentiates from military use).

## APPENDIX 24

# Acronyms

AAR After Action Report
ACEP American College of Emergency Physicians
AE All Employees
AEM Area Emergency Manager
ALS Advanced Life Support
AP Action Plan
ASTM American Society for Testing Materials (now known as "ASTM International")
APTR Association for Prevention Teaching and Research
BAA Business Area Analysis
BCO Business Continuity Office
BCP Business Continuity Program
BIA Business Impact Analysis
CD Civil Defense
CEM Comprehensive Emergency Management
CEMP Comprehensive Emergency Management Program
CEO Chef Executive Officer
CFO Chief Finance Officer
CFR Code of Federal Regulations
CIM Complex Incident Management

CMOPs Consolidated Mail Outpatient Pharmacies
COBRA Consolidated Omnibus Budget Reconciliation Act (1985)
CON OPS Concept of Operations
COO Chief Operations Officer
COOP Continuity of Operations Planning
CP Command Post
CRNA Certified Registered Nurse Anesthetist
CSP Clinical Support Personnel
DHHS Department of Health and Human Services
DECON Decontamination
DMAT Disaster Medical Assistance Team
DOC Department Operations Center
DoD US Department of Defense
DRC Disaster Recovery Center
ED Emergency Department
EEG Exercise Evaluator Guidance
EM Emergency Management
EMAC Emergency Management Assistance Compact
EMC Emergency Management Committee
EMI Emergency Management Institute
EMP Emergency Management Program
EMS Emergency Medical Services
EMSHG Emergency Management Strategic Healthcare Group
EMTALA Emergency Medical Treatment for Active Labor Act
EOC Emergency Operations Center
EOP Emergency Operations Plan
EPC Emergency Program Coordinator
EPM Emergency Program Manager
ERT Emergency Response Team
ERT-A Emergency Response Team- Advanced
ESAR-VHP Emergency System for Advance Registration of Volunteer Health Professionals

ESF Emergency Support Function
ESP Emergency Safety Procedures
EST Emergency Support Team
FBI Federal Bureau Investigation
FCC Federal Coordinating Center
FCO Federal Coordinating Officer
FEMA Federal Emergency Management Agency
FEP Facility Emergency Plan
FIRST Federal Incident Response Support Team
FL Facility Leader
FPC Federal Preparedness Circular
FRERP Federal Radiological Emergency Response Plan
FRP Federal Response Plan
GPMRC Global Patient Movements Requirements Center
GPRA Government Performance and Results Act (1993)
GSA General Services Administration
GWU George Washington University
HAZMAT Hazardous Materials
HCF Health Care Facility
HCFA Health Care Financing Administration
HCS Health Care System
HEICS Hospital Emergency Incident Command System
HHS Department of Health and Human Services
HICS Hospital Incident Command System
HIPAA Health Insurance Portability and Accountability Act
HPT Human Performance Technology
HRSA Health Resources and Services Administration
HSEEP Homeland Security Exercise and Evaluation Program
HSPD Homeland Security Presidential Directive
HVA Hazard Vulnerability Analysis
IAP Incident Action Plan
IC Incident Commander

ICDRM Institute for Crisis Disaster & Risk Management (George Washington University)
ICP Incident Command Post
ICS Incident Command System
IC/UC Incident Command or Unified Command
ID Identification
IEMS Integrated Emergency Management System
IMP Incident Management Post
IMS Incident Management System
IMT Incident Management Team
INCMCE International Nursing Coalition for Mass Casualty Education
IR Incident Review
IS Independent Study
ISC Installation Support Center
ISD Instructional Systems Development
IT Information Technology
JCAHO Joint Commission on Accreditation of Healthcare Organizations
JFO Joint Field Office
JIC Joint Information Center
JIS Joint Information System
LEPCs Local Emergency Planning Committees
LNO Liaison Officer
LO Learning Objective
NDMS National Disaster Medical System
NVOAD National Voluntary Organizations Active in Disasters
MAC Multi Agency Coordination
MACC Multi Agency Coordination Center
MACE Multi Agency Coordination Entity
MaHIM Medical and Health Incident Management
MCI Mass Casualty Incident

MCS Mission Critical Systems
MMI Modified Mercalli Intensity
MOU Memoranda of Understanding
MSCA Military Support to Civil Authorities
MSCC Medical Surge Capacity and Capability
MSEL Master Sequence of Events List
NAICS North American Industry Classification System
N/A Not Applicable
NCR National Capital Region
NFES National Fire Equipment System
NFPA National Fire Protection Association
NGO Nongovernmental Organization
NIMS National Incident Management System
NIIMS National Interagency Incident Management System
NRCC National Response Coordination Center
NRP National Response Plan
NSP Non-clinical Support Personnel
NVOAD National Voluntary Organizations Active in Disasters
NWCG National Wildfire Coordinating Group
OEP Occupant Emergency Pan
OES Office of Emergency Services
OSCAR Operating Status Checklist and Reports
OSHA Occupational Safety and Health Administration
PA Public Assistance
PCP Patient Care Provider
PM Program Manager
POLREP Pollution Report
PIO Public Information Officer
PNP Private Non-Profit
PPE Personal Protective Equipment
PRC Primary Receiving Center
PVO Private Voluntary Organizations

R&D Research & Development
RESTAT Resources Status
RF Radio Frequency
RNP Registered Nurse Practitioners
ROSS Resource Ordering and Status System
RRCC Regional Response Coordination Center
SARS Severe Acute Respiratory Syndrome
SBA Small Business Administration
SDO Standards Development Organizations
SEMS Standardized Emergency Management System
SIMCELL Simulation Cell
SITREP Situation Report
SO Safety Officer
SOP Standard Operating Procedure
SSC Supply Service Center
START Simple Triage and Rapid Treatment
TCL Target Capabilities List
TOPOFF Top Officials (an exercise designed to test top officials in the U.S. government)
TRAC2ES United States Transportation Command [USTRANSCOM] Command and
Control Evacuation System
UC Unified Command
UM Unified Management
UN United Nations
US&R Urban Search and Rescue
USC United States Code
USCA United States Code Annotated
USCG United States Coast Guard
USTRANSCOM United States Transportation Command
VA US Department of Veterans Affairs
VHA Veterans Health Administration

VAMC Veterans Affairs Medical Center
VISN Veteran's Integrated Service Network
WMD Weapons of Mass Destruction
WMO World Meteorological Organization
Ref: (*Emergency Management Principles and Practices for Healthcare Systems Unit 5. Appendices 5-71)*

## Authorities and References


- The Homeland Security Act of 2002, PL 107-296, enacted 11/25/02.
- The National Security Act of 1947, 50 U.S.C. 401 (as amended).
- Robert T. Stafford Disaster Relief and Emergency Assistance Act, as amended
(42 U.S.C. 5121, et seq.).
- Executive Order 12656, *Assignment of Emergency Preparedness Responsibilities*, dated November 18, 1988, as amended.
- Executive Order 12472, *Assignment of National Security and Emergency Preparedness Telecommunications Functions*, dated April 3, 1984.
- Executive Order 12148, *Federal Emergency Management*, dated July 20, 1979, as amended.
- PDD 62, *Combating Terrorism – Homeland Defense*, dated May 22, 1998.
- PDD 67, *Enduring Constitutional Government and Continuity of Government Operations*, dated October 21, 1998.
- White House Memorandum, Continuity Policy/ Department and Agency Essential Functions, dated January 10, 2005, by Francis Fragos Townsend
- White House Memorandum, Background paper on Essential Functions Concept and Implementation and Recommended Guidelines for Submitting Department/ Agencies Priority Mission Essential Functions Information, dated January 10, 2005, by David W. Howe

## References


- Title 44, Code of Federal Regulations (CFR) Part 2, Subpart A - *Organization, Functions, and Delegations of Authority*, dated October 1, 2002.
- Title 41, Code of Federal Regulations (CFR) 101.20.003, *Occupant Emergency Program*, revised on July 1, 2000.
- Title 36, Code of Federal Regulations (CFR) Part 1236, *Management of Vital Records*, revised on May 16. 2001.
- Homeland Security Presidential Directive 3 (HSPD 3), *Homeland Security Advisory System*, dated, March 11, 2002.
- HSPD 7, *Critical Infrastructure Identification, Prioritization, and Protection (CIP)*, dated Dec 17, 2003.
- HSPD 8, *National Preparedness*, dated December 17, 2003.
- Federal Preparedness Circular (FPC) 60, *Continuity of the Executive Branch of the Federal Government at the Headquarters Level during National Security Emergencies*, dated November 20, 1990.
- FPC 65, *Federal Executive Branch Continuity of Operations (COOP)*, dated June 15, 2004.


## ACTIVE Shooter

**http://www.fbi.gov/news/stories/2014/september/**

## BioTerrorism

Hospital Preparedness for Bioterrorism, Public Health Reports, 2001 Supplement, Vol. 10. American Hospital Association, Washington, D.C.

Bioterrorism – Preparedness Varied across State and Local Jurisdictions, United States General Accounting Office Report to Congressional Committees (GAO-03-373), April 2003

Bioterrorism: Healthcare Preparation and Response; Rickard, L.; Healthcare Weekly Review

Bioterrorism—Guidelines for Medical and Public Health Management, Henderson, Inglesby and O'Toole, JAMA, Chicago, Illinois, 2002.

Henderson, D.A et al

"Anthrax as a Biological Weapon," *JAMA*, May 12, 1999 (1735-1745).

"The Looming Threat of Bioterrorism," *Science*, February 26, 1999 (1279-1282).

"Smallpox as a Biological Weapon" *JAMA*, June 9, 1999 (2127-2137).

Inglesby, Thomas V. "Anthrax: A Possible Care History," *Emerging Infectious Diseases*, 5:4 (July-August 1999), 556-560.

Institute of Medicine Committee on R&D
Needs for Improving Civilian Medical Response to Chemical and Biological Terrorism Incidents. "Executive Summary," *Chemical and Biological Terrorism*. Washington, DC:

"Hospital Response to Bioterrorism: National Academy Press, 1999. O'Toole, Tara and Inglesby, Thomas.

Briefing Paper. Photocopied, no date. Baltimore: Johns Hopkins University Center for Civilian Biodefense Studies.

Stein, Aimee. "Bioterrorism: It could happen here." *Hospitals and Health Networks*, (January 1, 2000).

## DMAT

http://www.ndms.dhhs.gov

## Drill Evaluations

Tools for Evaluating Core Elements of Hospital Disaster Drills, Cosgrove, S. et.al John Hopkins University (AHRQ No 08-0019), June 2008

## Emergency Management

Emergency Management Principles and Practices for Healthcare Systems, The Institute for Crisis, Disaster and Risk Management, George Washington University, Unit 5
http://www.gwu.edu/icdm/index.html
http://www.1.va.gov/emshg

Emergency Management: Principles and Practice for Local Government, International City Management Association, Washington, D.C. 1991.

Standards on Disaster/Emergency Management and Business Continuity Programs; NFPA 1600, 2010 Edition (ISBN: 978-087765956-3), Quincy. MA

Principles of Emergency Management and EOC Operations, Fagel, M. et.al, CRC Press 2011.

Crisis Management and Emergency Planning, Fagel, M. et.al, CRC Press 2014

## EMAC

www.nccusl.org

## Emergency Operations Centers

EOC Design Considerations, Holdeman, E. Disaster Resource Guide, 2009

Principles of Emergency Management and EOC Operations, Fagel, M. CRC Press 2011

## Federal Emergency Management Agency

FEMA Independent Study **http://training.fema.gov/IS/**

FEMA Emmitsburg Training Courses **http://training.fema.gov/EMICourses/**

FEMA Center for Domestic Preparedness **https://cdp.dhs.gov/**

Local Mulit-Hazard Mitigation Planning Guidance

FEMA, July 2008 (44 CFR Part 201)

www.ready.gov

www.pandemicflu.gov.

Independent Study Courses: www.fema.gov/emi

- IS 29 PIO Awareness
- IS 100HCb Introduction to ICS for Hospitals
- IS 200HCa Advanced ICS for Hospitals
- IS 700 National Incident Management System (NIMS)
- IS 704 NIMS Communications & Information Management
- NIMS National Response Plan (NRP): www.dhs.gov.

## Federal Grants

Grant Writers Handbook for Successful Grant Proposals; Bradley, K., Stark, M., Philipott, D., 2006 www.GovernmentTrainingInc.com

## Financial

CMS Post-Katrina Provisions, September 2005

http://questions.cms.hhs.gov/cgi-bin/cmshhs.cfg/php/enduser/std_adp.php?p_faqid=5605

## Helicopter Safety

https://www.dir.ca.gov/title8/1938c.html

icacho.org/misc/**Helicopter**%20**Landing**%20Zone.

## Hospital Preparedness

http://www.gao.gov/new.items/d03924.pdf

Macintyre, E., Effective Planning for Health Care Facilities," *JAMA*, 283:2

(January 12, 2000, Anthony G et al. "Weapons of Mass Destruction with Contaminated Casualties.

## Hurricane Planning

Hurricane Planning for the Atlantic and Gulf of Mexico --Student Manual, Federal Emergency Management Agency, Emergency Management Institute, National Hurricane, National Weather Service. 2005.
www.nhc.gov
www.nhc.gov/gccalc.shtml

Hurricane Watch, Sheets, Bob and Williams, Jack, Vintage Books/ Random House Publishing, New York, 2001.

Hurricane Almanac, Norcross, Bryan, St Martin's Griffin, New York, 2007.

## Incident Command

Firescope Incident Command, October 15, 1999.
http://www.nimsonline.com/firescope_forms/ICS%20010-1.pdf

The Hospital Emergency Incident Command System, San Mateo County Department of Health Services, Third Edition, Vol. 1, June 1998.

Hospital Incident Command System Guidebook, August 2006 United States Guard Incident Management Handbook; U.S. Coast Guard COMDTPUB P3120.17, April 11, 2001; pp. 8–12, available at: http://www.uscg.mil/hq/nsfweb/download/IMH/IMH-2001.pdf.

Shaw, G. and Harrald J. The Identification of the Core Competencies Required of Executive Level Business Crisis and Continuity Managers. *The Electronic Journal of Homeland Security and Emergency Management. Berkeley Electronic Press*, January 2004.

## Influenza Planning

Statewide Pandemic Influenza Plan, Department of Health and Hospitals Office of Public Health, September 2006.

## The Joint Commission

Joint Commission Perspectives, Vol. 21, No. 12, December 2001

## Mass Causalities

Hospital Preparedness for Mass Causalities—Final Report, American Hospital Association/United States Department of Health and Human Services, March 2000

Management of Dead Bodies after Disaster, Pan American Health World Organization, Washington, D.C. 2006.

Mass Fatality Incident Response, Federal Emergency Management Institute, National Emergency Training Center, Emmitsburg, Maryland 1993.

## NIMS Sites:

www.fema.gov/emergency/nims

## Guidelines

http://www.fema.gov/emergency/nims/ResourceMngmnt.shtm#item3

http://www.fema.gov/pdf/emergency/nims/ng_0002.pdf

## Public Health

Public Health Emergency Response—A Guide for Leaders and Responders, United States Department of Health and Human Services, Washington, D.C. August 2007. http://www.hhs.gov/emergency

## Surge

Hospital Operational Tool Manual, California Department of Public Health Standards and Guidelines for Healthcare Surge During Emergencies

Guidelines for Managing Inpatient and Outpatient Surge Capacity, State of Wisconsin, November 2005 Toxic Substances Portal

## Toxic Substances

http://www.atsdr.cdc.gov/substances/index.asp
http://www.atsdr.cdc.gov/MHMI/mmg.html

## Waste Management

Occupational Safety and Health Administration, Department of Labor.

"Hazardous Waste Operations and Emergency Response" Fact Sheet 93-31, 1993.

## Wrist Bands:

http://www.pdcorp.com/en-us/crowd-control/index.html

www.ingramcontent.com/pod-product-compliance
Lightning Source LLC
Chambersburg PA
CBHW070218190526
45169CB00001B/7